Clinical Aspects of Breastfeeding

Clinical Aspects of Breastfeeding

Editor: Johanna Watts

hayle medical
New York

Hayle Medical,
750 Third Avenue, 9th Floor,
New York, NY 10017, USA

Visit us on the World Wide Web at:
www.haylemedical.com

ISBN 978-1-64647-564-3 (Hardback)

Cataloging-in-Publication Data

Clinical aspects of breastfeeding / edited by Johanna Watts.
p. cm.
Includes bibliographical references and index.
ISBN 978-1-64647-564-3
1. Breastfeeding. 2. Breast milk. 3. Infants--Nutrition. 4. Lactation--Nutritional aspects.
5. Breastfeeding--Physiological aspects. I. Watts, Johanna.
RJ216 .C55 2023
649.33--dc23

Contents

Preface VII

Chapter 1 **Factors Associated with the Early Initiation of Breastfeeding in Economic Community of West African States (ECOWAS)** 1
Osita Kingsley Ezeh, Felix Akpojene Ogbo, Garry John Stevens, Wadad Kathy Tannous, Osuagwu Levi Uchechukwu, Pramesh Raj Ghimire and Kingsley Emwinyore Agho

Chapter 2 **Zinc Deficiency among Lactating Mothers from a Peri-Urban Community of the Ecuadorian Andean Region: An Initial Approach to the Need of Zinc Supplementation** 17
Camila Narváez-Caicedo, Gabriela Moreano, Bernardo A. Sandoval and Miguel Á. Jara-Palacios

Chapter 3 **Human Milk Oligosaccharides in the Milk of Mothers Delivering Term versus Preterm Infants** 26
Sean Austin, Carlos A. De Castro, Norbert Sprenger, Aristea Binia, Michael Affolter, Clara L. Garcia-Rodenas, Lydie Beauport, Jean-François Tolsa and Céline J. Fischer Fumeaux

Chapter 4 **Determinants of Exclusive Breastfeeding Cessation in the Early Postnatal Period among Culturally and Linguistically Diverse (CALD) Australian Mothers** 42
Felix Akpojene Ogbo, Osita Kingsley Ezeh, Sarah Khanlari, Sabrina Naz, Praween Senanayake, Kedir Y. Ahmed, Anne McKenzie, Olayide Ogunsiji, Kingsley Agho, Andrew Page, Jane Ussher, Janette Perz, Bryanne Barnett AM and John Eastwood

Chapter 5 **Worldwide Variation in Human Milk Metabolome: Indicators of Breast Physiology and Maternal Lifestyle?** 58
Melvin C. L. Gay, Petya T. Koleva, Carolyn M. Slupsky, Elloise du Toit, Merete Eggesbo, Christine C. Johnson, Ganesa Wegienka, Naoki Shimojo, Dianne E. Campbell, Susan L. Prescott, Daniel Munblit, Donna T. Geddes and Anita L. Kozyrskyj

Chapter 6 **Hormones in Breast Milk and Effect on Infants' Growth** 70
Alessandra Mazzocchi, Maria Lorella Giannì, Daniela Morniroli, Ludovica Leone, Paola Roggero, Carlo Agostoni, Valentina De Cosmi and Fabio Mosca

Chapter 7 **What Evidence do we have for Pharmaceutical Galactagogues in the Treatment of Lactation Insufficiency?** 81
Luke E. Grzeskowiak, Mary E. Wlodek and Donna T. Geddes

Chapter 8 **Human Breast Milk NMR Metabolomic Profile across Specific Geographical Locations and its Association with the Milk Microbiota** 102
Carlos Gómez-Gallego, Jose Manuel Morales, Daniel Monleón, Elloise du Toit, Himanshu Kumar, Kaisa M. Linderborg, Yumei Zhang, Baoru Yang, Erika Isolauri, Seppo Salminen and Maria Carmen Collado

Chapter 9 **Lipid Profile, Lipase Bioactivity and Lipophilic Antioxidant Content in High Pressure Processed Donor Human Milk** 122
Aleksandra Wesolowska, Joanna Brys, Olga Barbarska, Kamila Strom, Jolanta Szymanska-Majchrzak, Katarzyna Karzel, Emilia Pawlikowska, Monika A. Zielinska, Jadwiga Hamulka and Gabriela Oledzka

Chapter 10 **Validation of the Breastfeeding Score—A Simple Screening Tool to Predict Breastfeeding Duration** 137
Hanne Kronborg and Michael Væth

Chapter 11 **Sex-Specific Human Milk Composition: The Role of Infant Sex in Determining Early Life Nutrition** 149
Laura Galante, Amber M. Milan, Clare M. Reynolds, David Cameron-Smith, Mark H. Vickers and Shikha Pundir

Chapter 12 **Do a Few Weeks Matter? Late Preterm Infants and Breastfeeding Issues** 160
Beatrice Letizia Crippa, Lorenzo Colombo, Daniela Morniroli, Dario Consonni, Maria Enrica Bettinelli, Irene Spreafico, Giulia Vercesi, Patrizio Sannino, Paola Agnese Mauri, Lidia Zanotta, Annalisa Canziani, Paola Roggero, Laura Plevani, Donatella Bertoli, Stefania Zorzan, Maria Lorella Giannì and Fabio Mosca

Chapter 13 **Exclusive Breastfeeding Rates and Associated Factors in 13 "Economic Community of West African States" (ECOWAS) Countries** 169
Kingsley Emwinyore Agho, Osita Kingsley Ezeh, Pramesh Raj Ghimire, Osuagwu Levi Uchechukwu, Garry John Stevens, Wadad Kathy Tannous, Catharine Fleming and Felix Akpojene Ogbo

Chapter 14 **Comparison of Human Milk Immunoglobulin Survival during Gastric Digestion between Preterm and Term Infants** 187
Veronique Demers-Mathieu, Mark A. Underwood, Robert L. Beverly, Søren D. Nielsen and David C. Dallas

Chapter 15 **Antenatal Influenza A-Specific IgA, IgM and IgG Antibodies in Mother's Own Breast Milk and Donor Breast Milk and Gastric Contents and Stools from Preterm Infants** 200
Veronique Demers-Mathieu, Robert K. Huston, Andi M. Markell, Elizabeth A. McCulley, Rachel L. Martin and David C. Dallas

Chapter 16 **The Impact of Maternal Diet during Pregnancy and Lactation on the Fatty Acid Composition of Erythrocytes and Breast Milk of Chilean Women** 211
Cynthia Barrera, Rodrigo Valenzuela, Rodrigo Chamorro, Karla Bascuñán, Jorge Sandoval, Natalia Sabag, Francesca Valenzuela, María-Paz Valencia, Claudia Puigrredon and Alfonso Valenzuela

Chapter 17 **Levels of Growth Factors and IgA in the Colostrum of Women from Burundi and Italy** 225
Daniel Munblit, Priya Abrol, Shreya Sheth, Li Yan Chow, Ekaterina Khaleva, Alan Asmanov, Silvana Lauriola, Ezio M. Padovani, Pasquale Comberiati, Attilio L. Boner, John O. Warner, Robert J. Boyle and Diego G. Peroni

Permissions

List of Contributors

Index

Preface

This book has been a concerted effort by a group of academicians, researchers and scientists, who have contributed their research works for the realization of the book. This book has materialized in the wake of emerging advancements and innovations in this field. Therefore, the need of the hour was to compile all the required researches and disseminate the knowledge to a broad spectrum of people comprising of students, researchers and specialists of the field.

Lactation is a process of milk secretion by the mammary glands in female mammals including humans. Breastfeeding refers to the action of feeding milk from the breast of a lactating female to a young child or a new born baby. Breastfeeding is helpful in reducing risk of several diseases including type-1 diabetes, asthma, childhood leukemia, allergies and obesity. Benefits of breastfeeding for the mother in the long term include reduced risk of rheumatoid arthritis, breast cancer, metabolic syndrome, cardiovascular disease, and diabetes. Some of the common problems associated with lactation include sore nipples, breast engorgement, too little or too much breast milk, and mastitis. This book on breastfeeding presents researches and studies performed by experts across the globe. It will also provide interesting topics for research which interested readers can take up. The extensive content of this book provides the readers with a thorough understanding of the subject.

At the end of the preface, I would like to thank the authors for their brilliant chapters and the publisher for guiding us all-through the making of the book till its final stage. Also, I would like to thank my family for providing the support and encouragement throughout my academic career and research projects.

Editor

1

Factors Associated with the Early Initiation of Breastfeeding in Economic Community of West African States (ECOWAS)

Osita Kingsley Ezeh [1], Felix Akpojene Ogbo [2], Garry John Stevens [3], Wadad Kathy Tannous [4], Osuagwu Levi Uchechukwu [5], Pramesh Raj Ghimire [1], Kingsley Emwinyore Agho [1,2,*] and Global Maternal and Child Health Research Collaboration (GloMACH) [†]

1 School of Science and Health, University of Western Sydney, Locked Bag 1797, Penrith, NSW 1797, Australia; Ezehosita@yahoo.com (O.K.E.); Prameshraj@hotmail.com (P.R.G.)

2 Translational Health Research Institute (THRI), School of Medicine, Western Sydney University, Campbelltown Campus, Locked Bag 1797, Penrith, NSW 2571, Australia; F.Ogbo@westernsydney.edu.au

3 Humanitarian and Development Research Initiative (HADRI), School of Social Sciences and Psychology, Western Sydney University, Locked Bag1797, Penrith, NSW 2751, Australia; G.Stevens@westernsydney.edu.au

4 School of Business, Western Sydney University, Locked Bag 1797, Penrith, NSW 2751, Australia; K.Tannous@westernsydney.edu.au

5 Diabetes, Obesity and Metabolism Translational Research Unit, Western Sydney University, Campbelltown, NSW 2560, Australia; L.osuagwu@westernsydney.edu.au

* Correspondence: K.agho@westernsydney.edu.au

† Members are listed at the end of Acknowledgments.

Abstract: The early initiation of breastfeeding (EIBF) within one hour after birth enhanced mother–newborn bonding and protection against infectious diseases. This paper aimed to examine factors associated with EIBF in 13 Economic Community of West African States (ECOWAS). A weighted sample of 76,934 children aged 0–23 months from the recent Demographic and Health Survey dataset in the ECOWAS for the period 2010 to 2018 was pooled. Survey logistic regression analyses, adjusting for country-specific cluster and population-level weights, were used to determine the factors associated with EIBF. The overall combined rate of EIBF in ECOWAS was 43%. After adjusting for potential confounding factors, EIBF was significantly lower in Burkina Faso, Cote d'Ivoire, Guinea, Niger, Nigeria, and Senegal. Mothers who perceived their babies to be average and large at birth were significantly more likely to initiate breastfeeding within one hour of birth than those mothers who perceived their babies to be small at birth. Mothers who had a caesarean delivery (AOR = 0.28, 95%CI = 0.22–0.36), who did not attend antenatal visits (ANC) during pregnancy, and delivered by non-health professionals were more likely to delay initiation of breastfeeding beyond one hour after birth. Male children and mothers from poorer households were more likely to delay introduction of breastfeeding. Infant and young child feeding nutrition programs aimed at improving EIBF in ECOWAS need to target mothers who underutilize healthcare services, especially mothers from lower socioeconomic groups.

Keywords: breastfeeding; infants; ECOWAS; antenatal care; pregnancy; infant mortality

---

1. Introduction

Globally, about 75% of all under-five deaths occur within the first year of life, and sub-Saharan African countries remain the hub of the world burden of all under-five deaths [1,2]. Early initiation of breastfeeding (EIBF) within one hour of birth remains a significant public health challenge, particularly in sub-Saharan African (SSA) countries, including the Economic Community of West African States (ECOWAS). In keeping with the Sustainable Development Goals, developing countries have committed to reducing under-five mortality by 25 deaths per 1000 live births by 2030 [3]. Global strategies, including the Baby-Friendly Hospital Initiative (BFHI), Community Integrated Management of Childhood Illness (C-IMCI), and Infant and Young Child Feeding (IYCF) guidelines have been developed by United Nations Children's Fund (UNICEF) and the World Health Organization (WHO). These aim to substantially reduce child mortality, morbidity, and undernutrition [4,5]. They have succeeded in some parts of the world but remain refractory in Africa. In addition, there is a strong epidemiological evidence to suggest that the nutritional benefits of EIBF may include a reduced risk of hypoglycemia in at-risk infants (e.g., small for gestational age and macrosomia infants), which can cause significant morbidity and mortality [6]. This is due to EIBF containing antibodies for natural immunity, which provide protection against infectious diseases (such as diarrheal and pneumonia) and other potentially life-threatening ailments [7,8]. ECOWAS is a regional political and economic union of 15 countries in West Africa, founded in 1975 with members including Benin, Burkina Faso, Cabo Verde, Cote d'Ivoire, The Gambia, Ghana, Guinea, Guinea-Bissau, Liberia, Mali, Niger, Nigeria, Senegal, Sierra Leone, and Togo. The main aim of this alliance is to promote socioeconomic integration among member states to raise living standards and promote economic development, with wider implications for judicial and health service cooperation [9].

There are numerous recognized advantages of EIBF, however, the rates of EIBF in ECOWAS are typically low and still suboptimal, ranging from 17% to 62% [10,11]. These low rates mean a substantial proportion of newborn babies are deprived of mother–newborn bonding, resistance against infection, and the early breastfeeding needed to fight disease [7,8]. Studies highlight that infants initiated to breastfeeding within an hour of birth have a reduced incidence of life-threatening conditions, such as serious systemic bacterial infections, diarrhea, respiratory infections, as well as less severe infections of the middle ear and urinary tract, and allergic conditions [12–14]. A cohort study conducted in rural Ghana indicated that 22% of neonatal deaths could be prevented if breastfeeding started within the first hour of birth [15]. Similarly, a community-based randomized trial conducted in southern Nepal revealed that approximately 8–19% of newborn deaths could be averted annually in developing countries if all newborns were breastfed within an hour of delivery [16]. EIBF is not only beneficial to neonates but also to mothers, as it reduces the risk of postpartum hemorrhage [17].

Published studies conducted on EIBF in SSA, including ECOWAS countries, have indicated that EIBF is associated with demographic, socioeconomic, and obstetric characteristics. A nationwide cross-sectional study on trends and factors associated with EIBF in Nigeria found that mothers who had four or more antenatal visits (ANC) visits during pregnancy, mothers from wealthier households, and mothers who delivered their babies at the health facility are more likely to initiate breastfeeding within one hour of birth [18,19]. Another population-based study conducted in Nigeria that examined urban–rural differences in the rates of EIBF concluded that EIBF rates were significantly lower in rural areas than urban areas [20]. The perception of a lack of breastmilk, perception that the mother and the baby need rest after birth, performing post-birth activities (such as bathing), and the baby not crying for milk were observed as barriers to EIBF among mothers in Ghana [11]. In that study, delivery in a health facility was a facilitator to EIBF, as health practitioners encouraged early breastfeeding [11]. A nationwide cross-sectional study in Zimbabwe found that skilled delivery assistants, multiparity, and postpartum skin to skin contact between mother and newborn babies immediately after birth were significantly related to EIBF [21]. Similarly, in a community-based cross-sectional study on EIBF conducted in Ethiopia, maternal education, delivery at a health facility and visiting antenatal care services during pregnancy were also significantly associated with EIBF within one hour of delivery [22]. The low rate of EIBF practice in ECOWAS could have potentially contributed to nearly half of all under-five deaths, such as those due to prematurity or malnutrition in sub-Saharan Africa region in the year 2017 [1]. Prior to the current study, no studies have used combined country-specific local data across ECOWAS countries to examine factors associated with EIBF within one hour of birth. Evidence based on collective data will provide region-specific targeted interventions to scale up EIBF practices to reduce morbidity and mortality.

Hence, this study aims to investigate the possible characteristics influencing EIBF in 13 of the ECOWAS member countries using the most recent Demographic and Health Survey (DHS) survey datasets conducted between 2010 and 2018. Recognition of factors associated with EIBF in ECOWAS countries is essential for building effective nutrition education and behavior change communication interventions in targeting women at heightened risk of sub-optimal feeding behaviors. In addition, the identification of modifiable associated factors will help public health nutrition program managers and policymakers develop strategies to support these contributory factors. ECOWAS would gain enormous health and economic benefits by improving EIBF. Thus, the findings from this study could assist in the planning and monitoring of effective infant and breastfeeding promotion programs in each ECOWAS country, which may contribute to achieving the child survival sustainable development goal.

2. Materials and Methods

The most recent ECOWAS DHS datasets between 2010 and 2018 were used for this study. Cabo Verde and Guinea-Bissau were not included in the study because their last DHS surveys were not within the study period. As a result, the most recent DHS datasets from 13 ECOWAS countries were used for this study. These data sets were obtained from standardized population-based cross-sectional surveys with a high response rate and trained interviewers [10]. The DHS surveys are publicly available for download [10,23]. Each ECOWAS National Bureau of Statistics collects the DHS Data in collaboration with the United States Agency for International Development [10]. The DHS surveys use identical questionnaires in all countries to collect information on diverse topics, including fertility, reproductive health, maternal and child health, mortality, nutrition, and self-reported health behaviors among adults [5]. In this study and to reduce recall bias, we restricted the analysis to the last born child at 23 months and living with the respondent. This yielded a weighted total of 76,934 children.

2.1. Outcome and Confounding Factors

The outcome variable was EIBF. Women were asked how long after birth the baby was put to the breast for the first time. Responses were recorded in minutes and/or hours. EIBF within one hour of birth was estimated using the World Health Organization recommendation [24,25]. This indicator includes the EIBF rate (the proportion of children born aged 0–23 months who were put to the breast within one hour of birth). EIBF was categorized into a binary form of the outcome variables: "Yes" (1 = if a child was given EIBF) and "No" (0 = if a child was not given EIBF). The potential confounding factors were organised into four distinct groups: demographic factors (countries, place of residence, mother's age, marital status, combined birth rank and birth interval, sex of baby, child's age in category, perceived size of the baby); socio-economic factors (household wealth index, maternal work in the last 12 months, maternal education, and maternal literacy); access to media factors (frequency of reading newspapers/magazine, frequency of listening to radio, and frequency of watching television); and healthcare utilization factors (place of delivery, mode of delivery, type of delivery assistance, and antenatal clinic visits). For the pooled dataset, the household wealth index was constructed using the 'hv271' variable. The hv271 is a household's wealth index value generated by the product of standardized scores (z-scores) and factor coefficient scores (factor loadings) of wealth indicators [26]. In the household wealth index categories, the bottom 20% of households was arbitrarily referred to as the poorest households and the top 20% as richest households, and they were divided into poorest, poor, middle, rich, and richest.

2.2. Statistical Analysis

For the combined 13 ECOWAS datasets, a population-level weight, unique country-specific clustering, and strata were created. This was to manage large country weights being greater than small country weights and also because clusters were different in each country. Population-level weights were used for survey (SVY) tabulation that adjusted for a unique country-specific stratum, and clustering was used to determine the percentage, frequency count, and univariate analysis of all selected characteristics. Country-specific weights were used for the Taylor series linearization method [27] in the surveys when estimating the rates and 95% confidence intervals of EIBF in each country.

Population-level weights were used in the multivariate analyses. In the multivariate analyses, a four-stage hierarchical model was carried out. In the first stage model, demographic factors were entered into the model. In the second stage model, demographic factors were added to the socio-economic factors. A similar procedure was employed for the third stage model, which included the demographic and socio-economic level factors, as well as access to media factors. The fourth and final stage model, healthcare utilization factors, were added to demographic, socio-economic, and media factors. All statistical analyses were conducted using (statistics and data) STATA/MP Version.14.1 (StataCorp, College Station, TX, USA) and adjusted odds ratios (AORs) and their 95% confidence intervals (CIs) obtained from the adjusted multivariate logistic regression model were used to measure the factors associated with EIBF.

3. Results

3.1. Characteristics of the Sample and Univariate Analyses for EIBF

The pooled rate of EIBF in the 13 ECOWAS was 43% and EIBF lay between 52% and 62% in Togo, Niger, Mali, Benin, Sierra Leone, Liberia, Ghana, and Gambia, as indicated in Figure 1. The highest rates of EIBF were observed in Togo and Liberia, and the lowest was in Guinea (17%).

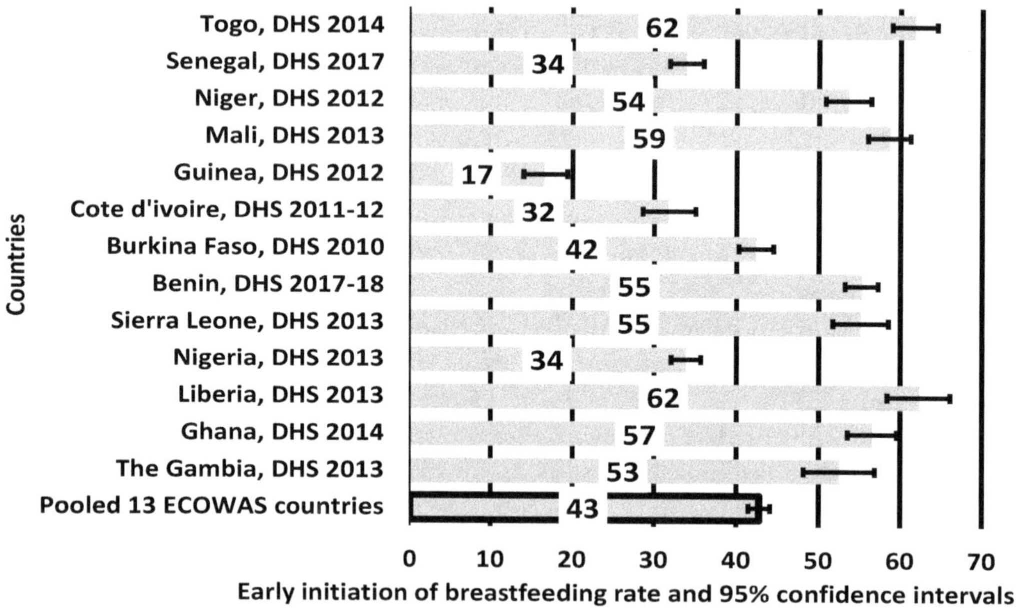

Figure 1. Rates of early initiation of breastfeeding in thirteen Economic Community of West African States. DHS = Demographic and Health Survey.

Table 1 illustrates the characteristics of the sample of children aged 0–23 months and the unadjusted odd ratios of EIBF in children aged 0–23 months. Overall, 21% of children aged 0–23 months were from Nigeria, and compared to Benin (7.7%), the odds of EIBF in Nigeria was reduced significantly, by 58% (OR = 0.42, 95% CI:0.36, 0.48). About 42% of EIBF babies were perceived by their mothers to be of average birth size compared to the 18% of EIBF babies perceived to be small at birth. The unadjusted odd ratios of EIBF were significant with babies perceived by their mothers to be the average birth size at birth, combined birth rank and birth interval, household wealth, frequency of listening to the radio, and watching television.

Table 1. Individual, household, and community level characteristics and unadjusted odds ratios (OR) (95% CI) of early initiation of breastfeeding (EIBF) among children aged 0–23 months in 13 Economic Community of West African States (ECOWAS).

Characteristic	*n* *	% *	%	EIBF			
				OR	95% CI		*p*-Value
Demographic factors							
Country							
Benin	5937	7.7	9.2	1.00			
Burkina Faso	6887	9.0	10.0	0.58	0.50	0.67	<0.001
Cote d'ivoire	4554	5.9	5.2	0.43	0.33	0.56	<0.001
The Gambia	5387	7.0	6.0	0.76	0.52	1.11	0.151
Ghana	3412	4.4	4.0	1.07	0.88	1.31	0.483
Guinea	3574	4.6	4.7	0.17	0.13	0.22	<0.001
Liberia	4241	5.5	5.1	1.30	0.96	1.77	0.093
Mail	4843	6.3	6.7	1.11	0.93	1.32	0.242
Niger	7044	9.2	8.1	0.90	0.75	1.08	0.262
Nigeria	15,993	20.8	20.7	0.42	0.36	0.48	<0.001
Senegal	5790	7.5	8.1	0.35	0.29	0.41	<0.001
Sierra Leone	6230	8.1	7.4	0.85	0.67	1.08	0.173
Togo	3042	4.0	4.8	1.49	1.23	1.79	<0.001
Residence							
Urban	27,769	36.1	31.0	1.00			
Rural	49,165	63.9	69.0	0.96	0.85	1.08	0.468
Mothers' age in years							
15–19	25,575	33.2	33.4	1.00			
20–34	36,855	47.9	46.9	1.09	1.02	1.17	0.012
35–49	14,503	18.9	19.8	1.08	0.99	1.17	0.084
Marital status							
Currently married	70,916	92.2	92.7	1.00			
Formerly married ^	1875	2.4	2.5	1.13	0.91	1.39	0.269
Never married	4142	5.4	4.8	0.98	0.83	1.17	0.863
Age of child (months)							
0–5	19,736	25.7	25.8	1.00			
6–11	20,308	26.4	26.9	1.02	0.93	1.12	0.657
12–17	20,402	26.5	26.0	1.07	0.98	1.16	0.138
18–23	16,488	21.4	21.3	1.10	1.00	1.21	0.047
Birth order or birth rank							
First-born	15,935	20.7	20.0	1.00			
Second–fourth	36,840	47.9	46.6	1.26	1.16	1.36	<0.001
Fifth or more	24,159	31.4	33.4	1.19	1.09	1.31	<0.001

Table 1. *Cont.*

Characteristic	n *	% *	%	EIBF			
				OR	95% CI		p-Value
Preceding birth interval (n = 76,748)							
No previous birth	15,935	20.7	20.0	1.00			
<24 months	8163	10.6	10.6	1.13	1.00	1.28	0.042
≥24 months	52,650	68.4	69.2	1.25	1.16	1.35	<0.001
Combined birth rank and birth interval							
Second/third birth rank, more than two years interval	30,717	39.9	39.0	1.00			
First birth rank	15,935	20.7	20.0	0.78	0.72	0.85	<0.001
Second/third birth rank, less than or equal to two years interval	6123	8.0	7.7	0.90	0.79	1.02	0.097
Fourth birth rank, more than two years interval	20,520	26.7	28.4	0.94	0.87	1.02	0.120
Fourth birth rank, less than or equal to two years interval	3638	4.7	5.0	0.89	0.77	1.02	0.103
Sex of baby							
Male	38,723	50.3	50.6	1.00			
Female	38,211	49.7	49.4	1.05	0.99	1.11	0.120
Size of baby (n = 76,255)							
Small	13,689	17.8	17.5	1.00			
Average	32,517	42.3	42.6	1.22	1.11	1.34	<0.001
Large	30,049	39.1	38.9	1.19	1.07	1.31	0.001
Socio-economic factors							
Household Wealth Index							
Poorest	12,753	16.6	20.1	1.00			
Poorer	13,520	17.6	19.7	1.35	1.19	1.54	<0.001
Middle	15,088	19.6	19.8	1.55	1.36	1.78	<0.001
Richer	14,854	19.3	20.1	1.33	1.16	1.52	<0.001
Richest	20,719	26.9	20.5	1.25	1.07	1.46	0.005
Work in the last 12 months (n = 76,918)							
Not working	30,637	39.8	38.2	1.00			
Working	46,281	60.2	61.8	0.94	0.86	1.02	0.150
Maternal education (n = 76,926)							
No education	45,527	59.2	61.6	1.00			
Primary	13,319	17.3	18.1	1.06	0.96	1.17	0.239
Secondary and above	18,080	23.5	20.4	1.03	0.93	1.14	0.549
Maternal Literacy (n = 76,549)							
Cannot read at all	57,292	74.5	77.4	1.00			
Able to read only part of sentences	19,257	25.0	22.1	0.96	0.88	1.04	0.341

Table 1. *Cont.*

Characteristic	n *	% *	%	EIBF			
				OR	95% CI		p-Value
Access to media							
Frequency of reading newspaper or magazine (n = 76,736)							
Not at all	68,490	89.0	91.5	1.00			
Less than once a week	4575	5.9	4.8	0.93	0.81	1.08	0.356
At least once a week	3644	4.7	3.7	1.10	0.92	1.32	0.281
Almost every day	27	0.0	0.0	2.13	0.80	5.69	0.132
Frequency of listening to radio (n = 76,808)							
Not at all	25,977	33.8	36.0	1.00			
Less than once a week	19,798	25.7	25.0	0.95	0.87	1.04	0.300
At least once a week	30,250	39.3	37.8	0.97	0.88	1.06	0.466
Almost every day	783	1.0	1.1	3.27	2.49	4.29	<0.001
Frequency of watching Television (n = 76,760)							
Not at all	42,468	55.2	59.8	1.00			
Less than once a week	12,287	16.0	15.1	1.01	0.90	1.13	0.861
At least once a week	21,294	27.7	24.1	0.84	0.76	0.93	0.001
Almost every day	711	0.9	0.8	2.60	1.97	3.44	<0.001
Healthcare utilization factors							
Place of delivery							
Home	31,183	40.5	41.3	1.00			
Health facility	45,751	59.5	58.7	1.34	1.23	1.47	<0.001
Mode of delivery (n = 76,729)							
Non-caesarean	73,763	95.9	96.3	1.00			
Caesarean section ‡	2966	3.9	3.5	0.39	0.32	0.49	<0.001
Type of delivery assistance (n = 63,553)							
Health professional	49,991	65.0	62.8	1.00			
Traditional birth attendant	1884	2.4	2.8	0.73	0.61	0.88	0.001
Other untrained	6959	9.0	10.7	0.76	0.64	0.90	0.001
No one	4699	6.1	6.0	0.61	0.51	0.72	<0.001
Antenatal clinic visits (n = 74,550)							
None	9478	12.3	12.6	1.00			
1–3	23,314	30.3	31.9	1.55	1.36	1.77	<0.001
4+	41,758	54.3	52.7	1.67	1.45	1.91	<0.001

^ divorce/separated/widowed; * Weighted sample sizes and percentages; ‡ Caesarean section is a combination of both general and regional anesthesia.

3.2. Factors Associated with Early Initiation of Breastfeeding

As shown in Table 2, EIBF within one hour of birth was significantly lower among children living in Nigeria, Cote d'Ivoire, Burkina Faso, Guinea, and Senegal. Mothers from poorest households, mothers' first birth, and delivery by non-health professionals were significantly associated with delayed initiation of breastfeeding. Mothers who underwent caesarean delivery were significantly more likely to delay the initiation of breastfeeding (adjusted OR = 0.28, 95% CI:0.22, 0.36; $p < 0.001$) than those who had non-caesarean delivery.

Mothers who perceived their babies to be average or larger at birth were more likely to initiate breastfeeding within one hour of delivery than mothers who perceived their babies to be small. EIBF was significantly higher among mothers who frequently listened to the radio, who delivered their babies at the health facilities, and those mothers who had four or more antenatal clinic visits. EIBF was significantly higher with female births (adjusted OR = 1.17, 95% CI:1.00, 1.37; $p = 0.046$) than male births.

Table 2. Adjusted odds ratio (AOR) (95% confidence intervals (CI)) of factors associated with the early initiation of breastfeeding (EIBF) among children aged 0–23 months in 13 Economic Community of West African States (ECOWAS).

Characteristic	Model 1				Model 2				Model 3				Model 4			
	AOR	95% CI		*p*-Value	AOR	95% CI		*p*-Value	AOR	95% CI		*p*-Value	AOR	95% CI		*p*-Value
Demographic factors																
Benin	1.00				1.00				1.00				1.00			
Burkina Faso	0.58	0.50	0.67	<0.001	0.56	0.48	0.65	<0.001	0.56	0.48	0.66	<0.001	0.58	0.48	0.69	<0.001
Cote d'ivoire	0.42	0.32	0.54	<0.001	0.43	0.33	0.56	<0.001	0.43	0.33	0.56	<0.001	0.43	0.33	0.55	<0.001
The Gambia	0.75	0.51	1.09	0.134	0.73	0.50	1.07	0.109	0.75	0.51	1.11	0.148	0.67	0.44	1.02	0.062
Ghana	1.08	0.88	1.34	0.460	1.11	0.89	1.38	0.351	1.15	0.92	1.43	0.212	1.33	1.03	1.72	0.028
Guinea	0.17	0.13	0.22	<0.001	0.17	0.13	0.23	<0.001	0.17	0.13	0.23	<0.001	0.19	0.14	0.25	<0.001
Liberia	1.30	0.95	1.79	0.106	1.34	0.96	1.87	0.081	1.34	0.96	1.87	0.085	1.44	1.04	1.98	0.028
Mali	1.10	0.93	1.32	0.271	1.30	1.07	1.58	0.009	1.34	1.09	1.63	0.005	1.36	1.09	1.71	0.006
Niger	0.94	0.78	1.13	0.520	0.86	0.71	1.04	0.132	0.87	0.72	1.05	0.144	0.98	0.80	1.22	0.882
Nigeria	0.41	0.36	0.48	<0.001	0.44	0.38	0.51	<0.001	0.44	0.38	0.52	<0.001	0.51	0.43	0.61	<0.001
Senegal	0.36	0.30	0.43	<0.001	0.37	0.31	0.45	<0.001	0.38	0.32	0.46	<0.001	0.40	0.33	0.48	<0.001
Sierra Leone	0.86	0.67	1.10	0.230	0.84	0.65	1.07	0.151	0.83	0.65	1.07	0.147	0.78	0.60	1.03	0.075
Togo	1.50	1.25	1.81	0.000	1.50	1.24	1.81	<0.001	1.29	1.05	1.59	0.015	1.56	1.25	1.94	<0.001
Residence																
Urban	1.00				1.00				1.00				1.00			
Rural	0.95	0.84	1.06	0.335	0.94	0.83	1.07	0.373	0.94	0.82	1.07	0.355	0.92	0.81	1.04	0.200
Mothers' age in years																
15–19	1.00				1.00				1.00				1.00			
20–34	0.98	0.90	1.07	0.732	0.99	0.91	1.08	0.777	0.98	0.90	1.07	0.605	0.98	0.90	1.08	0.731
35–49	0.98	0.86	1.11	0.725	0.98	0.86	1.11	0.727	0.96	0.85	1.09	0.538	0.94	0.82	1.08	0.372
Marital status																
Currently married	1.00				1.00				1.00				1.00			
Formerly married ^	0.99	0.79	1.26	0.957	0.99	0.78	1.26	0.940	0.99	0.78	1.26	0.952	0.98	0.76	1.26	0.894
Never married	0.96	0.78	1.18	0.692	0.93	0.76	1.14	0.501	0.95	0.77	1.17	0.610	0.98	0.79	1.21	0.843
Birth rank and birth interval																
Second/third birth rank, more than two years interval	1.00				1.00				1.00				1.00			
First birth rank	0.78	0.71	0.86	<0.001	0.78	0.70	0.86	<0.001	0.77	0.70	0.85	<0.001	0.78	0.69	0.87	<0.001
Second/third birth rank, less than or equal to two years interval	0.89	0.78	1.03	0.123	0.89	0.77	1.02	0.098	0.89	0.77	1.03	0.105	0.91	0.78	1.07	0.268
Fourth birth rank, more than two years interval	0.98	0.89	1.08	0.699	0.99	0.89	1.09	0.791	1.00	0.90	1.11	0.978	1.03	0.93	1.15	0.551
Fourth birth rank, less than or equal to two years interval	0.92	0.79	1.07	0.268	0.92	0.78	1.07	0.288	0.93	0.79	1.09	0.359	0.98	0.82	1.17	0.808
Sex of baby																
Male	1.00				1.00				1.00				1.00			
Female	1.07	1.01	1.13	0.027	1.07	1.01	1.13	0.024	1.07	1.01	1.13	0.025	1.08	1.01	1.16	0.021
Age of child (months)																
0–5	1.00				1.00				1.00				1.00			
6–11	1.03	0.94	1.13	0.546	1.03	0.94	1.13	0.538	1.03	0.93	1.13	0.570	1.02	0.92	1.14	0.664
12–17	1.09	1.00	1.20	0.056	1.10	1.00	1.20	0.045	1.09	0.99	1.19	0.071	1.10	0.98	1.22	0.096
18–23	1.10	1.00	1.21	0.048	1.10	1.00	1.21	0.047	1.10	1.00	1.21	0.052	1.10	0.99	1.23	0.075

Table 2. *Cont.*

Characteristic	Model 1			Model 2			Model 3			Model 4		
	AOR	95% CI	*p*-Value	AOR	95% CI	*p*-Value	AOR	95% CI	*p*-Value	AOR	95% CI	*p*-Value
Size of baby												
Small	1.00			1.00			1.00			1.00		
Average	1.21	1.09 1.33	<0.001	1.20	1.08 1.32	<0.001	1.20	1.09 1.32	<0.001	1.19	1.07 1.32	0.002
Large	1.23	1.11 1.37	<0.001	1.22	1.10 1.36	<0.001	1.22	1.10 1.36	<0.001	1.20	1.07 1.36	0.002
Socio-economic factors												
Household Wealth Index												
Poorest				1.00			1.00			1.00		
Poorer				1.29	1.13 1.48	<0.001	1.32	1.15 1.51	<0.001	1.19	1.02 1.38	0.028
Middle				1.38	1.20 1.59	<0.001	1.42	1.23 1.63	<0.001	1.22	1.03 1.43	0.018
Richer				1.34	1.17 1.55	<0.001	1.39	1.20 1.60	<0.001	1.17	0.98 1.39	0.077
Richest				1.16	0.98 1.36	0.083	1.19	1.00 1.43	0.052	1.03	0.84 1.26	0.782
Work in the last 12 months												
Not working				1.00			1.00			1.00		
Working				0.95	0.86 1.04	0.243	0.95	0.87 1.04	0.291	0.95	0.87 1.05	0.329
Maternal education												
No education				1.00			1.00			1.00		
Primary				1.02	0.92 1.13	0.732	1.03	0.92 1.14	0.627	1.00	0.90 1.12	0.992
Secondary and above				0.98	0.80 1.21	0.860	0.96	0.78 1.19	0.717	0.89	0.73 1.10	0.291
Maternal Literacy												
Cannot read at all				1.00			1.00			1.00		
Able to read only part of sentences				1.04	0.87 1.24	0.690	1.00	0.82 1.21	0.985	1.02	0.85 1.23	0.811
Access to media												
Frequency of reading newspaper or magazine												
Not at all							1.00			1.00		
Less than once a week							1.11	0.93 1.32	0.255	1.06	0.89 1.27	0.508
At least once a week							1.33	1.09 1.63	0.006	1.36	1.10 1.67	0.004
Almost every day							0.91	0.33 2.51	0.856	1.01	0.40 2.50	0.990
Frequency of listening to Radio												
Not at all							1.00			1.00		
Less than once a week							0.90	0.82 0.99	0.037	0.86	0.78 0.95	0.002
At least once a week							0.92	0.83 1.01	0.089	0.92	0.83 1.02	0.099
Almost every day							1.47	1.11 1.95	0.007	1.45	1.07 1.95	0.016
Frequency of watching Television												
Not at all							1.00			1.00		
Less than once a week							1.03	0.90 1.18	0.660	1.00	0.86 1.17	0.967
At least once a week							0.95	0.84 1.06	0.333	0.90	0.80 1.02	0.104
Almost every day							1.17	0.85 1.60	0.335	1.14	0.82 1.60	0.438
Healthcare utilization factors												
Place of delivery												
Home										1.00		
Health facility										1.38	1.21 1.57	<0.001
Mode of delivery												

Table 2. *Cont.*

Characteristic	Model 1			Model 2			Model 3			Model 4		
	AOR	95% CI	*p*-Value	AOR	95% CI	*p*-Value	AOR	95% CI	*p*-Value	AOR	95% CI	*p*-Value
Non-caesarean										1.00		
Caesarean section ‡										0.28	0.22 0.36	<0.001
Type of delivery assistance												
Health professional										1.00		
Traditional birth attendant.										0.77	0.60 0.98	0.037
Other untrained										0.96	0.79 1.16	0.663
No one										0.76	0.62 0.92	0.005
Antenatal Clinic visits												
None										1.00		
1–3										1.17	1.00 1.37	0.052
4+										1.20	1.01 1.41	0.034

^ divorce/separated/widowed.; ‡ Caesarean section is a combination of both general and regional anesthesia.

4. Discussion

Our results indicate that EIBF rates in the 13 ECOWAS are at a sub-optimum level, and need further improvement to fulfil the goal of optimal infant feeding in this subregion and the related Sustainable Development Goals (SDGs) of reducing neonatal mortality. During the study period (2010–2018), we noted the uneven prevalence of EIBF among infants aged between 0 and 23 months of age across the ECOWAS countries, ranging from a low of 17% (Guinea) to the highest of 61% (Togo). The reported rates of EIBF in this study are still well below the expected target of ≥70% recommended by the WHO [1] to further reduce infant mortality and morbidity in the sub-region by 25 deaths per 1000 live births by 2030. The wide variation in the rates of EIBF within the 13 ECOWAS countries may be due to socio-cultural, geographical location, and health inequalities, as well as economic issues among different populations. The study indicated that place of delivery (health institution), mode of delivery (vaginal delivery), ANC visits (≥4), and household wealth index (poorer or middle-class household) were significantly associated with EIBF within one hour of birth. Media exposure (newspaper/magazine or radio), baby size at birth (average and large), child's sex (female), and first birth order were also found to be positively related to EIBF. Delayed introduction to breastfeeding was significant in six ECOWAS member states (Gambia, Nigeria, Senegal, Guinea, Burkina Faso, and Cote d'Ivoire).

Child delivery at health facilities predicts EIBF practices within one hour of the birth. This finding is consistent with previous studies conducted in Nepal [28], Nigeria [29], Namibia [30], and Ethiopia [31]. However, this is not unexpected given that the majority of health institutions across ECOWAS countries have adopted BFHI, which is overseen by skilled health providers (midwife, nurse, or doctor) whose core aim is to encourage and assist mothers in achieving optimal breastfeeding practices, including EIBF. It has been suggested that the presence of trained breastfeeding and delivery assistants in health institutions improved mothers' EIBF practice [32]. This may have contributed to the substantial proportion (60%) of EIBF among mothers who gave birth at a hospital, as observed in the current study.

Similar to reports from earlier studies [22,29,30], the present study found that vaginal delivery was strongly correlated with EIBF practice when compared with caesarean birth. A plausible reason for this difference may be related to the adverse physical effects mothers and newborns often experience after CS surgery. Factors such as excruciating pain, anesthesia, prolonged labor, and related respiratory distress among newborns [33,34] may result in healthcare providers being preoccupied with helping both babies and mothers to stabilize rather than initiating breastfeeding [35,36].

Previously published studies indicated that pregnant women being unable to access or attend ANC services during pregnancy poses a significant barrier in initiating breastfeeding within one-hour post-birth [37,38]. However, in the present study, we found that mothers who had four or more ANC visits to a health institution prior to childbirth showed a greater likelihood of EIBF practice than those who had none or less than four ANC visits. This result is similar to that reported in past studies carried out in India [39] and Nepal [40]. Breastfeeding counseling and health messages received through the Baby-Friendly Hospital Initiative (BFHI) may have contributed to the increased likelihood of EIBF noted in the study. It has been suggested in previous work that breastfeeding counseling during ANC visits is positively related to the mother's adherence to the WHO optimal breastfeeding practices [41,42]. Therefore, promoting and supporting ANC uptake in ECOWAS countries could ensure remarkable improvement in EIBF practices.

Newborn babies whose mother perceived their size to be average or larger had an increased likelihood of EIBF within one hour of birth compared with those who were perceived to be small or smaller size. This finding is consistent with a cross-sectional study carried out in Nigeria in 2016, which indicated that newborn babies perceived by their mothers as average or larger size at birth were more likely to be EIBF [29]. Also, a cross-sectional study done in Nepal in 2014 reported that newborn babies whose size was large at birth were significantly more likely to receive EIBF within one hour of birth in comparison with babies whose size was small [28]. The significantly increased odds of EIBF practice among newborn babies perceived to be of average or larger size in ECOWAS countries may be attributed to their physical maturity and associated proper coordination of the suction–deglutination–respiratory cycle and breast-seeking reflex [28]. Conversely, the immaturity of small babies often hinders the abilities required to initiate breastfeeding within one hour of delivery due to poor breast-seeking reflex and sucking inability [43]. Additionally, illness often leads to newborn babies being kept away from their mothers [44], resulting in the early introduction of complementary drinks. Notably, female births were found to be associated with EIBF within one hour of delivery. This outcome is similar to earlier reports in Sri Lanka [45] and Ethiopia [46], which found that male babies were less likely to receive early breastfeeding than their female counterparts. This gender difference in EIBF practice may be influenced by socio-cultural beliefs and require further assessment. However, previous studies have suggested that the practice of prelacteal feeds (or the act of given foods to newborn babies before initiating breastfeeding) in male babies is common and acceptable in African [8,47] and Asian countries [47,48].

Newborn babies born to mothers from a poor household had significantly higher odds of initiating breastfeeding within one hour of birth compared with those from a wealthy household. This finding contradicts previous reports, which indicated that mothers from wealthy households were more likely to initiate breastfeeding in the first hour of delivery [28,35]. Nevertheless, our finding is similar to those reported from Nepal [49] and Namibia [30]. The significantly higher odds of EIBF practice among poor mothers noted in the current study may be attributed to lack of access to infant formula or inability to buy costly complementary substitutes to breast milk, which may result in poor mothers depending solely on breastfeeding. It has also been suggested that mothers from wealthy households were more likely have an elective caesarean section, resulting in delayed initiation of breastfeeding within one hour of birth [50]. It was not unexpected that mothers who frequently watch television or listen to radio were more likely to initiate breastfeeding within one hour of delivery. This finding is consistent with previous studies [51,52]. Apart from health facilities, exposure to other information sources regarding breastfeeding practices during antenatal and postnatal care can also play a key role in encouraging women to practice early initiation of breastfeeding.

Similar to previous reports [30,46], we found that mothers who were having their first child were less likely to initiate breastfeeding within one hour of birth compared with those with two or more deliveries. This may be related to inexperience regarding breastfeeding and relatively poor use of maternal health services by first time mothers. As shown in a past study, earlier breastfeeding experience is correlated with both intention and timely breastfeeding initiation [53].

5. Limitations and Strengths

The following limitations of this study should be considered when making specific conclusions about its findings: (a) the study was unable to establish a causal relationship between the study characteristics and EIBF, as cross-sectional data was used to identify the predictors of EIBF; (b) recall and measurement errors may have overestimated or underestimated the findings of this study, as data regarding some of the study factors was obtained from mothers up to five years after childbirth; (c) there were some unmeasured coexisting factors, such as instrumental vaginal birth, cultural beliefs, and health professionals' prior knowledge of EIBF or family dynamics, which may have also impacted the study findings. Additionally, detailed information concerning infant formula advertising via electronic or print media was not available at the time of the DHS survey. Despite the highlighted weaknesses, there are a number of strengths that should also be noted regarding this study. Firstly, the rate of EIBF was based on nationally representative data of 13 countries, and hence findings could be generalized across the subregion. Secondly, the results are comparable across the ECOWAS countries because all the variables used were similarly described across countries. Thirdly, the study used a combined nationally representative large sample size across the 13 ECOWAS, which meant that the potential impact of selection bias was minimal and unlikely to affect the estimates.

6. Conclusions

The findings of this study suggest that delivery in a hospital or health facility, vaginal delivery, frequent ANC visits (≥4), middle income household, access to electronic media (television or radio), average or larger baby size at birth, child's sex (female), and first birth order were significantly associated with EIBF within one hour of birth in the 13 ECOWAS countries. In the ECOWAS subregion, it is crucial that integrated nutritional health promotion campaigns be conducted both at the community and individual levels. At the community level, the role of midwives and community health officers (CHO) in promoting breastfeeding practices appeared evident, with CHO antenatal home visits contributing to the early initiation of breastfeeding and empowering the community with greater knowledge of the nutrition and health requirements of children under two years of age. At the individual level, interventions to promote the involvement of family members during pregnancy and child birth are needed in ECOWAS and should particularly target young mothers and families from lower socioeconomic groups with lower rates of EIBF.

Author Contributions: Conceptualization, K.E.A. and F.A.O.; methodology, K.E.A. and O.K.E.; software, K.E.A.; validation, O.L.U., F.A.O. and O.K.E.; formal analysis, K.E.A. and P.R.G.; investigation, O.K.E., P.R.G.; resources, W.K.T.; data curation, F.A.O., P.R.G. and O.L.U.; writing—original draft preparation, K.E.A. and O.K.E.; writing—review and editing, O.L.U., W.K.T., G.J.S.; visualization, G.J.S., O.L.U.; supervision, K.E.A., W.K.T. and G.J.S.; project administration, O.K.E., P.R.G. and K.E.A.

Acknowledgments: The authors are grateful to Measure DHS, ICF International, Rockville, Marylands, USA for providing the data for this study. GloMACH: Members are Kingsley E Agho, Felix A Ogbo, Thierno Diallo, Osita E Ezeh, Osuagwu L Uchechukwu, Pramesh R Ghimire, Blessing Akombi, Paschal Ogeleka, Tanvir Abir, Abukari I Issaka, Kedir Yimam Ahmed, Rose Victor, Deborah Charwe, Abdon Gregory Rwabilimbo, Daarwin Subramanee, Mehak Mehak, Nilu Nagdev and Mansi Dhami.

References

1. Collective, G.B.; UNICEF; World Health Organization. *Global Breastfeeding Scorecard, 2017: Tracking Progress for Breastfeeding Policies and Programmes*; World Health Organization: Geneva, Switzerland, 2017.
2. UNICEF. *Levels and Trends in Child Mortality: Report 2011*; WHO Estimates Developed by the UN Inter-Agency Group for Child Mortality Estimation: New York, NY, USA, 2011.
3. United Nations. *Population Facts*; United Nations, Department of Economic and Social Affairs, Population Division: New York, NY, USA, 2017; Volume 6, pp. 1–2.
4. WHO; UNICEF. *Planning Guide for National Implementation of the Global Strategy for Infant and Young Child Feeding*; World Health Organization: Geneva, Switzerland, 2007.
5. WHO; UNICEF; Health WHODoCA. *Handbook IMCI: Integrated Management of Childhood Illness*; World Health Organization: Geneva, Switzerland, 2005.
6. Smith, E.R.; Hurt, L.; Chowdhury, R.; Sinha, B.; Fawzi, W.; Edmond, K.M.; Neovita Study Group. Delayed breastfeeding initiation and infant survival: A systematic review and meta-analysis. *PLoS ONE* **2017**, *12*, e0180722. [CrossRef]
7. Horta, B.L.; Victora, C.G. *Long-Term Effects of Breastfeeding*; World Health Organization: Geneva, Switzerland, 2013; Volume 74.
8. Agho, K.E.; Ogeleka, P.; Ogbo, F.A.; Ezeh, O.K.; Eastwood, J.; Page, A. Trends and Predictors of Prelacteal Feeding Practices in Nigeria (2003–2013). *Nutrients* **2016**, *8*, 462. [CrossRef]
9. Turner, B. Economic Community of West African States (ECOWAS). In *The Statesman's Yearbook*; Springer: Berlin, Germany, 2012; pp. 59–60.
10. DHS. *The Demographic and Health Survey Program*, 2016 ed.; United States Agency for International Development: Washington, DC, USA, 2016.
11. Tawiah-Agyemang, C.; Kirkwood, B.; Edmond, K.; Bazzano, A.; Hill, Z. Early initiation of breast-feeding in Ghana: Barriers and facilitators. *J. Perinatol.* **2008**, *28*, S46–S52. [CrossRef]
12. Leung, A.K.C.; Sauve, R.S. Breast is best for babies. *J. Nat. Med. Assoc.* **2005**, *97*, 1010–1019.
13. Hanieh, S.; Ha, T.T.; Simpson, J.A.; Thuy, T.T.; Khuong, N.C.; Thoang, D.D.; Tran, T.D.; Tuan, T.; Fisher, J.; Biggs, B.-A. Exclusive breast feeding in early infancy reduces the risk of inpatient admission for diarrhea

and suspected pneumonia in rural Vietnam: A prospective cohort study. *BMC Public Health* **2015**, *15*, 1166. [CrossRef] [PubMed]

14. Arifeen, S.; Black, R.E.; Antelman, G.; Baqui, A.; Caulfield, L.; Becker, S. Exclusive breastfeeding reduces acute respiratory infection and diarrhea deaths among infants in Dhaka slums. *Pediatrics* **2001**, *108*, e67. [CrossRef] [PubMed]
15. Edmond, K.M.; Zandoh, C.; Quigley, M.A.; Amenga-Etego, S.; Owusu-Agyei, S.; Kirkwood, B.R. Delayed breastfeeding initiation increases risk of neonatal mortality. *Pediatrics* **2006**, *117*, e380–e386. [CrossRef] [PubMed]
16. Mullany, L.C.; Katz, J.; Li, Y.M.; Khatry, S.K.; LeClerq, S.C.; Darmstadt, G.L.; Tielsch, J.M. Breast-feeding patterns, time to initiation, and mortality risk among newborns in southern Nepal. *J. Nutr.* **2008**, *138*, 599–603. [CrossRef]
17. Exavery, A.; Kanté, A.M.; Hingora, A.; Phillips, J.F. Determinants of early initiation of breastfeeding in rural Tanzania. *Int. Breastfeed. J.* **2015**, *10*, 27. [CrossRef] [PubMed]
18. Ogbo, F.A.; Page, A.; Agho, K.E.; Claudio, F. Determinants of trends in breast-feeding indicators in Nigeria, 1999–2013. *Public Health Nutr.* **2015**, *18*, 3287–3299. [CrossRef]
19. Ogbo, F.A.; Agho, K.E.; Page, A. Determinants of suboptimal breastfeeding practices in Nigeria: Evidence from the 2008 demographic and health survey. *BMC Public Health* **2015**, *15*, 259. [CrossRef] [PubMed]
20. Adewuyi, E.O.; Zhao, Y.; Khanal, V.; Auta, A.; Bulndi, L.B. Rural-urban differences on the rates and factors associated with early initiation of breastfeeding in Nigeria: Further analysis of the Nigeria demographic and health survey, 2013. *Int. Breastfeed. J.* **2017**, *12*, 51. [CrossRef] [PubMed]
21. Mukora-Mutseyekwa, F.; Gunguwo, H.; Mandigo, R.G.; Mundagowa, P. Predictors of early initiation of breastfeeding among Zimbabwean women: Secondary analysis of ZDHS 2015. *Matern. Health Neonatol. Perinatol.* **2019**, *5*, 2. [CrossRef] [PubMed]
22. Bisrat, Z.; Kenzudine, A.; Bossena, T. Factors associated with early initiation and exclusive breastfeeding practices among mothers of infant's age less than 6 months. *J. Pediatr. Neonatal Care* **2017**, *7*, 00292.
23. Corsi, D.J.; Neuman, M.; Finlay, J.E.; Subramanian, S. Demographic and health surveys: A profile. *Int. J. Epidemiol.* **2012**, *41*, 1602–1613. [CrossRef]
24. UNICEF; World Health Organization. *Capture the Moment: Early Initiation of Breastfeeding: The Best Start for Every Newborn*; UNICEF: New York, NY, USA; World Health Organization: Geneva, Switzerland, 2018.
25. Bortz, K. WHO, UNICEF: 78 million newborns not breastfed within first hour after birth. *Infect. Dis. Child.* **2018**, *31*, 19.
26. Rutstein, S.O.; Johnson, K. The DHS Wealth Index. DHS Comparative Reports No. 6. (ORC Macro, Calverton, MD, 2004). Available online: https://dhsprogram.com/pubs/pdf/CR6/CR6.pdf (accessed on 20 August 2019).
27. Rutstein, S.O.; Rojas, G. *Guide to DHS Statistics*; ORC Macro: Calverton, MD, USA, 2006.
28. Adhikari, M.; Khanal, V.; Karkee, R.; Gavidia, T. Factors associated with early initiation of breastfeeding among Nepalese mothers: Further analysis of Nepal Demographic and Health Survey, 2011. *Int. Breastfeed. J.* **2014**, *9*, 21. [CrossRef]
29. Berde, A.S.; Yalcin, S.S. Determinants of early initiation of breastfeeding in Nigeria: A population-based study using the 2013 demograhic and health survey data. *BMC Pregnancy Childbirth* **2016**, *16*, 32. [CrossRef]
30. Ndirangu, M.; Gatimu, S.; Mwinyi, H.; Kibiwott, D. Trends and factors associated with early initiation of breastfeeding in Namibia: Analysis of the demographic and health surveys 2000–2013. *BMC Pregnancy Childbirth* **2018**, *18*, 171. [CrossRef]
31. Liben, M.L.; Gemechu, Y.B.; Adugnew, M.; Asrade, A.; Adamie, B.; Gebremedin, E.; Melak, Y. Factors associated with exclusive breastfeeding practices among mothers in dubti town, afar regional state, northeast Ethiopia: A community based cross-sectional study. *Int. Breastfeed. J.* **2016**, *11*, 4. [CrossRef]
32. Okafor, I.; Olatona, F.; Olufemi, O. Breastfeeding practices of mothers of young children in Lagos, Nigeria. *Niger. J. Paediatr.* **2014**, *41*, 43–47. [CrossRef]
33. Awi, D.; Alikor, E. Barriers to timely initiation of breastfeeding among mothers of healthy full-term babies who deliver at the University of Port Harcourt Teaching Hospital. *Niger. J. Clin. Pract.* **2006**, *9*, 57–64. [PubMed]
34. Liben, M.L.; Yesuf, E.M. Determinants of early initiation of breastfeeding in Amibara district, Northeastern Ethiopia: A community based cross-sectional study. *Int. Breastfeed. J.* **2016**, *11*, 7. [CrossRef] [PubMed]
35. Tilahun, G.; Degu, G.; Azale, T.; Tigabu, A. Prevalence and associated factors of timely initiation of

breastfeeding among mothers at Debre Berhan town, Ethiopia: A cross-sectional study. *Int. Breastfeed. J.* **2016**, *11*, 27. [CrossRef] [PubMed]

36. Hobbs, A.J.; Mannion, C.A.; McDonald, S.W.; Brockway, M.; Tough, S.C. The impact of caesarean section on breastfeeding initiation, duration and difficulties in the first four months postpartum. *BMC Pregnancy Childbirth* **2016**, *16*, 90. [CrossRef] [PubMed]
37. Goldie, S.J.; Sweet, S.; Carvalho, N.; Natchu, U.C.M.; Hu, D. Alternative strategies to reduce maternal mortality in India: A cost-effectiveness analysis. *PLoS Med.* **2010**, *7*, e1000264. [CrossRef] [PubMed]
38. Darmstadt, G.L.; Bhutta, Z.A.; Cousens, S.; Adam, T.; Walker, N.; De Bernis, L. Evidence-based, cost-effective interventions: How many newborn babies can we save? Lancet Neonatal Survival Steering Team. *Lancet* **2005**, *365*, 977–988. [CrossRef]
39. Senanayake, P.; O'Connor, E.; Ogbo, F.A. National and rural-urban prevalence and determinants of early initiation of breastfeeding in India. *BMC Public Health* **2019**, *19*, 896. [CrossRef]
40. Subedi, N.; Paudel, S.; Rana, T.; Poudyal, A. Infant and young child feeding practices in Chepang communities. *J. Nepal Health Res. Counc.* **2012**, *10*, 141–146.
41. El Shafei, A.M.H.; Labib, J.R. Determinants of exclusive breastfeeding and introduction of complementary foods in rural Egyptian communities. *Glob. J. Health Sci.* **2014**, *6*, 236–244. [CrossRef]
42. Mekuria, G.; Edris, M. Exclusive breastfeeding and associated factors among mothers in Debre Markos, Northwest Ethiopia: A cross-sectional study. *Int. Breastfeed. J.* **2015**, *10*, 1. [CrossRef]
43. Walker, M. Breastfeeding the late preterm infant. *J. Obstet. Gynecol. Neonatal Nurs.* **2008**, *37*, 692–701. [CrossRef]
44. Mulready-Ward, C.; Sackoff, J. Outcomes and factors associated with breastfeeding for <8 weeks among preterm infants: Findings from 6 states and NYC, 2004–2007. *Matern. Child Health J.* **2013**, *17*, 1648–1657. [CrossRef]
45. Senarath, U.; Siriwardena, I.; Godakandage, S.S.; Jayawickrama, H.; Fernando, D.N.; Dibley, M.J. Determinants of breastfeeding practices: An analysis of the Sri Lanka Demographic and Health Survey 2006–2007. *Matern. Child Nutr.* **2012**, *8*, 315–329. [CrossRef]
46. John, J.R.; Mistry, S.K.; Kebede, G.; Manohar, N.; Arora, A. Determinants of early initiation of breastfeeding in Ethiopia: A population-based study using the 2016 demographic and health survey data. *BMC Pregnancy Childbirth* **2019**, *19*, 69. [CrossRef]
47. Nguyen, P.H.; Keithly, S.C.; Nguyen, N.T.; Nguyen, T.T.; Tran, L.M.; Hajeebhoy, N. Prelacteal feeding practices in Vietnam: Challenges and associated factors. *BMC Public Health* **2013**, *13*, 932. [CrossRef]
48. Khanal, V.; Adhikari, M.; Sauer, K.; Zhao, Y. Factors associated with the introduction of prelacteal feeds in Nepal: Findings from the Nepal demographic and health survey 2011. *Int. Breastfeed. J.* **2013**, *8*, 9. [CrossRef]
49. Khanal, V.; Scott, J.; Lee, A.; Karkee, R.; Binns, C. Factors associated with early initiation of breastfeeding in Western Nepal. *Int. J. Environ. Res. Public Health Nutr.* **2015**, *12*, 9562–9574. [CrossRef]
50. Rowe-Murray, H.J.; Fisher, J.R. Baby friendly hospital practices: Cesarean section is a persistent barrier to early initiation of breastfeeding. *Birth* **2002**, *29*, 124–131. [CrossRef]
51. Tamiru, D.; Mohammed, S. Maternal knowledge of optimal breastfeeding practices and associated factors in rural communities of Arba Minch Zuria. *Int. J. Nutr. Food Sci.* **2013**, *2*, 122–129. [CrossRef]
52. Hailemariam, T.W.; Adeba, E.; Sufa, A. Predictors of early breastfeeding initiation among mothers of children under 24 months of age in rural part of West Ethiopia. *BMC Public Health* **2015**, *15*, 1076. [CrossRef]
53. Lessen, R.; Crivelli-Kovach, A. Prediction of initiation and duration of breast-feeding for neonates admitted to the neonatal intensive care unit. *J. Perinat. Neonatal Nurs.* **2007**, *21*, 256–266. [CrossRef]

2

Zinc Deficiency among Lactating Mothers from a Peri-Urban Community of the Ecuadorian Andean Region: An Initial Approach to the Need of Zinc Supplementation

Camila Narváez-Caicedo [1], Gabriela Moreano [1], Bernardo A. Sandoval [1,2] and Miguel Á. Jara-Palacios [1,*]

[1] Escuela de Medicina, Facultad de Ciencias Médicas de la Salud y de la Vida, Universidad Internacional del Ecuador, 170113 Quito, Ecuador; camilanarvaezca@gmail.com (C.N.-C.); gaby.moreano94@gmail.com (G.M.); bsandoval@uide.edu.ec (B.A.S.)

[2] Servicio de Cirugía, Hospital Metropolitano, 170521 Quito, Ecuador

* Correspondence: migueljarapalacios@gmail.com

Abstract: Zinc is an important mineral for biological and physiological processes. Zinc deficiency (ZD) is one of the most common micronutrient deficiencies worldwide and a crucial determinant of pregnancy outcomes and childhood development. Zinc levels and the zinc supplementation rate among lactating women have not been assessed neither in Ecuador nor in the Andean region. We conducted a pilot study including 64 mothers of infants between eight days to seven months old from a primary care center located in Conocoto, a peri-urban community of Quito, Ecuador. The mothers were interviewed and a fasting blood sample was taken to determine plasma zinc levels. The prevalence of ZD was calculated and compared with the prevalence of ZD among Ecuadorian non-pregnant non-lactating women, and the sample was analysed considering zinc supplementation during pregnancy. The prevalence of ZD among the participants was 81.3% (95% CI: 71.7–90.9), higher than the reported among non-pregnant non-lactating women ($G^2 = 18.2$; $p < 0.05$). Zinc supplementation rate was 31.2%. No significant differences were found comparing the groups considering zinc supplementation. The insights obtained from this study encourage extending studies to document zinc levels and its interactions among breastfeeding women in areas with a high prevalence of ZD in order to determine the need of zinc supplementation.

Keywords: zinc deficiency; plasma zinc; lactating women; zinc supplementation; Quito; Ecuador; Andean region

---

1. Introduction

Zinc is an ubiquitous mineral within the body that has catalytic, structural, and regulatory biological functions [1]. This mineral is known to be an essential micronutrient for development and normal cell activity [2]. Zinc deficiency (ZD) is one of the most common micronutrient deficiencies worldwide, affecting around 2 billion people, especially among developing countries. ZD has important consequences especially during pregnancy, lactation, and childhood development [3,4].

In spite of the physiological adjustment, which increases the zinc absorption during pregnancy and lactation, women and children are still affected by zinc deficiency due to increased nutrient requirements [5,6]. During pregnancy, ZD can affect multiple systems and could increase the risk of infections, preeclampsia, miscarriages, and adverse fetal outcomes, such as fetal growth restriction, low weight at birth, neurological malformations, and/or neurological impairment [2,4–11]. If ZD in the mothers persists after birth, particularly if their infants are exclusively breastfed, adverse infant development outcomes may occur [2,8].

Approximately 82% of mothers around the world do not have an adequate zinc intake in their diet, but the prevalence of ZD during pregnancy worldwide has not been determined [12]. It has been reported a higher prevalence of zinc deficiency among pregnant, compared to non-pregnant, women in India (65; 41%), Ethiopia (56; 34%), and Pakistan (48; 42%) [13–16]. In lactating women, the prevalence of ZD varied widely among small cohorts from different countries, such as Indonesia (25%) and Vietnam (55%) [17,18].

In Ecuador, according to the Ecuadorian National Health and Nutrition Survey (ENSANUT-ECU, 2014), 56.1% (95% CI: 54.9–57.1) of women of reproductive age have ZD. Pregnant and lactating women were not sampled in this survey [19]. On the other hand, a study conducted previously by our research group, found a prevalence of ZD of 31.4% (95% CI: 17.1–48.6) in a small cohort of mothers of children with non-syndromic cleft lip with or without cleft palate. It is important to clarify that these women did not exclusively breastfed their babies due to the oral malformation [20].

Micronutrient deficiencies have been observed in Ecuador for at least two decades, particularly in vulnerable segments of the population [21]; in part, it could be affected by globalization through multiple pathways, such as urbanization, economic growth, trade, and investments [21,22]. Processes of urbanization are associated with higher inequality and changes in the food environment, subsequently affecting the nutritional status, especially in poor people who cannot afford food of high nutritional quality [22]. Nowadays, peri-urban areas of Quito are suffering accelerated urbanization, growing in population at a higher index than the urban area [23,24].

The suggested association between maternal zinc depletion and poor outcomes of pregnancy and lactation have raised the possibility of prevention by using supplementary zinc, but results of previous studies have not been conclusive and still need to be assessed, especially focusing on populations with low dietary zinc intake [25].

The objective of the present study was to assess plasma zinc (PZn) levels and zinc supplementation rate during pregnancy, among lactating women attending to a public care center from a peri-urban Andean community of Quito, Ecuador in order to make an initial approach to the zinc status of lactating women in the region.

2. Materials and Methods

2.1. Study Setting and Participants

Between October 2015 and July 2016, a case study series was conducted in order to determine the rate of ZD among Ecuadorian mothers who have a breastfeeding infant, lived in Conocoto, and attended to the Primary Health Centre of Conocoto for regular paediatric and/or gynaecological check-ups. This health center belongs to the Ministry of Public Health which offers its services to the general population especially to people who have no private or social insurance [26].

Conocoto is one of the 33 rural parishes of Quito, the capital of Ecuador, located in the Andean region. Today, it is a heterogeneous territory with extensively urbanized areas and a few rural neighbourhoods pressed by growing urbanization. According to the last national census conducted in 2010, in Conocoto there were 82,072 inhabitants of whom 42,381 were women, with a population density of 1594 people/km^2 and a birth rate of 16.98 [27]. Of the 33 rural parishes of Quito, eight have been characterised as peri-urbans [23].

We collected pertinent clinical information and a single blood sample to quantify zinc levels from the mothers; after they read and signed an informed consent.

Inclusion criteria were women who lived in Conocoto and had a child who was being fed mainly with breast milk. By mainly, we mean that at the time of the interview at least 90% of the children's diet was breast milk, but three or fewer times a week some of them received other types of foods, such as "coladas" (a beverage made out of water and any kind of cereal flour), water, or formula.

As exclusion criteria, we considered the following: diagnosis of any chronic disease, any malformation in the index child, use of oral contraceptives, consumption of alcohol, cigarettes or any recreational drug at any time, any respiratory or gastrointestinal infection during the fifteen days prior to sampling and use of pharmacological therapy within this period. Additionally, we excluded pregnant women, non-fasting women, women with any disability that interferes with sample collection, and women who consumed alcohol or performed extreme exercise the night before sampling, factors that were contemplated by ENSANUT-ECU. We followed these guidelines following the methodology of a previous report of our research group [20].

This study was conducted following the Declaration of Helsinki, approved by the Bioethics Committee of the Universidad Internacional del Ecuador and registered it under the number 04-2013.

2.2. Measurements

Maternal variables recorded were age, educational level, number of pregnancy check-ups, and intake of vitamin and mineral supplements. In regards to vitamin and mineral supplements, we asked at what time during pregnancy they started consuming it, doses, frequency, and the form of the supplement ingested. Infant variables registered were age at the time of the interview, sex, weight at birth, length at birth, and gestational age at birth. The weight, length, and gestational age at birth were obtained from hospital records. All other information was based on self-report by the mothers.

2.3. Collection of Blood Samples and Determination of Zinc Levels

A single blood sample was obtained between 8 and 10 a.m. from fasting mothers using tubes coated with lithium heparin and a gel separator (BD Vacutainer® PST™, Becton-Dickinson Inc, Franklin Lakes, NJ, USA). The tubes were centrifuged for 10 min and refrigerated at 2–8 °C during 3–6 h. In the laboratory, the plasma was separated into additional tubes and stored at −80 °C. Plasma samples contaminated with lysed red blood cells were discarded. Then, prior to zinc quantification, the refrigerated samples were thawed at room temperature (20–24 °C), and mixed with a vortex. PZn were measured by flame-atomic-absorption spectrophotometry (AAnalyst 400, PerkinElmert, Billerica, MA, USA), the coefficient of variation for the essay was 6.2%. A standard solution of zinc in 1000 ± 4 mg/L of nitric acid (Fluka™ Analytical, Steinheim, Germany) (2% p/p) was used for the calibration curve with dilutions from 25 to 300 ppb. All chemicals were of analytical grade purity (Type I water, nitric acid 69%). Zinc quantification of all the samples was performed at the same time in dust-free fume hoods with minimal contact with air. We followed the same criteria that in our previous report [20].

Previous reports suggest 10.70 µmol/L as the cut-off point for zinc deficiency in fasting females over 10 years-old [6,28], and this value was utilized as the cut-off point by ENSANUT-ECU [19]. Therefore, we adopted this cut-off point in order to determine ZD in the present study and to compare it with the general population of Ecuadorian women of reproductive age.

2.4. Data Processing

The sample was evaluated as one group and divided in two subgroups based on the mothers' declaration of zinc consumption during pregnancy. The data were analyzed using the Statistical Package for Social Science (SPSS) Statistics for Windows, version 20.0 (IBM Corp., Armonk, NY, USA). Correlations were assessed by Spearman's rho, and $p < 0.05$ was considered as statistical significant. The t-test was used to compare the plasma zinc level means of the supplemented and non-supplemented groups.

In order to compare the prevalence of ZD in our sample with the reported among women of reproductive age by ENSANUT-ECU, we used the likelihood ratio and its corresponding statistic (G^2); $p < 0.05$ was considered as statistical significant.

3. Results

We collected data and blood samples from 64 mothers, 3.2 (1.8) months postpartum. The mothers were between 15 and 39 years old with a mean age of 26.8 (6.4) years old. The majority of their infants were full-term (93.8%), and had adequate weight (76.6%) and length (62.5%) at birth (Table 1).

Table 1. Plasma zinc levels, maternal and infant characteristics of zinc supplemented and non-supplemented women during their pregnancies (n = 64).

Recorded Variables	All the Sample n = 64	Women Who Did Not Received Zinc Supplements n = 44	Women Who Received Zinc Supplements n = 20	ρ (Rho) de Spearman	p−Value
Maternal variables					
Age (years, mean ± SD) *	26.8 ± 6.5	26.1 ± 6.8	28.4 ± 5.7	0.17	0.17
Level of education (%)					
Elementary school only	21.9	22.7	20.0	0.03	0.81
High school or any superior level	78.1	77.3	80.0		
Number of prenatal check−ups (%)					
<5	6.2	6.8	5.0	0.04	0.79
≥5	93.8	93.2	95.0		
Consumption of iron during pregnancy (%)					
Yes	93.8	90.9	100	0.17	0.17
No	6.2	9.1	0		
Consumption of folic acid during pregnancy (%)					
Yes	96.9	95.5	100	0.12	0.34
No	3.1	4.5	0		
PZn (μmol/L, mean ± SD) *	9.3 ± 1.8	9.07 ± 1.7	9.72 ± 2.0		
Zinc deficiency n (%)	52 (81.2)	37 (84.1)	15 (75)	−0.11	0.40
Infant variables					
Infants' age (months, mean ± SD) *	3.2 ± 1.8	3.3 ± 1.8	3.0 ± 1.7		
Sex (Male/Female)	32/32	22/22	10/10		
Gestational age at birth (%)					
37 weeks or more	92.2	90.9	95.0	0.07	0.58
Less than 37 weeks	7.8	9.1	5.0		
Weight at birth					
2500 g or more	78.1	79.5	75.0	−0.05	0.69
Less than 2500 g	21.9	20.5	25.0		
Length at birth (%)					
48 cm or more	62.5	61.4	65.0	0.04	0.79
Less than 48 cm	37.5	38.6	35.0		

* t was calculated with non-statistical significant results. SD: Standard deviation.

The percentages of women who consumed folic acid, iron, and zinc during pregnancy were 96.9%, 93.8%, and 31.2%, respectively (Table 1). The participants who reported ingesting zinc during pregnancy affirmed to have consumed zinc as part of a multivitamin supplement, but the majority of them were not able to accurately provide the doses and frequency of the supplements consumed and it was not possible to analyze this data.

The PZn levels were between 3.9 to 13.0 μmol/L, the mean PZn concentration was 9.3 (1.8) μmol/L. The first, second, third, and fourth quartiles were 8.1, 9.2, 10.3, and 13.0 μmol/L, respectively. We found ZD in 52 women with a prevalence of ZD of 81.2% (95% CI: 71.7–90.9), which is statically different to the reported among women of reproductive age by ENSANUT-ECU of 56.1% (95% CI: 54.9–57.1) ($G^2 = 18.23$; $p < 0.05$) [19]. There was no difference between the means of plasma zinc levels of the supplemented and non-supplemented groups ($t = 1.34$; $p > 0.05$).

4. Discussion

The prevalence of ZD worldwide is unknown. Nevertheless, a global inadequate zinc intake rate of 17.3% has been estimated with a high geographical variation. The Andean region, which Ecuador is part of, has an estimated inadequate zinc intake of 17.0% [29]. ZD is widespread especially among developing countries affecting mainly children, and pregnant and lactating women [2,3,5,9], and it is expected to especially affect people living in areas of high urbanization that have been associated with higher levels of inequality and subsequent micronutrient deficiencies [21,22].

Many studies have found that ZD is higher among pregnant than non-pregnant women [13–16] and that zinc levels between pregnancy and postpartum periods do not differ significantly [30], which raises the need to evaluate zinc status among pregnant and lactating women in Ecuador, where high rates of ZD have been reported [19].

In Ecuador, the prevalence of ZD reported by ENSANUT-ECU among women of reproductive age from the general population is 56.1% and varies across the country, being higher in the urban coast (62.9%) and lower in the rural highlands (46.6%). In Quito, the prevalence of ZD is 55.6% [19].

Our results showed a higher prevalence of ZD among lactating women than in non-pregnant non-lactating women of reproductive age reported by ENSANUT-ECU [19], which agrees with previous reports from India, Ethiopia, and Pakistan. However, it is worth clarifying that the studies performed in Ethiopia and Pakistan evaluated zinc deficiency in both groups which were part of the same cohort [14–16]. Additionally, it is important to note that we are comparing two groups with different physiological status because lactating women are in a period of high metabolic demand in order to supply milk for their offspring [5,6].

Another factor that could be related to the high prevalence of ZD in our sample is the fact that nearly all the participants received iron supplements during pregnancy. The competition between iron and zinc absorption is well known, which means that PZn levels will be lower when iron is concurrently supplemented [6,31,32].

Although a mother with ZD most likely would have breast milk with a normal zinc concentration due to a physiological adjustment that tries to supply enough zinc for their offspring, it has been found that children of mothers with profound ZD are at risk of ZD and its consequences [17,31,33]. Therefore, an adequate zinc nutrition is necessary for normal pregnancy outcomes, child growth, adequate immune function and neurocognitive development [2,4,5,7–11]. We could not find any association between maternal zinc levels, zinc supplementation, and the anthropometry of their infants at birth, probably because our sample was small with the majority having ZD; nevertheless, the rates of ZD, premature delivery, and low weight and length at birth are not negligible [11]. Despite this, comparing the groups based on the declaration of zinc ingestion during pregnancy, we observed a slightly lower prevalence of zinc deficiency among the supplemented group than the non-supplemented group which was not statistically significant. The aforementioned statements raise the necessity to extend studies in order to assess the need of zinc supplementation among lactating women in disadvantaged groups with similar conditions.

Zinc supplementation has proven to reduce the rate of premature delivery, and improve linear growth and weight gain, especially in children of short stature, and decrease morbidity, duration, and severity of diarrhea and acute lower respiratory infection [1,8,34]. Supplementing zinc during pregnancy and lactation increases the mothers' PZn concentration by 3% and 1%, respectively, which could protect the mothers' nutritional status and, therefore, their children during these periods of life [35].

In spite of the aforementioned health zinc benefits, the World Health Organization (WHO) recommends zinc supplementation for pregnant women only in the context of rigorous research due to the moderate to low certainty evidence related to maternal, fetal, and neonatal outcomes, and no guidelines for zinc supplementation during lactation exist [7,36]. Nevertheless, we found that 31.2% of the participants were supplemented with zinc during pregnancy and suspended after delivery. Maternal zinc supplementation during lactation has yielded inconsistent results regarding the improvement of breast milk zinc concentrations or to demonstrate benefits for mothers and their infants [37,38]; however, considering the high rates of ZD among lactating women, it is worth extending studies to address the need of zinc supplementation identifying a profile of mothers that could benefit from this.

It is important to mention that in a previous report following the same methodology, we evaluated PZn levels in a cohort of 35 women who had a child between 1 and 12-months-old with an oral malformation, reporting a prevalence of ZD of 31.4; these results were probably due to the use of formula to feed the children because the oral malformation causes breastfeeding difficulties [20]. Lactation is a risk factor for zinc deficiency and the recommended dietary allowance is higher among pregnant and lactating women than in non-pregnant non-lactating women [6]. Therefore, the use of formula could have protected the mothers of children with the oral malformation from developing ZD in the postpartum period and could explain its lower ZD prevalence compared with the women of the present study.

Our study had several limitations. First, the sample corresponds to a small group of women from a single peri-urban community of Quito which does not allow extending these results, as the prevalence of zinc deficiency could differ by taking into account differences in socio-economic status or geographical location, however, this could be an example of what is happening among women from communities under pressure of accelerated urbanization where inequality levels are high [21,22].

Second, even though women who were going through any type of clinical infection or disease were excluded from the study, we did not assess any inflammatory marker, such as alpha 1 glycoprotein, C-reactive protein and interleukin-6; that would allow exclusion of women with an inflammatory process that could be related to decreased PZn [39,40]. It is also important to note that postpartum women, in general, have a more active immune system and higher serum levels of proinflammatory cytokines, and it is somewhat more active among breastfeeding than formula-feeding women [41]. Third, we were unable to register the doses, frequency, and forms of zinc ingested as, most of time, it was part of a multivitamin and mineral supplement; this did not allow for a deep analysis regarding zinc supplementation. Finally, we included only healthy women, therefore, this prevalence would likely increase if women with any comorbidity were included.

The results of this study raise the necessity to evaluate zinc supplementation during pregnancy and the extension to the lactation period in breastfeeding women who attend public care centers for their controls after delivery living in communities experiencing accelerated urbanization, such as Conocoto. Furthermore, we recommend extending studies in the Andean region and in areas with a suspected or confirmed high prevalence of ZD to document levels of zinc among breastfeeding women.

Author Contributions: M.Á.J.-P. conceived the study, analyzed and interpreted the results, helped draft the manuscript, and provided overall coordination of the study. C.N.-C. collected data, analyzed the results, and drafted the manuscript. G.M. collected data and helped draft the manuscript. B.A.S. participated in the study design and analyzed the results. All authors read and approved the final manuscript.

Acknowledgments: The authors wish to thank Angélica C. Cornejo for the critical review and Andrés A. Galvis for his help with the statistical analysis. We also thank David Acosta and the staff of the Public Medical Center of Conocoto who helped us planning the sampling, and to the mothers who participated in the study; contributing considerably.

References

1. Brown, K.H.; Wuehler, S.E.; Peerson, J.M. The importance of zinc in human nutrition and estimation of the global prevalence of zinc deficiency. *Food Nutr. Bull.* **2001**, *22*, 113–125. [CrossRef]
2. Colombo, J.; Zavaleta, N.; Kannass, K.; Lazarte, F.; Albornoz, C.; Kapa, L.; Caulfield, L. Zinc supplementation sustained normative neurodevelopment in a randomized, controlled trial of peruvian infants aged 6–18 months. *J. Nutr.* **2014**, *144*, 1298–1305. [CrossRef] [PubMed]
3. Bailey, R.L.; West, K.P.; Black, R.E. The epidemiology of global micronutrient deficiencies. *Ann. Nutr. Metab.* **2015**, *66*, 22–33. [CrossRef] [PubMed]
4. Institute of Medicine (US) Committee on Micronutrient Deficiencies; Howson, C.P.; Kennedy, E.T.; Horwitz, A. *Prevention of Micronutrient Deficiencies: Tools for Policymakers and Public Health Workers*; National Academies Press (US): Washington, DC, USA, 1998. Available online: https://www.ncbi.nlm.nih.gov/books/NBK230107/ (accessed on 3 July 2018).
5. Ejezie, F.E.; Nwagha, U.I. Zinc Concentration During pregnancy and Lactation in Enugu, South-East Nigeria. *Ann. Med. Health Sci. Res.* **2011**, *1*, 69–76. [PubMed]
6. King, J.C.; Brown, K.H.; Gibson, R.S.; Krebs, N.F.; Lowe, N.M.; Siekmann, J.H.; Raiten, D.J. Biomarkers of Nutrition for Development (BOND)—Zinc Review. *J. Nutr.* **2016**, *146*, 858S. [CrossRef] [PubMed]
7. Ota, E.; Mori, R.; Middleton, P.; Tobe-Gai, R.; Mahomed, K.; Bhutta, Z. Zinc supplementation for improving pregnancy and infant outcome. *Cochrane Database Syst. Rev.* **2012**, 1–97. [CrossRef] [PubMed]
8. Black, M. Zinc deficiency and child development. *Am. J. Clin. Nutr.* **1998**, *68*, 464S–469S. [CrossRef] [PubMed]
9. Liu, J.; Hanlon, A.; Ma, C.; Zhao, S.R.; Cao, S.; Compher, C. Low blood zinc, iron, and other sociodemographic factors associated with behavior problems in preschoolers. *Nutrients* **2014**, *6*, 530–545. [CrossRef] [PubMed]
10. Tamura, T.; Goldenberg, R.L.; Ramey, S.L.; Nelson, K.G.; Chapman, V.R. Effect of zinc supplementation of pregnant women on the mental and psychomotor development of their children at 5 years of age. *Am. J. Clin. Nutr.* **2003**, *77*, 1512–1516. [CrossRef] [PubMed]
11. Wang, H.; Hu, Y.-F.; Hao, J.-H.; Chen, Y.-H.; Su, P.-Y.; Wang, Y.; Yu, Z.; Fu, L.; Xu, Y.-Y.; Zhang, C.; et al. Maternal zinc deficiency during pregnancy elevates the risks of fetal growth restriction: A population-based birth cohort study. *Sci. Rep.* **2015**, *5*, 11262. [CrossRef] [PubMed]
12. Caulfield, L.E.; Zavaleta, N.; Shankar, A.H.; Merialdi, M. Potential contribution of maternal zinc supplementation during pregnancy to maternal and child survival 1–3. *Am. J. Clin. Nutr.* **1998**, *68*, 499S–508S. [CrossRef] [PubMed]
13. Pathak, P.; Kapil, U.; Dwivedi, S.N.; Singh, R. Serum zinc levels amongst pregnant women in a rural block of Haryana state, India. *Asia Pac. J. Clin. Nutr.* **2008**, *17*, 276–279. [PubMed]
14. Harika, R.; Faber, M.; Samuel, F.; Kimiywe, J.; Mulugeta, A.; Eilander, A. Micronutrient status and dietary intake of iron, Vitamin A, iodine, folate and zinc in women of reproductive age and pregnant women in Ethiopia, Kenya, Nigeria and South Africa: A systematic review of data from 2005 to 2015. *Nutrients* **2017**, *9*, 1096. [CrossRef] [PubMed]
15. Akhtar, S. Zinc status in South Asian populations—An update. *J. Health Popul. Nutr.* **2013**, *31*, 139–149. [CrossRef] [PubMed]
16. Bhutta, Z. Pakistan National Nutrition Survey 2011. *Natl. Nutr. Surv.* **2012**, 1–84. Available online: http://www.mhinnovation.net/sites/default/files/downloads/innovation/research/Pakistan%20National%20Nutrition%20Survey%202011.pdf (accessed on 3 July 2018).
17. Dijkhuizen, M.A.; Wieringa, F.T.; West, C.E.; Muherdiyantiningsih; Muhilal. Concurrent micronutrient deficiencies in lactating mothers and their infants in Indonesia. *Am. J. Clin. Nutr.* **2001**, *73*, 786–791. [PubMed]

18. Nakamori, M.; Ninh, N.X.; Isomura, H.; Yoshiike, N.; Hien, V.T.T.; Nhug, B.T.; Nhien, N.V.; Nakano, T.; Khan, N.C.; Yamamoto, S. Nutritional status of lactating mothers and their breast milk concentration of iron, zinc and copper in rural Vietnam. *J. Nutr. Sci. Vitaminol.* **2009**, *55*, 338–345. [CrossRef] [PubMed]
19. Freire, W.B.; Ramírez-Luzuriaga, M.J.; Belmont, P.; Mendieta, M.J.; Silva-Jaramillo, K.; Romero, N.; Sáenz, K.; Piñeiros, P.; Gómez, L.F.; Monge, R. *Tomo I: Encuesta Nacional de Salud y Nutrición de la población ecuatoriana de cero a 59 años*; ENSANUT-ECU 2012; Ministerio de Salud Pública/Instituto Nacional de Estadísticas y Censos: Quito, Ecuador, 2014. Available online: http://www.ecuadorencifras.gob.ec/documentos/web-inec/Estadisticas_Sociales/ENSANUT/MSP_ENSANUT-ECU_06-10-2014.pdf (accessed on 3 July 2018).
20. Jara-Palacios, M.A.; Cornejo, A.C.; Narváez-Caicedo, C.; Moreano, G.; Vásquez, K.P.; Moreno-Izquierdo, C.; Romero-Sandoval, N. Plasma zinc levels in Ecuadorian mothers of infants with nonsyndromic cleft lip with or without cleft palate: A case series. *Birth Defects Res.* **2018**, 495–501. [CrossRef] [PubMed]
21. Freire, W.; Silva-jaramillo, K.; Ramírez-Luzuriaga, M.; Belmont, P.; Waters, W. The double burden of undernutrition and excess body weight in Ecuador. *Am. J. Clin. Nutr.* **2014**, *100*, 1636–1643. [CrossRef] [PubMed]
22. Schram, A.; Labonté, R.; Sanders, D. Urbanization and international trade and investment policies as determinants of noncommunicable diseases in sub-saharan Africa. *Prog. Cardiovasc. Dis.* **2013**, *56*, 281–301. [CrossRef] [PubMed]
23. Pinto-Valencia, P. Las parroquias rurales de Quito y sus interrelaciones con el espacio urbano. *Revista del Instituto de la Ciudad* **2013**, *2*, 71–119. Available online: http://repositorio.flacsoandes.edu.ec/bitstream/10469/6454/1/REXTN-QUR5-03-Pinto.pdf (accessed on 3 July 2018).
24. *Diagnóstico del Territorio del Distrito Metropolitano de Quito*. Unidad del Plan de Desarrollo y Ordenamiento Territorial del DMQ. Municipio del Distrito Metropolitano de Quito: Diagnóstico Estratégico-Eje Territorial. 2014. Available online: http://gobiernoabierto.quito.gob.ec/wp-content/uploads/documentos/pdf/diagnosticoterritorio.pdf (accessed on 3 July 2018).
25. Mahomed, K.; James, D.K.; Golding, J.; McCabe, R. Zinc supplementation during pregnancy: A double blind randomised controlled trial. *Br. Med. J.* **1989**, *299*, 826–830. [CrossRef]
26. Lucio, R.; Villacrés, N.; Henríquez, R. Sistema de salud de Ecuador. *Salud Pub. Mex.* **2011**, *53*, 177–187. [CrossRef]
27. Gobierno Autónomo Descentralizado Parroquial de Conocoto. *Plan De Desarrollo y Ordenamiento Territorial de Conocoto 2012–2025*; Dirección de Gestión de Desarrollo Comunitario e Inclusión Social/Dirección de Gestión de Planificación: Quito, Ecuador, 2012. Available online: http://181.112.151.230:8081/attachments/download/558/PDOT%20CONOCOTO%202012.pdf (accessed on 3 July 2018).
28. Hotz, C.; Peerson, J.M.; Brown, K.H. Suggested lower cutoffs of serum zinc concentrations for assessing zinc status: Reanalysis of the second National Health and Nutrition Examination Survey data (1976–1980). *Am. J. Clin. Nutr.* **2003**, *78*, 756–764. [CrossRef] [PubMed]
29. Wessells, K.R.; Brown, K.H. Estimating the Global Prevalence of Zinc Deficiency: Results Based on Zinc Availability in National Food Supplies and the Prevalence of Stunting. *PLoS ONE* **2012**, *7*, e50568. [CrossRef] [PubMed]
30. Severi, C.; Hambidge, M.; Krebs, N.; Alonso, R.; Atalah, E. Zinc in plasma and breast milk in adolescents and adults in pregnancy and pospartum: A cohort study in Uruguay. *Nutr. Hosp.* **2013**, *28*, 223–228. [CrossRef] [PubMed]
31. Donangelo, C.M.; King, J.C. Maternal zinc intakes and homeostatic adjustments during pregnancy and lactation. *Nutrients* **2012**, *4*, 782–798. [CrossRef] [PubMed]
32. Swanson, C.A.; King, J.C. Zinc utilization in pregnant and nonpregnant women fed controlled diets providing the zinc RDA. *J. Nutr.* **1982**, *112*, 697–707. [CrossRef] [PubMed]
33. Donangelo, C.M.; Vargas-Zapata, C.L.; Woodhouse, L.R.; Shames, D.M.; Mukherjea, R.; King, J.C. Zinc absorption and kinetics during pregnancy and lactation in Brazilian women. *Am. J. Clin. Nutr.* **2005**, *82*, 118–124. [CrossRef] [PubMed]
34. Bhutta, Z.A.; Black, R.E.; Brown, K.H.; Meeks-Gardner, J.; Gore, S.; Hidayat, A.; Khatun, F.; Martorell, R.; Ninh, N.X.; Penny, M.E.; et al. Prevention of diarrhea and pneumonia by zinc supplementation in children in developing countries: Pooled analysis of randomized controlled trials. *J. Pediatr.* **1999**, *135*, 689–697. [CrossRef]

35. Moran, V.H.; Skinner, A.L.; Medina, M.W.; Patel, S.; Dykes, F.; Souverein, O.W.; Dullemeijer, C.; Lowe, N.M. The relationship between zinc intake and serum/plasma zinc concentration in pregnant and lactating women: A systematic review with dose-response meta-analyses. *J. Trace Elem. Med. Biol.* **2012**, *26*, 74–79. [CrossRef] [PubMed]
36. World Health Organization (WHO). *WHO Recommendation on Antenatal Care for a Positive Pregnancy Experience*; WHO: Geneva, Switzerland, 2016.
37. Krebs, N. Zinc supplementation during lactation. *Am. J. Clin. Nutr.* **1998**, 510S–512S. [CrossRef] [PubMed]
38. Sazawal, S.; Black, R.E.; Dhingra, P.; Jalla, S.; Krebs, N.; Malik, P.; Dhingra, U.; Bhan, M.K. Zinc Supplementation does not Affect the Breast Milk Zinc Concentration of Lactating Women Belonging to Low Socioeconomic Population. *J. Hum. Nutr. Food Sci.* **2013**, *1*, 1–6.
39. Karakochuk, C.D.; Barr, S.I.; Boy, E.; Bahizire, E.; Tugirimana, P.L.; Akilimali, P.Z.; Houghton, L.A.; Green, T.J. The effect of inflammation on serum zinc concentrations and the prevalence estimates of population-level zinc status among Congolese children aged 6–59 months. *Eur. J. Clin. Nutr.* **2017**, *71*, 1467–1470. [CrossRef] [PubMed]
40. MacDonell, S.O.; Miller, J.C.; Harper, M.J.; Reid, M.R.; Haszard, J.J.; Gibson, R.S.; Houghton, L.A. A comparison of methods for adjusting biomarkers of iron, zinc, and selenium status for the effect of inflammation in an older population: A case for interleukin 6. *Am. J. Clin. Nutr.* **2018**, 932–940. [CrossRef] [PubMed]
41. Groer, M.W.; Davis, M.W.; Smith, K.; Casey, K.; Kramer, V.; Bulovsky, E. Immunity, inflammation and infection in post-partum breast and formula feeders. *Am. J. Reprod. Immunol.* **2005**, *54*, 222–231. [CrossRef] [PubMed]

3

Human Milk Oligosaccharides in the Milk of Mothers Delivering Term versus Preterm Infants

Sean Austin [1,*], Carlos A. De Castro [2], Norbert Sprenger [1], Aristea Binia [1], Michael Affolter [1], Clara L. Garcia-Rodenas [1], Lydie Beauport [3], Jean-François Tolsa [3] and Céline J. Fischer Fumeaux [3]

1 Nestlé Research, Vers-Chez-Les-Blanc, 1000 Lausanne, Switzerland; norbert.sprenger@rdls.nestle.com (N.S.); Aristea.Binia@rdls.nestle.com (A.B.); michael.affolter@rdls.nestle.com (M.A.); Clara.Garcia@rdls.nestle.com (C.L.G.-R.)

2 Nestle Research Singapore, 29 Quality Road, 618802 Singapore, Singapore; CarlosAntonio.DeCastro@rdsg.nestle.com

3 Centre Hospitalier Universitaire Vaudois, 1011 Lausanne, Switzerland; Lydie.Beauport@chuv.ch (L.B.); Jean-Francois.Tolsa@chuv.ch (J.-F.T.); Celine-Julie.Fischer@chuv.ch (C.J.F.F.)

* Correspondence: sean.austin@rdls.nestle.com

Abstract: Human milk oligosaccharides (HMOs) are a major component of human milk, and play an important role in protecting the infant from infections. Preterm infants are particularly vulnerable, but have improved outcomes if fed with human milk. This study aimed to determine if the HMO composition of preterm milk differed from that of term milk at equivalent stage of lactation and equivalent postmenstrual age. In all, 22 HMOs were analyzed in 500 samples of milk from 25 mothers breastfeeding very preterm infants (< 32 weeks of gestational age, < 1500 g of birthweight) and 28 mothers breastfeeding term infants. The concentrations of most HMOs were comparable at equivalent postpartum age. However, HMOs containing α-1,2-linked fucose were reduced in concentration in preterm milk during the first month of lactation. The concentrations of a number of sialylated oligosaccharides were also different in preterm milk, in particular 3′-sialyllactose concentrations were elevated. At equivalent postmenstrual age, the concentrations of a number of HMOs were significantly different in preterm compared to term milk. The largest differences manifest around 40 weeks of postmenstrual age, when the milk of term infants contains the highest concentrations of HMOs. The observed differences warrant further investigation in view of their potential clinical impact.

Keywords: 2′-fucosyllactose (2′FL); 3′-sialyllactose (3′SL); disialyllacto-N-tetraose (DSLNT); human milk oligosaccharides (HMO); milk group; secretor; Lewis; lactation; preterm

---

1. Introduction

Human milk is the optimal source of nutrition for infants, and it is widely recommended that infants are exclusively or predominantly breastfed for the first 6 months of life [1,2]. In preterm neonates, human milk feeding is known to have several important specific protective actions and it is strongly encouraged too [1,3,4]. Preterm infants consuming human milk have notably improved immunity [5], are less likely to develop necrotizing enterocolitis (NEC) [6], have improved neurodevelopmental outcomes [1,7] and a better long term health outcome [8,9].

However, as nutritional needs of preterm infants are higher compared to those of term infants, human milk composition may not match the nutritional needs of very preterm infants (< 32 weeks of gestational age, < 1500g of birthweight) during the first weeks of life. In this context, human milk fortification in energy, proteins and minerals is commonly recommended in routine nutritional neonatal care of very preterm infants [4]. To optimize current practices, additional knowledge on human milk composition and opportunities in nutrient supplementation remain to be further explored.

While the composition of preterm milk has been investigated [10], and it is reported to be slightly different from that of term milk [11,12], there are relatively few studies focusing on the human milk oligosaccharide (HMO) composition of preterm milk.

HMOs are the 4th most abundant component of human milk after water, lipids and lactose, and may be present at concentrations up to 25 g/L in colostrum and between 10 to 15 g/L in mature milk [13–15]. This family of over 160 compounds [16] is postulated to play an important role in protecting infants from infection, by acting as decoy receptors or through modulation of the gut microbiota. They may also modulate the immune system through direct interactions [17–20]. Furthermore, HMOs may act as a dietary source of sialic acid [21,22], potentially important for learning and memory [23,24]. Recent evidence from animal studies suggests non-sialylated HMOs may also be important for learning and memory [25]. Today, randomized placebo controlled trials with HMO supplementation are scarce and only done with individual HMOs. Trials that have been carried out indicate that 2′FL is associated with infant immunity [26] and 2′FL together with lacto-N-neotetraose (LNnT) relate to protection from illnesses of the lower respiratory tract and a reduction in antibiotic use [27].

Of specific relevance to preterm infants, HMOs have been linked to the prevention of gut dysfunction [28] and development of NEC [28,29]. Disialyllacto-N-tetraose (DSLNT) and 2′FL have been shown to protect against the development of NEC in rat models [30,31]. It was also observed that DSLNT was present in lower concentrations in the milk fed to preterm infants who developed NEC compared to those who did not [32], leading to the proposal that DSLNT could be used as a marker to predict the likelihood of an infant developing NEC [32].

HMOs are built from lactose, the lactose can be elongated with residues of galactose and N-acetylglucosamine to produce at least 13 different core oligosaccharides [16,33,34]. The core oligosaccharides can be further decorated with sialic acid residues by the action of sialylltransferases, and fucose residues by the action of fucosyltransferases. Due to genetic polymorphisms, two fucosyltransferases, fucosyltransferase-2 (FUT2) and fucosyltransferase-3 (FUT3) are not active in 100% of the population. Fucosyltransferase-2 (FUT2) is responsible for the attachment of fucose to core oligosaccharides through an α-1,2-linkage creating HMOs such as 2′-fucosyllactose (2′FL) or lacto-N-fucopentaose-I (LNFP-I). When FUT2 is inactive such HMOs are absent from the milk. Fucosyltransferase-3 (FUT3), attaches fucose to the core oligosaccharides through an α-1,4 linkage creating oligosaccharides such as LNFP-II, and along with other fucosyltransferases HMOs containing α-1,3 linkages. When FUT3 is inactive HMOs containing α-1,4 linkages are absent from the milk. This results in there being four major milk groups with differing HMO compositions depending on the activities of the FUT2 and FUT3 enzymes:

- Milk group 1, in which both enzymes are active
- Milk group 2, in which FUT3 is active but FUT2 is not
- Milk group 3, in which FUT2 is active but FUT3 is not
- Milk group 4, in which both enzymes are inactive.

In general, milk group 1 seems to be the most common milk group, and milk group 4 is rare [35], however the distribution of milk groups in different populations varies depending on genetic background [36]. Based on the HMO composition of different milk samples, there is also evidence that further subgroups may exist [37,38].

There have been a few previous investigations looking at the HMO composition of preterm milk [17,32,36,39–43], in most cases it is reported that the HMO composition of preterm milk is comparable to that of term milk. However, Coppa [39] reported that preterm milk contained a higher total HMO concentration compared to term milk and De Leoz [36] reported that some HMO features were more variable in preterm milk than in term milk. Kunz [43] pointed out that the Lewis and secretor status should be taken in to account when making studies on HMOs, since these are important factors determining the HMO composition, but milk group has been considered in only a few studies [40–42].

Here we report the composition and trajectories of several different HMOs analyzed in milk collected from mothers of preterm infants and term infants. The HMO composition was compared at equivalent stage of lactation (i.e., equivalent infant postnatal age) and at equivalent postmenstrual age (i.e., equivalent infant developmental stage). In addition the milk group for each donor could be identified from the HMO composition of the milk, thus comparisons could be performed on samples with matched milk groups.

2. Materials and Methods

2.1. Trial Design

This research is part of a prospective cohort study to compare the nutritional composition of human milk from mothers giving birth at term or preterm. The detailed study design has already been published [44].

The study was conducted at the Neonatal Intensive Care Unit (NICU) and at the maternity ward of the University Hospital in Lausanne (CHUV), Switzerland, between October 2013 and July 2014. In this cohort, human milk was longitudinally collected from mothers of preterm infants (gestational age 28 0/7 weeks to 32 6/7 weeks) and mothers of term infants (gestational age 37 0/7 weeks to 41 6/7 weeks). A dedicated research nurse, qualified as a lactation consultant, followed and supported the subjects during the study period. Neonatal demographic and delivery data were collected from the medical charts upon enrollment.

2.2. Milk Collection & Storage

Preterm human milk samples were collected once per week at 7 ± 1 day intervals during the first 8 weeks after delivery. An additional 4 samples were collected until 16 weeks after delivery with sample collection at 14 ± 1 day intervals. Term human milk samples were collected once per week at 7 ± 1 day intervals during the first 8 weeks after delivery (Figure 1). With such a sampling design, it was possible to compare preterm milk with term milk at the same stage of lactation (in Figure 1 the preterm sample at wk1 with the term sample at wk1, etc) or at the equivalent postmenstrual age of the infant (in Figure 1 samples at 42, 44 and 46 weeks would be compared ie. preterm wk12 with term wk2, preterm wk14 with term wk4, etc.)

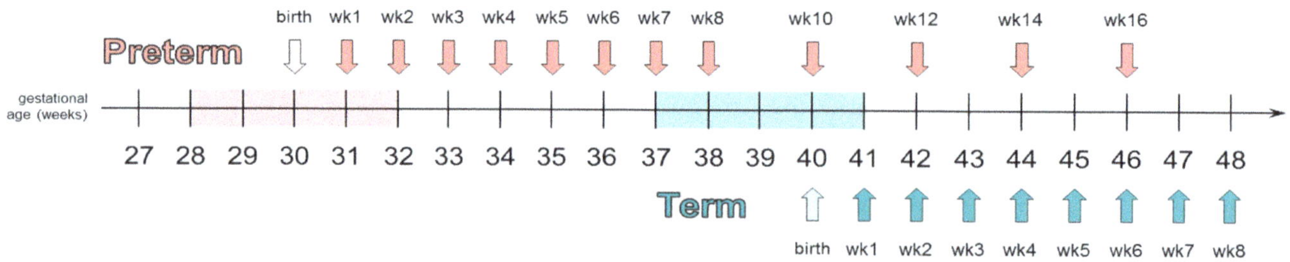

Figure 1. Example of milk sampling scheme from term and preterm mothers delivering at postmenstrual weeks 40 and 30 respectively. Reprinted from Garcia-Rodenas, et al. Clinical Nutrition, 2018 [44] with kind permission from Elsevier.

Samples were collected at the first milk expression in the morning between 06:00 and 12:00 using an electric, double breast pump (Symphony®, Medela, 6340 Baar Switzerland). Full milk expression from a single breast was collected, homogenized, and a 10 mL sample was taken for analysis (except for the first 2 visits, when the volume of sample for analysis was 1–3 mL). Milk for analysis was transferred to a 15 mL polypropylene tube and stored at −18 °C for up to 1 week until hospital transfer and then at −80 °C. Samples were thawed once, homogenized, and split in to 15 different aliquots for different analyses. Those aliquots were then stored at −80 °C until analysis or shipment. Aliquots for HMO analysis were shipped to Neotron S.p.A, Modena, Italy on dry ice.

2.3. Ethical & Legal Considerations

The study was conducted according to the guidelines in the Declaration of Helsinki. The study was approved by the local ethics committee (Commission cantonale d'éthique de la recherche sur l'être humain du Canton de Vaud, Switzerland; Protocol 69/13, clinical study 11.39.NRC). Written informed consent was obtained from all subjects participating in the study. The study was registered on ClinicalTrials.gov with the identifier NCT02052245.

2.4. Analytical Method

HMOs were analyzed by liquid chromatography with fluorescence detection after labelling with 2-aminobenzamide using the protocol described by Austin & Benet [45]. Ten HMOs were quantified against genuine standards with known purity; 2′-fucosyllactose (2′FL), 3-fucosyllactose (3FL), A-tetrasaccharide (A-Tetra), Lacto-N-tetraose (LNT), Lacto-N-neotetraose (LNnT), 3′-sialyllactose (3′SL), 6′-sialyllactose (6′SL), Lacto-N-fucopentaose-I (LNFP-I), LNFP-V and Lacto-N-neofucopentaose (LNnFP). All other HMOs were quantified against maltotriose with known purity, assuming equimolar response factors (graphical representations of the HMOs studied can be found in supplementary Figure S1). A pooled human milk sample (Lee Biosolutions, St Louis, USA) was analyzed with every batch of analysis and at least every 25 injections as a quality control (QC) sample to ensure the method was performing consistently between analytical batches.

2.5. Assignment to FUT2 and FUT3-Dependant Milk Group

The milk samples were assigned to one of 4 milk groups depending on the levels of 2′FL (a marker for FUT2 activity) and LNFP-II (a marker for FUT3 activity) in the sample at visit 2 (2 weeks postpartum). Samples in milk group 1 have high levels (> 25 mg/L) of 2′FL and (>35 mg/L) LNFP-II, samples in milk group 2 have high levels (> 35 mg/L) of LNFP-II and low levels (< 25 mg/L) of 2′FL, samples in milk group 3 have high levels (> 25 mg/L) of 2′FL and low levels (< 35mg/L) of LNFP-II, samples in milk group 4 have low levels (< 25mg/L) of 2′FL and (< 35 mg/L) LNFP-II.

2.6. Data Analysis

All statistical analyses were done with the statistical software R 3.2.3. Prior to statistical analysis all results below the method limit of quantification (LoQ) were set to a value of $0.5 \times$ LoQ. A mixed linear model was used in comparing the two groups (preterm and term) in which the group, infant age (postpartum or postmenstrual) and mode of delivery were considered as fixed effects. The "within subject" variability is taken into account by declaring the subjects as random effects. The main point of comparison is preterm vs term infants. An adjustment for mode of delivery was made because it is a confounding effect with term status given that there are higher proportion of preterm infants delivered by C-section. A logarithmic transformation was applied to some of the HMO concentrations when modelling as the distribution was skewed and according to Box-Cox and QQ plots a log-transformation seemed adequate. Contrast estimates of the model were used to assess significant differences between preterm and term infants at specified lactation and postmenstrual weeks.

3. Results

3.1. Subject Characteristics

This study included 27 mothers with a total of 33 preterm infants, and 34 mothers with a total of 34 term infants. Two of the 27 mothers with preterm infants and six of the 34 mothers with term infants dropped out of the study before completion. No serious adverse events were reported during the study. A total of 500 milk samples were collected and analyzed for HMO content; 280 preterm samples and 220 term samples. The study flow chart and detailed demographic and anthropometric data have already been reported [44]. In summary, baseline maternal characteristics were not different between the two groups, and all mothers in both groups were healthy. Delivery by cesarean section was more common in the preterm group, as were multiple deliveries (twins). Unsurprisingly, term and preterm infants differed in gestational age, birth weight, height and head circumference. There was no difference in gender distribution.

3.2. Milk Groups

The milk samples were assigned to one of 4 milk groups. Overall, 75% of samples were assigned to milk group 1, 19% to milk group 2, 4% to milk group 3 and 2% (1 individual) to milk group 4 (Figure 2). Milk group distribution was similar in the preterm and term populations.

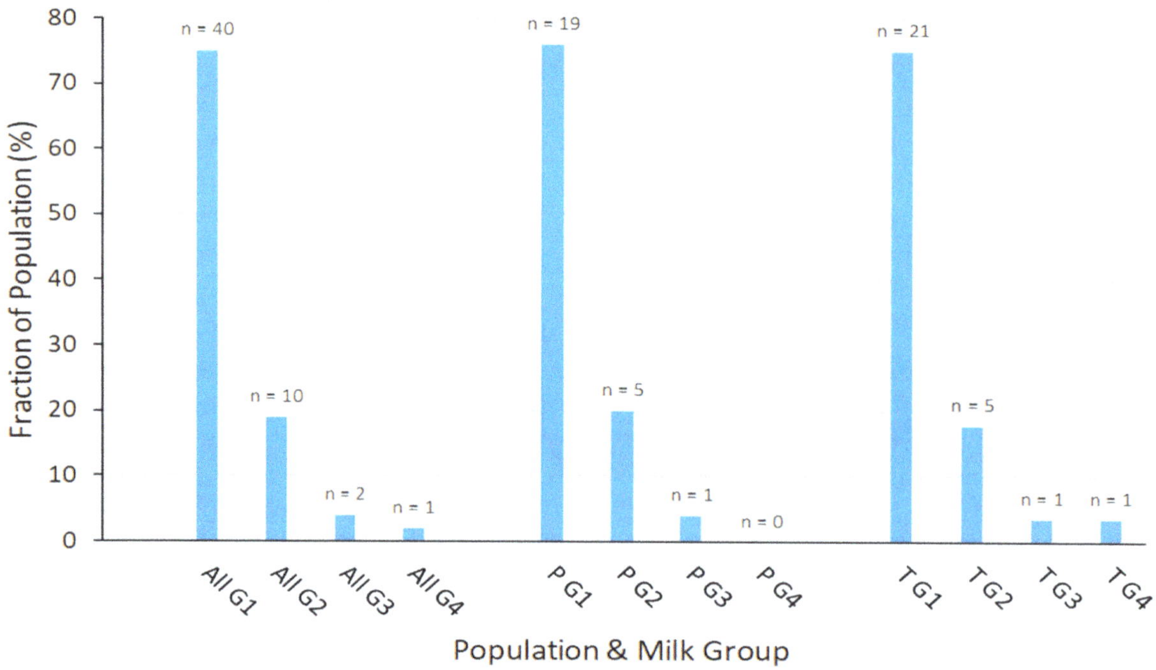

Figure 2. Distribution of milk groups in the different populations: All = all participants, P = participants with preterm infants, T = participants with term infants, G1 = milk group 1, G2 = milk group 2, G3 = milk group 3, G4 = milk group 4.

3.3. Changes in HMO Concentration During Lactation

For both term and preterm milk, the concentration of many of the HMOs decreased at later stages of lactation (Figure 3, and Supplementary Table S1), of those LNT, DSLNT, LNDFH-I, MFLNH-III and DFLNHa reached their maximum concentration after the first week postpartum (i.e., at weeks 2 or 3 postpartum). The only HMO to increase in concentration at later stages of lactation was 3FL.

3.4. HMO Concentration in Term versus Preterm Milk at Equivalent Postpartum Age (Lactation Stages)

Considering all samples, when the children were the same age postpartum, the concentration of each HMO in the mother's milk was generally comparable between term and preterm groups (Figure 3 and Supplementary Table S1). The main exceptions to this were 3′SL, LSTb and DSLNT all of which were at significantly higher concentrations in the preterm milk at postpartum weeks 2 to 8. The concentrations of LSTc (at weeks 1 to 4) and 6′SL (at weeks 2 to 4) were higher in term milk during the first month, but were not significantly different at later time points.

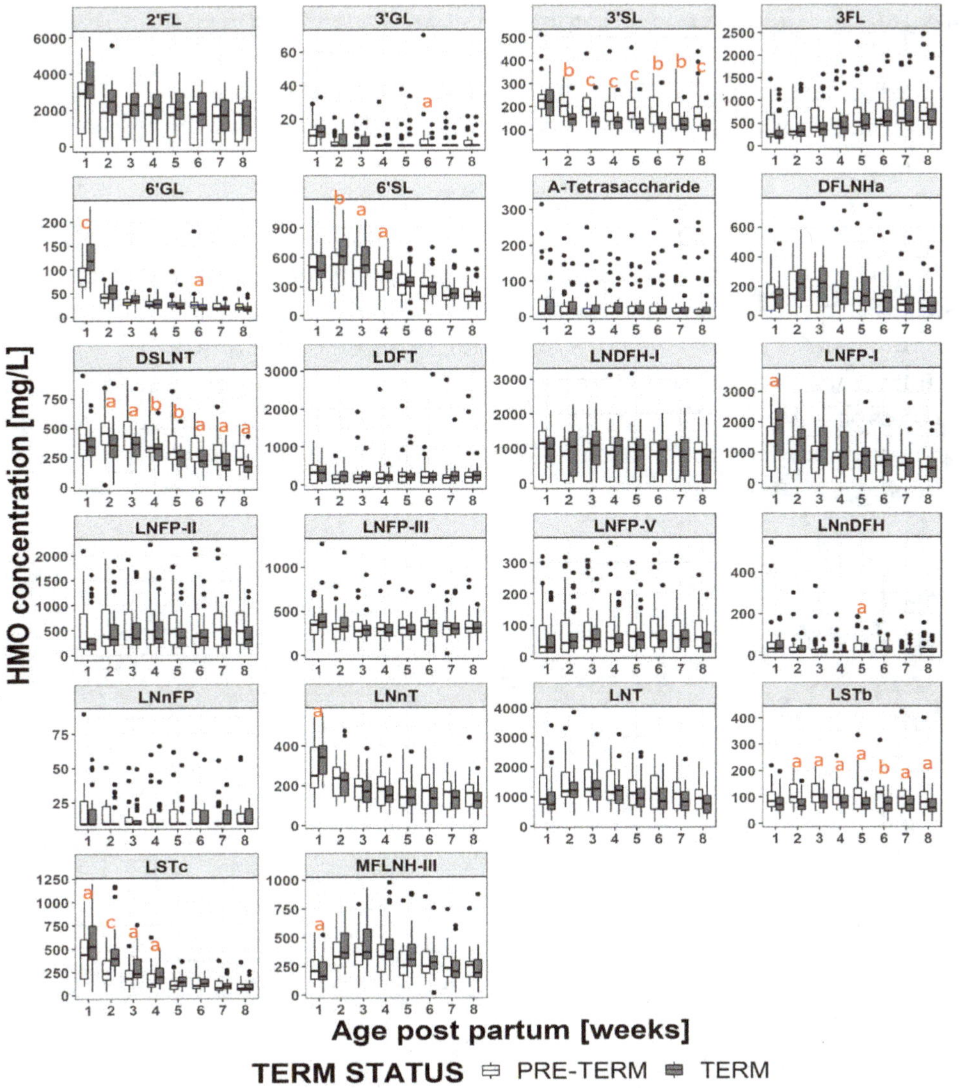

Figure 3. Mean concentration of each HMO at each visit for term (grey) and preterm (white) infants, letters indicate if difference between term and preterm is significant; a: $p < 0.05$, b: $p < 0.005$, c: $p < 0.0005$.

Comparing term and preterm milk at the same age postpartum, but restricting the comparison to milks within the same milk group the picture changes slightly (Figure 4, Figure 5, Supplementary Figure S2, and Supplementary Table S2). Within samples from milk group 1, LNFP-I concentrations are significantly higher in term milk at weeks 1-4, 2′FL concentrations are significantly higher in term milk samples at weeks 1-3 and DFLNHa concentrations are significantly higher in term milk samples at weeks 3-4 (Figure 4). These three HMO do not occur in group 2 or group 4 milks. The concentration of 3′SL remains significantly higher in group 1 preterm milk at weeks 2-8, but for DSLNT the difference between term and preterm milk is only significant at weeks 5 and 8 and for LSTb only at weeks 5, 6 and 8 (Figure 5). For 6′SL, the differences observed between term and preterm is lost when considering only group 1 milk and for LSTc the difference between term and preterm group 1 milk is only significant at weeks 2 to 3 (Figure 5). For the group 2 milks (Supplementary Figure S2) there are only 5 subjects in the term and 5 subjects in the preterm group so statistical significance was not tested at each visit. However from Figure 5 it can be seen that LNFP-V, 3′SL, 6′SL and DSLNT concentrations appear numerically much higher in preterm group 2 milk than term group 2 milk, while 6′SL and LSTc, appear numerically higher in term group 2 milk, especially in the first month. For group 3 milk there was only 1 subject in the term group and 1 subject in the preterm group so a comparison was not made, and for group 4 milk we had only one subject in the whole study.

3.5. HMO Concentration in Term versus Preterm Milk at Equivalent Postmenstrual Age (Developmental Status)

When the milks are compared at infants' equivalent postmenstrual age (Figure 6 and Supplementary Table S3), the concentrations of several HMOs (2′FL, 3′GL, 3′SL, 3FL, 6′GL, 6′SL, DFLNHa, DSLNT, LNFP-I, LNnDFH, LNnT, LNT, LSTc, MFLNH-III) are different at 2 or more visits in the preterm milk compared to term milk. The differences tend to manifest at weeks 38-41 where the concentration of several HMOs in term milk are at their maximum, and the concentration of 3FL is at the minimum. Thus, at equivalent developmental status, preterm infants consume higher concentrations of 3FL in their milk than term infants. However the preterm infants consume lower concentrations of most other HMOs. Making the same exercise only on milk group 1 samples (Figure 7 and Supplementary Table S4) doesn't change this a lot although the magnitude and the duration of some differences (especially for 2′FL and LNFP-I) does change. Similar plots for milk group 2 are reported in Supplementary Figure S3, but no statistical analyses have been performed due to the low number of subjects.

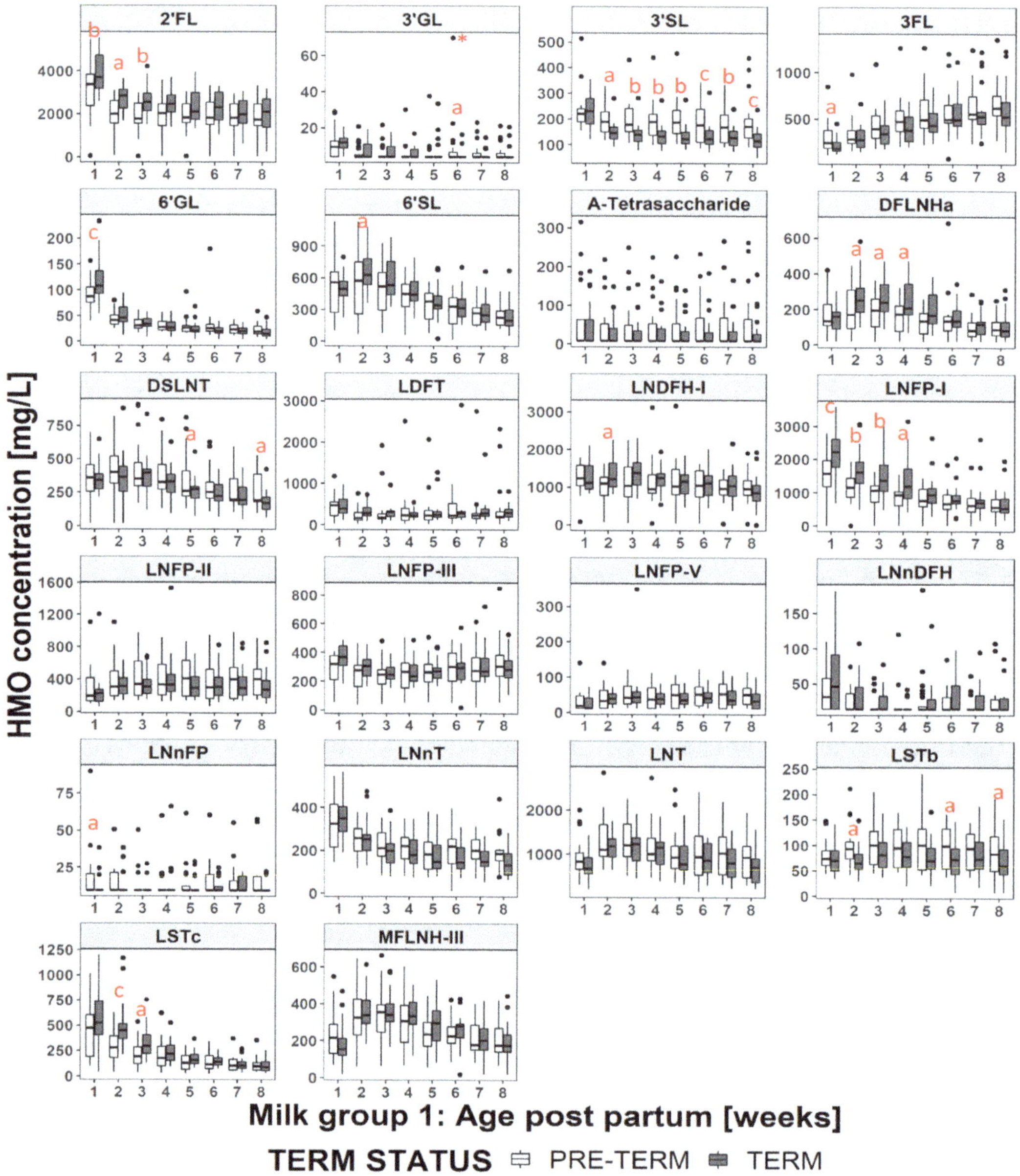

Figure 4. Comparison of HMO concentrations in group 1 term (grey bars) and preterm (white bars) milk. a: $p < 0.05$, b: $p < 0.005$ c: $p < 0.0005$.

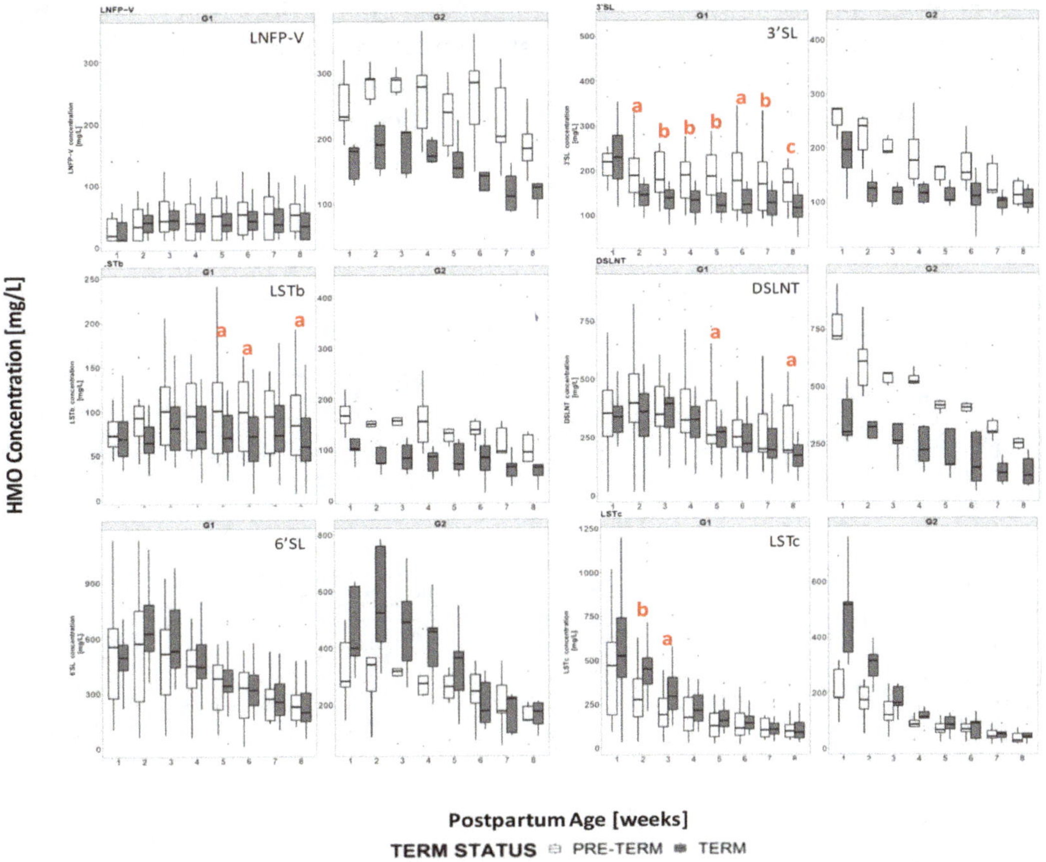

Figure 5. Comparison of selected HMO concentrations in group 1 (G1) and group 2 (G2) term (grey bars) and preterm (white bars) milk. a: $p < 0.05$, b: $p < 0.005$ c: $p < 0.0005$. Significance not tested in G2 milk due to low number of subjects (5 for each arm).

4. Discussion

In this study we have compared the content of 22 HMOs of 500 breast milk samples from mothers of preterm infants and term infants over time. The comparison has been performed both by equivalent stage of lactation (postpartum age) or equivalent postmenstrual age (developmental stage).

4.1. HMO in Term vs Preterm Milk at Equivalent Postpartum Age (Lactation Stages)

The HMO concentrations and trajectories over lactation were generally comparable in the milk of mothers giving birth preterm and term, but several important differences were observed, in particular for the sialylated oligosaccharides. This contrasts some of the previous studies [40,43,46] in which no significant differences were observed in HMO concentrations between term and preterm milk. Coppa et al. [39] reported that the sum of the measured HMOs in preterm milk was significantly higher than that of term milk at day 4 postpartum, but not at days 10 or 30 postpartum. Gabrielli et al. [41] also reported that concentrations of HMOs were higher in preterm milk, but did not go in to details. In this study, we observed the HMOs carrying sialic acid residues, 3'SL, LSTb and DSLNT, were present at significantly higher concentrations in preterm milk between weeks 2-8, while 6'SL (at weeks 2-4) and LSTc (at weeks 1-4) were higher in term milk. Wang et al. [47] reported that the total sialic acid content of preterm milk was significantly higher than that of term milk up to 45 days postpartum, but not beyond 92 days postpartum. In this study we did not collect milk from term infants beyond 56 days postpartum. Although our data appear to be in line with the observations of Wang et al. [47], they contradict the data of Kunz et al. [43] and Spevacek et al. [46] who did not report differences in concentrations of sialylated HMO between term and preterm milk. Variability in HMO concentration between individuals is high, and both of these studies were slightly smaller than ours, which is itself rather small. As pointed out by Kunz et al. [43] it is difficult to compare quantitative HMO results between studies, due to the lack of standardized methods of analysis, milk collection timing and milk collection methodology. Further, although some studies have considered the impact of milk group and stage of lactation on HMO concentrations, they have not matched both stage of lactation and milk group prior to comparing term vs preterm milk, which could mask (or enhance) any compositional differences.

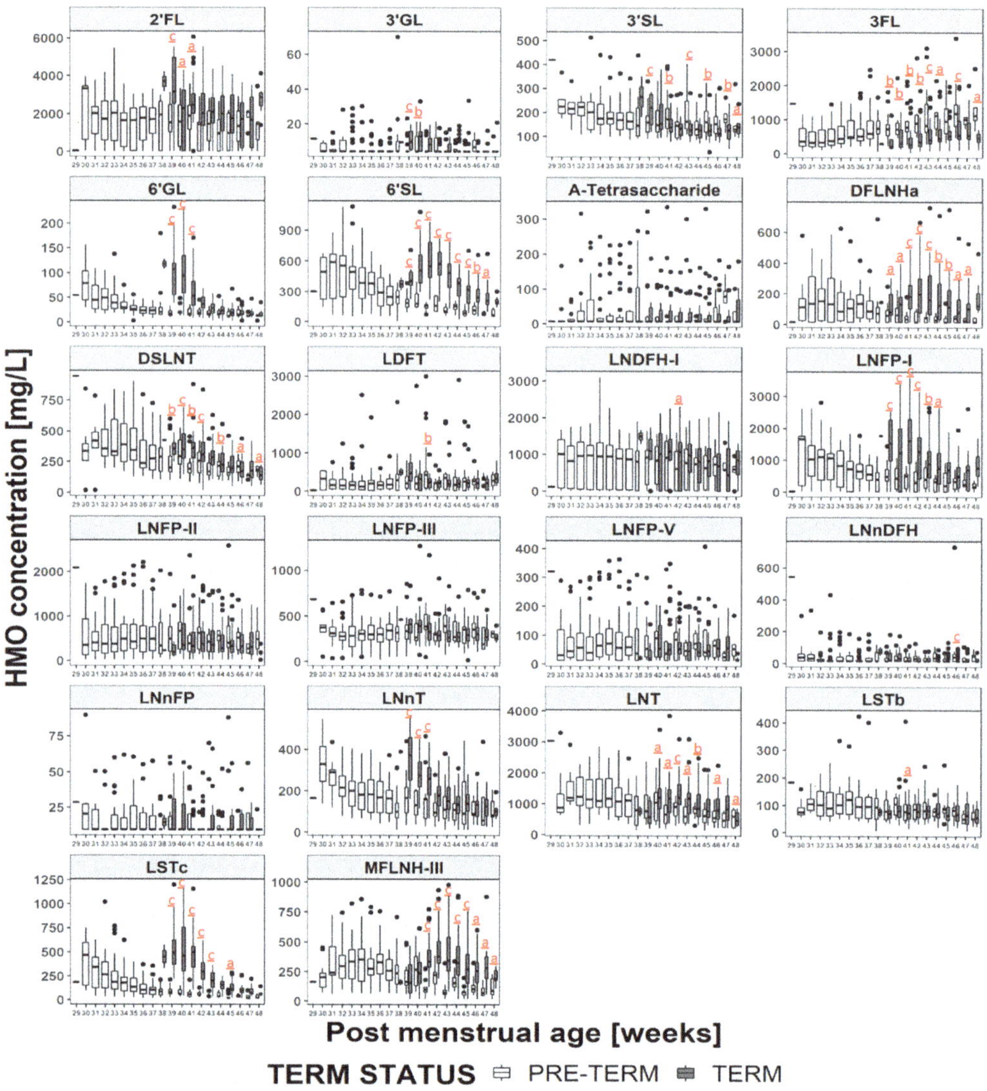

Figure 6. Comparison of the HMO concentration in the milk of mothers giving birth to term (grey bars) or preterm (white bars) infants at equivalent postmenstrual age. a: $p < 0.05$, b: $p < 0.005$ c: $p < 0.0005$.

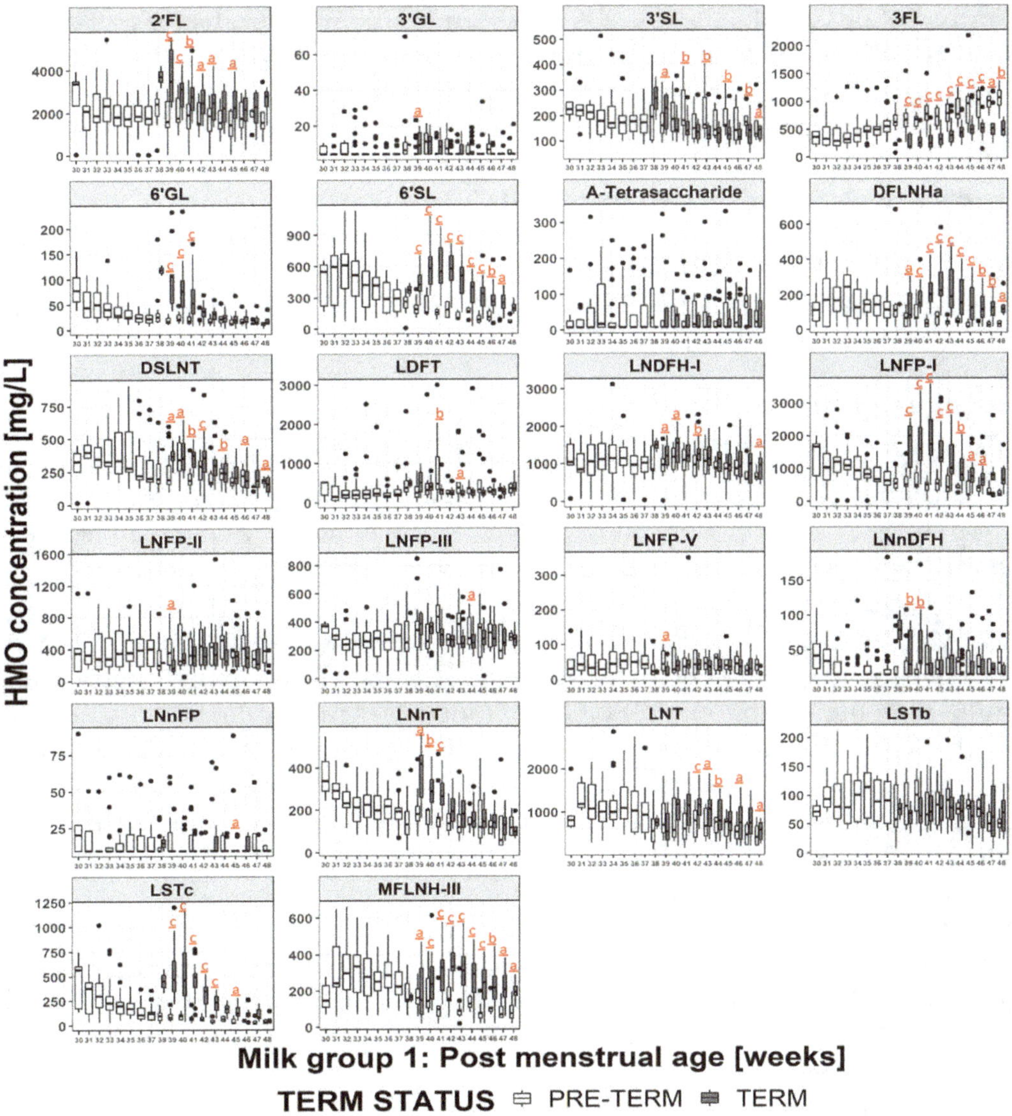

Figure 7. Comparison of the HMO concentration in group 1 milk of mothers giving birth to term (grey bars) or preterm (white bars) infants at equivalent gestational age. a: $p < 0.05$, b: $p < 0.005$ c: $p < 0.0005$.

As to why we observed higher concentrations of several sialylated HMOs in preterm milk and lower concentrations of other sialylated HMOs, we can only speculate. From a structural viewpoint, 6'SL and LSTc, both at higher concentrations in term milk, both contain the structural motif α-Neu5Ac(2→6)β-D-Gal- which is absent from 3'SL, LSTb and DSLNT. 3'SL, LSTb and DSLNT all contain the structural motifs α-Neu5Ac(2→6)β-D-GlcNAc- and/or α-Neu5Ac(2→3)β-D-Gal-. Therefore we may envisage that the sialyltransferase responsible for attaching sialic acid to galactose through an α-1,6-linkage has reduced activity after preterm delivery while those responsible for attaching sialic acid through an α-1,3 linkage to galactose or an α-1,6-linkage to N-acetylglucosamine have increased activity. During the final trimester of gestation, the ganglioside density of the cerebral cortex increases significantly [48], and sialic acids are an important component of the gangliosides. One may also postulate that at this stage of gestation the mother has an increased production of sialic acid to help with the baby's brain development. If the baby is born prematurely, and lactation begins early, the upregulation of the system to produce sialic acids may result in an increased production of sialylated HMOs. Dietary sources of sialic acid have been demonstrated to be processed by the body and the sialic acids incorporated in to glycoproteins [49]. Data from Wang et al. [24] have also demonstrated that supplementing pigs' diets with a dietary source of sialic acid improves learning and memory.

The higher concentration of sialylated HMOs in preterm milk may be a factor that contributes to the important benefits experienced by preterm infants consuming their own mothers' milk.

DSLNT has been observed to protect neonatal rats from development of NEC [30]. An observational study in preterm human infants also observed that infants receiving milk with higher levels of DSLNT were less likely to develop NEC [32] leading to the proposition that DSLNT concentrations could be used as a possible marker for risk of developing NEC. This work demonstrates that the mothers own milk of preterm infants is probably a good source of DSLNT. Our data also suggest children receiving group 2 milk may receive higher concentrations of DSLNT than those receiving group 1 milk, but a larger study would be needed to test if the difference is significant, and to determine if infants receiving group 2 milk may be better protected from NEC.

4.2. HMO at Equivalent Postmenstrual Age (Developmental Status)

As shown above, when comparisons were made at equivalent postpartum age, there were few differences in concentrations of most HMOs between term milk and preterm milk and the trajectories of concentration during lactation were comparable. This can indicate that birth sets off a program that defines the HMO trajectory with most HMOs showing a decrease in concentration with stage of lactation with the exception of 3FL, which increases.

Since the HMO concentration varies with stage of lactation, when the milk is compared at infants' equivalent postmenstrual age, the concentrations of most of the HMOs in preterm milk are lower than in the term milk, with the exception of 3FL (since it increases during lactation) and 3'SL (since it is generally in higher concentrations in preterm milk). The largest differences manifest around 40 weeks of postmenstrual age, which is when the milk for term infants contains the highest concentrations of HMOs. Interestingly, as the postmenstrual age increases, the differences reduce, and for some HMOs the concentrations are equivalent by 44-46 weeks postmenstrual age, while for some others a significant difference was maintained for the duration of the study. The biological relevance of these differences is unclear, and would be worthy of future investigation. Making the hypothesis that infants need to be exposed to a certain amount of HMOs at specific stages of their development, we can presume that preterm infants may be losing out by being exposed to lower amounts of HMOs than term infants as similar stages of development. In such a case supplementing preterm milk with HMOs is likely to be beneficial. Alternatively, perhaps the HMOs help the infant adjust to life outside the womb, and the concentrations in the mothers' milk are appropriate. However a very preterm infant may not receive full enteral feeding until several days or even weeks after delivery, meaning that the actual amount of HMOs they receive will be below what they would be receiving if they could be immediately fully breast fed. In such cases HMO supplementation may also be beneficial. Clinical evidence shows that premature infants greatly benefit from being fed own mother's milk [3,50], or, alternatively, being fed donor human milk [50]. For very preterm infants the milk needs to be fortified with energy, proteins and minerals [3]. Now that HMOs start to be commercially available, HMO fortification is also possible, but further work is needed to confirm the potential benefits and the appropriate timing and dosages for intervention.

4.3. Impact of Milk Group

In general, when comparing HMO compositions, it is important to consider the milk group. In this study the distribution of milk groups is comparable between mothers giving birth term or preterm, with the majority of mothers producing group 1 milk (milk containing oligosaccharides indicating both FUT2 and FUT3 were active). Milk group 2 was next most common with 5 mothers in each group. The equal distributions suggest that there is no link between the genetic factors controlling the milk groups, and the likelihood of giving birth prematurely, although this study is too small to properly address this question.

In this study, when combining data from all milk groups at the same postpartum stages it appears that there was relatively little difference in the concentrations of the neutral HMOs between term or preterm milk, similar to what has been observed previously [40,43,46]. However when only the group 1 milks were compared, three neutral HMOs, 2′FL, LNFP-I, and DFLNHa, were at significantly lower concentrations in preterm milk during the first month of lactation. 2′FL was 700-800 mg/L (20–27%) lower, LNFP-I was 420–590 mg/L (27–32%) lower and DFLNHa was 60-70 mg/L (26–30%) lower. These differences were hidden by the increased variability introduced by the inclusion of the data from the other milk groups, especially milk group 2 with inactive FUT2. All of these structures contain α-1,2-linked fucose residues and are present in significant concentrations only in milk of groups 1 and 3. The observation that these structures are at lower concentrations in group 1 preterm milk implies that the fucosyltransferase-2 enzyme (FUT2) is not fully active during the first month of lactation when an infant is born very preterm as suggested previously [36]. Higher levels of fucosylation have been shown to increase protection against infection [18] but the clinical relevance of the magnitude of the differences remains to be assessed.

Interestingly in group 1 milk, 3′SL is the only sialylated HMO that remains higher in preterm milk across weeks 2-8 (as observed when studying all milk groups together). The differences in concentrations of LSTb and DSLNT between term and preterm milks are largely lost, the differences being significant only at 2 or 3 non-consecutive time points. Likewise for 6′SL and LSTc, which were observed as being significantly higher in term milk when all milk groups were combined, the significance is largely lost when considering only milk group 1 data. Most of the differences in concentrations of sialylated structures appears to be driven by their concentrations in the group 2 milks (Figure 5). The reasons for this are not clear, but one may postulate that FUT2 outcompetes the other enzymes for access to the core structures, and so when FUT2 is active (even if slightly less active than normal for preterm milks), the difference in activity of the sialyltransferases is masked. However, when FUT2 is not active, the difference in sialyltransferase activities becomes more apparent.

Looking at differences in HMO concentrations at equivalent postmenstrual age, and considering only milk group 1 (Figure 7), does not much change the observations made considering all milk groups (Figure 6) with most of the differences being driven by the stage of lactation. However, it does emphasize the differences in the HMOs containing α-1,2-linked fucose. For example looking at all milk groups, 2′FL concentrations appear significantly different only between weeks 39-41, but when considering only milk group 1 then the concentration differences are significant between weeks 39-43 and at week 45. Similar phenomena can be observed for LNFP-I and LNDFH-I. This highlights the importance of considering milk group when making comparisons between different milk samples.

4.4. Strengths and Limitations of the Study

The main limitations of this study are the limited sample size and the monocentric design of the study. One may also argue that collecting milk at only one time of the day, the first milk expression in the morning, may mean the data are not representative of the milk composition during the whole day. Conversely one may see this as a strength of the study, since the main aim was to compare term versus preterm milk and sampling at different times of the day could have introduced additional variation not specifically related to the comparison of term versus preterm milk. Certainly a strength of the study was the very tight collection windows at each stage of lactation, each window being only ±1 day. It is well established that the HMO concentration changes at different stages of lactation [51–56], especially during the first few months of lactation. Keeping the milk collection window tight reduces variability due to differences in sampling day. The study protocol places quite a burden on the mothers who need to collect the full milk expression from a single breast at every sampling point. Despite this, we had very few drop outs from the study, the support provided to the mothers by the lactation nurse was surely a key factor in the successful retention of the volunteers. Importantly, the analytical method used for determination of the HMOs has been extensively validated [45]. To ensure the method performance was maintained day to day, a reference sample of pooled human milk was analysed with every batch of analyses, and at least every 25 samples. Such rigor assured that the variability introduced by the analytical method was also kept to a minimum. Milk group assignments have been done based on the concentrations of 2′FL and LNFP-II in the milk. Appropriate cut-off concentrations for making milk group assignments have not yet been established, so we have based our cut-offs based on the performance of the analytical method. Unfortunately, due to the small sample size, it was not possible to make statistical comparisons between term and preterm milk of milk groups 2,3 or 4. In this study we have only determined the concentrations of 22 out of over 160 HMOs. Although those 22 include the most abundant HMOs, concentrations of a large number of HMOs and how they are impacted by preterm birth remains unknown.

5. Conclusions

The HMO composition and concentration trajectory of term and preterm milk are largely comparable at equivalent infant postpartum age, suggesting that birth triggers a program that defines the HMO trajectory during lactation. Consequently, significant differences exist between preterm and term infants milk when comparing HMO concentrations at equivalent postmenstrual ages. Nevertheless some differences were observed when the comparison was made at the same postpartum age, in particular for the sialylated oligosaccharides and oligosaccharides containing α-1,2-linked fucose. The data suggest that when an infant is born preterm, FUT2 is not fully active during the first month of lactation, leading to reduced concentrations of HMOs such as 2′FL and LNFP-I. In addition the expression of enzymes responsible for sialyllation of HMOs is also perturbed leading to differences in concentrations of the sialylated HMOs. Interestingly, these observations are not fully consistent with previous studies in preterm infants. This study was small, thus the observations need corroboration in larger cohorts. The possible physiological significance of the observations remain to be determined.

Supplementary Materials:
Figure S1: Structures of the Determined HMO Depicted Using Symbol Nomenclature, Figure S2: Mean Concentration of each HMO in Group 2 Milk for Term and Preterm Infants at Equivalent Stage of Lactation, Figure S3: Mean Concentration of each HMO in Group 2 Milk for Term and Preterm Infants at Equivalent Postmenstrual Age, Table S1: Concentration of Human Milk Oligosaccharides in Term or Preterm Milk At Different Weeks Postpartum, Table S2: Concentration of Human Milk Oligosaccharides in Term or Preterm Milk At Different Weeks Postpartum Separated By Milk Group, Table S3: Concentration of Human Milk Oligosaccharides in Term or Preterm Milk At Specified Postmenstrual Age, Table S4: Concentration of Human Milk Oligosaccharides in Term or Preterm Milk At Specified Postmenstrual Age Separated By Milk Group.

Author Contributions: Conceptualization, C.L.G.-R., M.A., S.A., L.B., J.-F.T. and C.J.F.F.; Formal Analysis, C.A.D.C.; Investigation, L.B., J.-F.T., C.J.F.F., S.A., N.S. and A.B.; Resources, L.B., J.-F.T. and C.J.F.F.; Writing-Original Draft Preparation, S.A. Writing-Review & Editing, S.A., C.A.D.C., N.S., A.B., M.A., C.L.G.-R., L.B., J.-F.T., and C.J.F.F.; Visualization, C.A.D.C. and S.A.; Supervision, C.L.G.-R., M.A., and C.J.F.F.; Project Administration, M.A.; Funding Acquisition, C.L.G.-R. and M.A.

Acknowledgments: The authors would like to thank all the mothers and their infants who kindly donated their milk for this study, Nassima Grari, the study lactation nurse who cared for all mothers for the duration of the study, and the staff at Neotron S.p.A., in particular Marco Meschiari for performing the analysis of all the milk samples in their laboratory. Thanks also to Céline Romagny and Emilie Darcillon who managed the organizational and operational part of the clinical study and the data management.

References

1. Eidelman, A.I.; Schanler, R.J. Breastfeeding and the use of human milk. *Pediatrics* **2012**, *129*, e827–e841. [CrossRef]
2. Fewtrell, M.; Bronsky, J.; Campoy, C.; Domellof, M.; Embleton, N.; Fidler Mis, N.; Hojsak, I.; Hulst, J.M.; Indrio, F.; Lapillonne, A.; et al. Complementary feeding: A position paper by the european society for paediatric gastroenterology, hepatology, and nutrition (espghan) committee on nutrition. *J. Pediatr. Gastroenterol. Nutr.* **2017**, *64*, 119–132. [CrossRef] [PubMed]
3. Boquien, C.Y. Human milk: An ideal food for nutrition of preterm newborn. *Front. Pediatr.* **2018**, *6*, 295. [CrossRef]

4. Agostoni, C.; Buonocore, G.; Carnielli, V.P.; De Curtis, M.; Darmaun, D.; Decsi, T.; Domellof, M.; Embleton, N.D.; Fusch, C.; Genzel-Boroviczeny, O.; et al. Enteral nutrient supply for preterm infants: Commentary from the european society of paediatric gastroenterology, hepatology and nutrition committee on nutrition. *J. Pediatr. Gastroenterol. Nutr.* **2010**, *50*, 85–91. [CrossRef] [PubMed]
5. Lewis, E.D.; Richard, C.; Larsen, B.M.; Field, C.J. The importance of human milk for immunity in preterm infants. *Clin. Perinatol.* **2017**, *44*, 23–47. [CrossRef]
6. Corpeleijn, W.E.; Kouwenhoven, S.M.; Paap, M.C.; van Vliet, I.; Scheerder, I.; Muizer, Y.; Helder, O.K.; van Goudoever, J.B.; Vermeulen, M.J. Intake of own mother's milk during the first days of life is associated with decreased morbidity and mortality in very low birth weight infants during the first 60 days of life. *Neonatology* **2012**, *102*, 276–281. [CrossRef]
7. Lechner, B.E.; Vohr, B.R. Neurodevelopmental outcomes of preterm infants fed human milk: A systematic review. *Clin. Perinatol.* **2017**, *44*, 69–83. [CrossRef]
8. Lucas, A. Long-term programming effects of early nutrition—Implications for the preterm infant. *J. Perinatol.* **2005**, *25* (Suppl. 2), S2–S6. [CrossRef]
9. Lewandowski, A.J.; Lamata, P.; Francis, J.M.; Piechnik, S.K.; Ferreira, V.M.; Boardman, H.; Neubauer, S.; Singhal, A.; Leeson, P.; Lucas, A. Breast milk consumption in preterm neonates and cardiac shape in adulthood. *Pediatrics* **2016**, *138*. [CrossRef]
10. Boyce, C.; Watson, M.; Lazidis, G.; Reeve, S.; Dods, K.; Simmer, K.; McLeod, G. Preterm human milk composition: A systematic literature review. *Br. J. Nutr.* **2016**, *116*, 1033–1045. [CrossRef]
11. Ballard, O.; Morrow, A.L. Human milk composition: Nutrients and bioactive factors. *Pediatr. Clin. N. Am.* **2013**, *60*, 49–74. [CrossRef]
12. Gidrewicz, D.A.; Fenton, T.R. A systematic review and meta-analysis of the nutrient content of preterm and term breast milk. *BMC Pediatr.* **2014**, *14*, 216. [CrossRef]
13. Urashima, T.; Asakuma, S.; Leo, F.; Fukuda, K.; Messer, M.; Oftedal, O.T. The predominance of type I oligosaccharides is a feature specific to human breast milk. *Adv. Nutr.* **2012**, *3*, 473S–482S. [CrossRef]
14. Kunz, C.; Rodriguez-Palmero, M.; Koletzko, B.; Jensen, R. Nutritional and biochemical properties of human milk, part i: General aspects, proteins, and carbohydrates. *Clin. Perinatol.* **1999**, *26*, 307–333. [CrossRef]
15. Coppa, G.V.; Gabrielli, O.; Pierani, P.; Catassi, C.; Carlucci, A.; Giorgi, P.L. Changes in carbohydrate composition in human milk over 4 months of lactation. *Pediatrics* **1993**, *91*, 637–641.
16. Urashima, T.; Hirabayashi, J.; Sato, S.; Kobata, A. Human milk oligosaccharides as essential tools for basic and application studies on galectins. *Trends Glycosci. Glycotechnol.* **2018**, *30*, SE51–SE65. [CrossRef]
17. Kunz, C.; Rudloff, S. Biological functions of oligosaccharides in human milk. *Acta Paediatr.* **1993**, *82*, 903–912. [CrossRef]
18. Newburg, D.S.; Ruiz-Palacios, G.M.; Morrow, A.L. Human milk glycans protect infants against enteric pathogens. *Annu. Rev. Nutr.* **2005**, *25*, 37–58. [CrossRef]
19. Morozov, V.; Hansman, G.; Hanisch, F.G.; Schroten, H.; Kunz, C. Human milk oligosaccharides as promising antivirals. *Mol. Nutr. Food Res.* **2018**, *62*, 1700679. [CrossRef]
20. Bode, L. The functional biology of human milk oligosaccharides. *Early Hum. Dev.* **2015**, *91*, 619–622. [CrossRef]
21. Jacobi, S.K.; Yatsunenko, T.; Li, D.; Dasgupta, S.; Yu, R.K.; Berg, B.M.; Chichlowski, M.; Odle, J. Dietary isomers of sialyllactose increase ganglioside sialic acid concentrations in the corpus callosum and cerebellum and modulate the colonic microbiota of formula-fed piglets. *J. Nutr.* **2016**, *146*, 200–208. [CrossRef]
22. Sprenger, N.; Duncan, P.I. Sialic acid utlization. *Adv. Nutr.* **2012**, *3*, 392S–397S. [CrossRef]
23. Oliveros, E.; Vazquez, E.; Barranco, A.; Ramirez, M.; Gruart, A.; Delgado-Garcia, J.M.; Buck, R.; Rueda, R.; Martin, M.J. Sialic acid and sialylated oligosaccharide supplementation during lactation improves learning and memory in rats. *Nutrients* **2018**, *10*, 1519. [CrossRef]
24. Wang, B.; Yu, B.; Karim, M.; Hu, H.; Sun, Y.; McGreevy, P.; Petocz, P.; Held, S.; Brand-Miller, J. Dietary sialic acid supplementation improves learning and memory in piglets. *Am. J. Clin. Nutr.* **2007**, *85*, 561–569. [CrossRef]
25. Oliveros, E.; Ramirez, M.; Vazquez, E.; Barranco, A.; Gruart, A.; Delgado-Garcia, J.M.; Buck, R.; Rueda, R.; Martin, M.J. Oral supplementation of 2′-fucosyllactose during lactation improves memory and learning in rats. *J. Nutr. Biochem.* **2016**, *31*, 20–27. [CrossRef]

26. Goehring, K.C.; Marriage, B.J.; Oliver, J.S.; Wilder, J.A.; Barrett, E.G.; Buck, R.H. Similar to those who are breastfed, infants fed a formula containing 2′-fucosyllactose have lower inflammatory cytokines in a randomized controlled trial. *J. Nutr.* **2016**, *146*, 2559–2566. [CrossRef]
27. Puccio, G.; Alliet, P.; Cajozzo, C.; Janssens, E.; Corsello, G.; Sprenger, N.; Wernimont, S.; Egli, D.; Gosoniu, L.; Steenhout, P. Effects of infant formula with human milk oligosaccharides on growth and morbidity: A randomized multicenter trial. *J. Pediatr. Gastroenterol. Nutr.* **2017**, *64*, 624–631. [CrossRef]
28. Bering, S.B. Human milk oligosaccharides to prevent gut dysfunction and necrotizing enterocolitis in preterm neonates. *Nutrients* **2018**, *10*, 1461. [CrossRef]
29. Moukarzel, S.; Bode, L. Human milk oligosaccharides and the preterm infant a journey in sickness and in health. *Clin. Perinatol.* **2017**, *44*, 193–207. [CrossRef]
30. Jantscher-Krenn, E.; Zherebtsov, M.; Nissan, C.; Goth, K.; Guner, Y.S.; Naidu, N.; Choudhury, B.; Grishin, A.V.; Ford, H.R.; Bode, L. The human milk oligosaccharide disialyllacto-N-tetraose prevents necrotising enterocolitis in neonatal rats. *Gut* **2012**, *61*, 1417–1425. [CrossRef]
31. Autran, C.A.; Schoterman, M.H.; Jantscher-Krenn, E.; Kamerling, J.P.; Bode, L. Sialylated galacto-oligosaccharides and 2′-fucosyllactose reduce necrotising enterocolitis in neonatal rats. *Br. J. Nutr.* **2016**, *116*, 294–299. [CrossRef]
32. Autran, C.A.; Kellman, B.P.; Kim, J.H.; Asztalos, E.; Blood, A.B.; Spence, E.C.; Patel, A.L.; Hou, J.; Lewis, N.E.; Bode, L. Human milk oligosaccharide composition predicts risk of necrotising enterocolitis in preterm infants. *Gut* **2017**, *67*, 1064–1070. [CrossRef]
33. Blank, D.; Dotz, V.; Geyer, R.; Kunz, C. Human milk oligosaccharides and Lewis blood group: Individual high-throughput sample profiling to enhance conclusions from functional studies. *Adv. Nutr.* **2012**, *3*, 440S–449S. [CrossRef]
34. Kobata, A. Structures and application of oligosaccharides in human milk. *Proc. Jpn. Acad. Ser. B Phys. Biol. Sci.* **2010**, *86*, 731–747. [CrossRef]
35. Thurl, S.; Henker, J.; Siegel, M.; Tovar, K.; Sawatzki, G. Detection of four human milk groups with respect to Lewis blood group dependent oligosaccharides. *Glycoconj. J.* **1997**, *14*, 795–799. [CrossRef]
36. de Leoz, M.L.; Gaerlan, S.C.; Strum, J.S.; Dimapasoc, L.M.; Mirmiran, M.; Tancredi, D.J.; Smilowitz, J.T.; Kalanetra, K.M.; Mills, D.A.; German, J.B.; et al. Lacto-N-tetraose, fucosylation, and secretor status are highly variable in human milk oligosaccharides from women delivering preterm. *J. Proteome Res.* **2012**, *11*, 4662–4672. [CrossRef]
37. van Leeuwen, S.S.; Stoutjesdijk, E.; ten Kate, G.A.; Schaafsma, A.; Dijck-Brouwer, J.; Muskiet, F.A.J.; Dijkhuizen, L. Regional variations in human milk oligosaccharides in vietnam suggest FucTx activity besides FucT2 and FucT3. *Sci. Rep.* **2018**, *8*, 16790. [CrossRef]
38. Elwakiel, M.; Hageman, J.A.; Wang, W.; Szeto, I.M.; van Goudoever, J.B.; Hettinga, K.A.; Schols, H.A. Human milk oligosaccharides in colostrum and mature milk of Chinese mothers: Lewis positive secretor subgroups. *J. Agric. Food Chem.* **2018**, *66*, 7036–7043. [CrossRef]
39. Coppa, G.V.; Pierani, P.; Zampini, L.; Gabrielli, O.; Carlucci, A.; Catassi, C.; Giorgi, P.L. Lactose, oligosaccharide and monosaccharide content of milk from mothers delivering preterm newborns over the first month of lactation. *Minerva Pediatr.* **1997**, *49*, 471–475.
40. Nakhla, T.; Daotian, F.; Zopf, D.; Brodsky, N.L.; Hurt, H. Neutral oligosaccharide content of preterm human milk. *Br. J. Nutr.* **1999**, *82*, 361–367. [CrossRef]
41. Gabrielli, O.; Zampini, L.; Galeazzi, T.; Padella, L.; Santoro, L.; Peila, C.; Giuliani, F.; Bertino, E.; Fabris, C.; Coppa, G.V. Preterm milk oligosaccharides during the first month of lactation. *Pediatrics* **2011**, *128*, e1520–e1531. [CrossRef]
42. Van Niekerk, E.; Autran, C.A.; Nel, D.G.; Kirsten, G.F.; Blaauw, R.; Bode, L. Human milk oligosaccharides differ between HIV-infected and HIV-uninfected mothers and are related to necrotizing enterocolitis incidence in their preterm very-low-birth-weight infants. *J. Nutr.* **2014**, *144*, 1227–1233. [CrossRef]
43. Kunz, C.; Meyer, C.; Collado, M.C.; Geiger, L.; Garcia-Mantrana, I.; Bertua-Rios, B.; Martinez-Costa, C.; Borsch, C.; Rudloff, S. Influence of gestational age, secretor and Lewis blood group status on the oligosaccharide content of human milk. *J. Pediatr. Gastroenterol. Nutr.* **2017**, *64*, 789–798. [CrossRef]
44. Garcia-Rodenas, C.L.; De Castro, C.A.; Jenni, R.; Thakkar, S.K.; Beauport, L.; Tolsa, J.F.; Fischer-Fumeaux, C.J.; Affolter, M. Temporal changes of major protein concentrations in preterm and term human milk. A prospective cohort study. *Clin. Nutr.* **2018**, *38*, 1844–1852. [CrossRef]

45. Austin, S.; Benet, T. Quantitative determination of non-lactose milk oligosaccharides. *Anal. Chim. Acta* **2018**, *1010*, 86–96. [CrossRef]
46. Spevacek, A.R.; Smilowitz, J.T.; Chin, E.L.; Underwood, M.A.; German, J.B.; Slupsky, C.M. Infant maturity at birth reveals minor differences in the maternal milk metabolome in the first month of lactation. *J. Nutr.* **2015**, *145*, 1698–1708. [CrossRef]
47. Wang, B.; Brand-Miller, J.; McVeagh, P.; Petocz, P. Concentration and distribution of sialic acid in human milk and infant formulas. *Am. J. Clin. Nutr.* **2001**, *74*, 510–515. [CrossRef]
48. Schnaar, R.L.; Gerardy-Schahn, R.; Hildebrandt, H. Sialic acids in the brain: Gangliosides and polysialic acid in nervous system development, stability, disease, and regeneration. *Physiol. Rev.* **2014**, *94*, 461–518. [CrossRef]
49. Tangvoranuntakul, P.; Gagneux, P.; Diaz, S.; Bardor, M.; Varki, N.; Varki, A.; Muchmore, E. Human uptake and incorporation of an immunogenic nonhuman dietary sialic acid. *Proc. Natl. Acad. Sci. USA* **2003**, *100*, 12045–12050. [CrossRef]
50. Bhatia, J. Human milk and the premature infant. *Ann. Nutr. Metab.* **2013**, *62* (Suppl. 3), 8–14. [CrossRef]
51. Chaturvedi, P.; Warren, C.D.; Altaye, M.; Morrow, A.L.; Ruiz-Palacios, G.; Pickering, L.K.; Newburg, D.S. Fucosylated human milk oligosaccharides vary between individuals and over the course of lactation. *Glycobiology* **2001**, *11*, 365–372. [CrossRef]
52. Kunz, C.; Rudloff, S.; Baier, W.; Klein, N.; Strobel, S. Oligosaccharides in human milk: Structural, functional, and metabolic aspects. *Annu. Rev. Nutr.* **2000**, *20*, 699–722. [CrossRef]
53. Xu, G.; Davis, J.C.; Goonatilleke, E.; Smilowitz, J.T.; German, J.B.; Lebrilla, C.B. Absolute quantitation of human milk oligosaccharides reveals phenotypic variations during lactation. *J. Nutr.* **2017**, *147*, 117–124. [CrossRef]
54. Austin, S.; De Castro, C.A.; Benet, T.; Hou, Y.; Sun, H.; Thakkar, S.K.; Vinyes-Pares, G.; Zhang, Y.; Wang, P. Temporal change of the content of 10 oligosaccharides in the milk of Chinese urban mothers. *Nutrients* **2016**, *8*, 346. [CrossRef]
55. Erney, R.M.; Malone, W.T.; Skelding, M.B.; Marcon, A.A.; Kleman-Leyer, K.M.; O'Ryan, M.L.; Ruiz-Palacios, G.; Hilty, M.D.; Pickering, L.K.; Prieto, P.A. Variability of human milk neutral oligosaccharides in a diverse population. *J. Pediatr. Gastroenterol. Nutr.* **2000**, *30*, 181–192. [CrossRef]
56. Sprenger, N.; Lee, L.Y.; De Castro, C.A.; Steenhout, P.; Thakkar, S.K. Longitudinal change of selected human milk oligosaccharides and association to infants' growth, an observatory, single center, longitudinal cohort study. *PLoS ONE* **2017**, *12*, e0171814. [CrossRef]

4

Determinants of Exclusive Breastfeeding Cessation in the Early Postnatal Period among Culturally and Linguistically Diverse (CALD) Australian Mothers

Felix Akpojene Ogbo [1,2,*], Osita Kingsley Ezeh [3], Sarah Khanlari [4,5], Sabrina Naz [1], Praween Senanayake [1], Kedir Y. Ahmed [1], Anne McKenzie [6], Olayide Ogunsiji [7], Kingsley Agho [1,3], Andrew Page [1], Jane Ussher [1], Janette Perz [1], Bryanne Barnett AM [8] and John Eastwood [4,9,10,11,12,13]

1 Translational Health Research Institute, School of Medicine, Western Sydney University, Campbelltown Campus, Locked Bag 1797, Penrith, NSW 2571, Australia
2 General Practice Unit, Prescot Specialist Medical Centre, Welfare Quarters, Makurdi, Benue State 972261, Nigeria
3 School of Science and Health, Western Sydney University, Campbelltown Campus, Locked Bag 1797, Penrith, NSW 2571, Australia
4 Department of Community Paediatrics, Sydney Local Health District, Croydon Community Health Centre, 24 Liverpool Street, Croydon, NSW 2132, Australia
5 School of Medicine and Public Health, University of Newcastle, University Drive, Callaghan, NSW 2308, Australia
6 Child and Family Health Nursing, Primary & Community Health, South Western Sydney Local Health District, Narellan, NSW 2567, Australia
7 School of Nursing and Midwifery, Western Sydney University, Liverpool Campus, Locked Bag 1797, Penrith, NSW 2571, Australia
8 St John of God Raphael Services, Blacktown, NSW 2148, Australia
9 Ingham Institute for Applied Medical Research, 1 Campbell Street, Liverpool, NSW 2170, Australia
10 School of Women's and Children's Health, The University of New South Wales, Kensington, Sydney, NSW 2052, Australia
11 Menzies Centre for Health Policy, Charles Perkins Centre, School of Public Health, Sydney University, Sydney, NSW 2006, Australia
12 School of Public Health, Griffith University, Gold Coast, QLD 4222, Australia
13 Sydney Institute for Women, Children and their Families, Sydney Local Health District, Camperdown, NSW 2050, Australia
* Correspondence: f.ogbo@westernsyndey.edu.au

Abstract: There are limited epidemiological data on exclusive breastfeeding (EBF) among culturally and linguistically diverse (CALD) Australian mothers to advocate for targeted and/or culturally-appropriate interventions. This study investigated the determinants of EBF cessation in the early postnatal period among CALD Australian mothers in Sydney, Australia. The study used linked maternal and child health data from two local health districts in Australia (N = 25,407). Prevalence of maternal breastfeeding intention, skin-to-skin contact, EBF at birth, discharge, and the early postnatal period (1–4 weeks postnatal), were estimated. Multivariate logistic regression models were used to investigate determinants of EBF cessation in the early postnatal period. Most CALD Australian mothers had the intention to breastfeed (94.7%). Skin-to-skin contact (81.0%), EBF at delivery (91.0%), and at discharge (93.0%) were high. EBF remained high in the early postnatal period (91.4%). A lack of prenatal breastfeeding intention was the strongest determinant of EBF cessation (adjusted odds ratio [aOR] = 23.76, 95% CI: 18.63–30.30, for mothers with no prenatal breastfeeding intention and aOR = 6.15, 95% CI: 4.74–7.98, for those undecided). Other significant determinants of EBF cessation included a lack of partner support, antenatal and postnatal depression, intimate partner violence, low socioeconomic status, caesarean birth, and young maternal age (<20 years). Efforts to improve breastfeeding among women of CALD backgrounds in Australia should focus on women with vulnerabilities to maximise the benefits of EBF.

Keywords: exclusive breastfeeding; Australia; skin-to-skin; culturally and linguistically diverse (CALD)

1. Introduction

Global health organisations (such as the World Health Organization and the United Nations Children's Fund, WHO/UNICEF) recommend exclusive breastfeeding (EBF) for the first six months of life [1]. EBF is defined as providing the infant human breastmilk only, and when needed, oral rehydration solution, or drops/syrups of vitamins, minerals, or medicines [2]. Breast milk has a high proportion of fat, protein, sugar, and water that is required for infant growth and development compared to formula milk, as well as the immunologic substances to effectively protect against infectious diseases for the infant [3–5]. Appropriate EBF protects against childhood obesity [6] and has the potential to increase infant cognitive functioning [7]. EBF not only benefits the infant but is also associated with improved maternal health (e.g., a reduced risk developing of type 2 diabetes mellitus) [8] and improved household productivity due to no cost of human milk [9].

In Australia, culturally and linguistically diverse (CALD) is a term used for communities with diverse ethnic backgrounds, traditions, food, nationality, language, dress, societal structures, art, and religious characteristics [10]. While it may be debatable that such a 'label' exists to characterize such diverse populations, it is nevertheless one measure that can identify a sub-group in the Australian population who are often socioeconomically vulnerable, and for the purpose of focused research and programmatic interventions [11,12]. Past research suggests that CALD subgroups are more likely to experience adverse health outcomes, including depressive symptoms [13] and poor uptake of cancer screening [14], compared to the non-CALD populations.

Many qualitative studies conducted in Australia have reported that most CALD women value optimal breastfeeding practices, but a lack of access to traditional post-birth practices [15], stigma, and shame around public breastfeeding and ambivalence towards breastfeeding support [16,17], were barriers to appropriate breastfeeding. However, there is limited epidemiological data on the determinants of inappropriate EBF among CALD subgroups to inform targeted interventions. Quantitative research in the general Australian population suggests that intimate partner violence [18], a lack of partner support [18], assisted delivery [18,19], low socioeconomic status [20], lower maternal age (<25 years) [19], a mother not having intention to breastfeeding [21–23], and self-reported depressive symptoms [21] were associated with cessation of EBF. Notably, it is unclear whether these factors are relevant to mothers from CALD backgrounds as culturally-appropriate and focused intervention strategies are potentially more effective and less costly than traditional interventional approaches [12].

Understanding the factors that influence a mother's decision to initiate, cease, or continue EBF in the early postnatal period is essential as it can provide important information and opportunities for specific interventions. In addition to providing relevant data on EBF among CALD Australian mothers, this study seeks to provide an evidence base on EBF among CALD mothers for breastfeeding policy advocacy and/or evaluation of relevant social and health services for mothers of CALD backgrounds in Australia. This study aimed to investigate the determinants of EBF cessation in the early postnatal period among CALD Australian mothers in Sydney, New South Wales.

2. Materials and Methods

2.1. Data Source

The study was conducted based on retrospective maternal and child health data of all live births in public health facilities in Sydney Local Health District (SLHD) and South Western Sydney Local Health District (SWSLHD) between 2014 and 2016 (N = 25,407). These data were routinely collected as part of standard care provided during pregnancy and the postnatal period. Antenatal information that included socio-demographic characteristics, history of any previous pregnancy, probable depression based on the Edinburgh Postnatal Depression Scale (EPDS), and mothers' breastfeeding intention were collected by qualified midwives at the first prenatal care visit. Birth and postnatal data such as information on skin-to-skin contact, EBF at discharge and postnatally, were also obtained immediately after birth and during postnatal visits by qualified child and family health nurses (CFHN). During the first prenatal visit, women were asked to identify whether they belong to CALD, non-CALD, or Aboriginal or Torres Strait Islander subpopulations, and this information was entered into the database. CALD population was defined based on the Australian Bureau of Statistics description for the subgroup [10]. These maternal child health (MCH) data were stored in the local health district's Information Management & Technology Division (IM&TD) database. We obtained the perinatal data from the IM&TD, which were cleaned and linked using individual identifiers, and coded for analysis.

2.2. Study Setting

In Sydney, the SLHD and SWSLHD cover 52% of the metropolitan area, with an estimated population of 1.6 million people of different cultural backgrounds [24,25]. SLHD is located in the centre and inner west of Sydney, while SWSLHD is located in the south-western region of Sydney. A number of maternal and child health services are provided to all communities across both districts, including the most socioeconomically disadvantaged populations.

2.3. Outcome Variables

The main outcome variable was EBF in the early postnatal period (defined as 1–4 weeks post-birth). EBF was measured using the National Health and Medical Research Council (NHMRC) infant feeding guidelines [26], consistent with the WHO/UNICEF definitions for assessing infant and young child feeding practices [1]. EBF was defined as the proportion of infants who received only breast milk (including expressed milk) but allowed oral rehydration solution, syrups of vitamins/medicines. The prevalence of mothers' breastfeeding intention, skin-to-skin contact, EBF at delivery and discharge by the determining factors were also measured in the study.

EBF at delivery was defined as the proportion of infants who received only breast milk in the first 24 h post-birth, while EBF at discharge was measured as the proportion of infants who received only breast milk 24 h preceding discharge from the maternity unit. EBF in the early postnatal visit (1–4 weeks postnatal) referred to the proportion of infants who received only breast milk 24 h prior to this postnatal health visit by the CFHN. To assess mothers' breastfeeding intention, they were asked the following question: "Do you plan to breastfeed your child?" The study also considered skin-to-skin contact as past studies have indicated that skin-to-skin contact is the most effective strategy to promote, protect, and support EBF in early life, irrespective of the mode of birthing (vaginal or caesarean births) [27–29]. Skin-to-skin contact (SSC) was defined as placing the naked baby on the mother's bare chest or abdomen immediately or less than 10 min after birth or soon afterwards [30].

In each local health district, assessment of both the mother and baby is conducted between the first and fourth week post-birth by a CFHN during a universal health home visit. Relevant health information (including anthropometric measurement of the baby and assessment of infant feeding practices of the mother) are obtained and entered into the IM&TD database.

2.4. Study Factors

The exposure variables were broadly categorised into socio-demographic and health factors, which were selected based on previous studies [18,19,22,23] and data availability. Socio-demographic factors included maternal age (categorised as <20 years, 20–34 years or ≥35 years), socioeconomic status (SES, categorised as high, middle or low), maternal cigarette smoking in pregnancy (categorised as yes or no), partner support (categorised as yes, not sure or no), and major nationality groups (categorised as Oceania, North-West Europe, Southern-Eastern Europe, North Africa and The Middle East, South-East Asia, North-East Asia, Southern and Central Asia, Americas or Sub-Saharan Africa).

Health factors included pre-existing maternal health problems (such as diabetes mellitus and/or hypertension, categorised as yes or no), history of intimate partner violence (IPV, categorised as yes or no), type of delivery (categorised as normal vaginal, assisted vaginal or caesarean), and self-reported antenatal and postnatal depressive symptoms (categorised as score ≥13 or score <13 on the EPDS) [31]. Maternal breastfeeding intention was also considered a potential factor for the cessation of EBF in the early post-birth period based on past studies [21–23].

SES was calculated using the Socio-Economic Index for Areas (SEIFA). SEIFA is an indicator created by the Australian Bureau of Statistics using principal component analysis. It ranks areas (including a mother's address provided) in Australia according to relative socio-economic advantage and disadvantage [32]. In this study, deciles of SES were categorised into high (top 10% of the population), middle (middle 80%), and low (bottom 10%) groups, in line with previously published studies [13,31]. In accordance with NSW Health policy [33], IPV information was collected from mothers based on the following questions: (i) "within the last year have you been hit, slapped or hurt in other ways by your partner or ex-partner?", physical IPV; and (ii) "are you frightened of your partner or ex-partner?", psychological IPV.

2.5. Statistical Analysis

The analytical approach followed previously published studies [18,31]. Briefly, preliminary analyses were conducted to calculate frequencies of the study outcomes (i.e., breastfeeding intention, skin-to-skin contact, and EBF at delivery, discharge and postnatally) and cross-tabulations with study factors. This was followed by univariate regression models to examine the association between each study factor and cessation of EBF in the early postnatal period. Multivariate logistic regression analyses that adjusted for confounders was conducted to investigate the potential study factors that were associated with cessation of EBF in the early postnatal period among CALD mothers. Models adjusted for the potential confounding factors of birthing facility, the gender of the baby, maternal alcohol intake, and maternal body mass index, as well as socio-economic and health factors [21,34]. Odds ratios, with 95% confidence intervals, were calculated as the measure of association between the risk factors and cessation of EBF.

Our study also investigated the potential effect of missing data on the estimated odds ratios in sensitivity analyses that used an imputed dataset, based on the original data, which comprised complete information for EBF in the early postnatal period. Multiple imputations by chained equations were employed, which assume that data were missing at random [35]. This analytical approach also assumes that the known characteristics of study respondents can be used to examine the characteristics of participants with missing data [36]. All study factors and the outcome variable in the main analysis were included in the multiple imputation models. Revised odds ratios from the imputed data were generated using the *mim* command, for comparison with the complete case analyses. Sensitivity analyses were conducted based on 25 multiple imputations [37], and all analyses were conducted in Stata (Stata Corp, version 15.0, College Station, TX, USA).

2.6. Ethics

The Sydney Local Health District and South Western Sydney Local Health District Human Research Ethics Committees approved the collection of the data from the IM&TD database and subsequent analysis. Approval numbers HREC: LNR/11/LPOOL/463; SSA: LNRSSA/11/LPOOL/464 and Project No: 11/276 LNR; Protocol No X12-0164 and LNR/12/RPAH/266.

3. Results

3.1. Characteristics of the Study Population

The majority of mothers were from South-East Asia (24.5%) and North Africa and The Middle East (23.0%), while the lowest proportion of mothers were from North-West Europe (1.5%) (Table 1).

Table 1. Characteristics of the study population (N = 25,407).

Variables	N	(%)
Sociodemographic factors		
Maternal age group	25,407	
20–34 years	23,812	93.7
<20 years	124	0.5
≥35 years	1471	5.8
SES category	23,786	
Low	12,548	52.8
Middle	9377	39.4
High	1861	7.8
Smoking status	23,750	
No	23,170	97.6
Yes	580	2.4
Supportive partner	21,672	
Yes	21,061	97.2
No	611	2.8
Major nationality group	25,407	
Oceania	1481	5.8
North-West Europe	384	1.5
Southern-Eastern Europe	1316	5.2
North Africa and The Middle East	5846	23.0
South-East Asia	6222	24.5
North-East Asia	3512	13.8
Southern and Central Asia	5127	20.2
Americas	634	2.5
Sub-Saharan Africa	885	3.5
Health factors		
Antenatal health problems	24,603	
No	20,517	83.4
Yes	4086	16.6
Psychosocial intimate partner violence	21,583	
No	21,238	98.4
Yes	345	1.6
Physical intimate partner violence	21,523	
No	21,240	98.7
Yes	283	1.3
Type of delivery	25,378	
Normal vaginal	15,004	59.1
Assisted vaginal	2924	11.5
Caesarean section	7450	29.4

Table 1. *Cont.*

Variables	N	(%)
Antenatal depressive symptoms	20,560	
EPDS ≤ 9	16,972	82.6
EPDS 10–12	2078	10.1
EPDS ≥ 13	1510	7.3
Postnatal depressive symptoms	19,342	
EPDS ≤ 9	17,425	90.1
EPDS 10–12	1194	6.2
EPDS ≥ 13	723	3.7

N = Sample size; EPDS: Edinburgh Postnatal Depression Scale; SES: Socioeconomic status.

3.2. *Breastfeeding Patterns by Study Factors*

The proportion of CALD Australian mothers who exclusively breastfed in the early postnatal period varied by global regions, with mothers from South-East Asia (26.9%), North Africa and the Middle East (33.8%), and Oceania (12.2%) representing the highest percentage (Table 2). Mothers from the high SES category had a higher proportion of EBF (63.1%) compared to those from middle and low SES categories (33.4% and 3.5%, respectively).

Table 2. Prevalence of breastfeeding among culturally and linguistically diverse (CALD) mothers from South Western Sydney and Sydney Local Health Districts in Sydney, Australia, 2014–2016 (N = 25,407).

Variables	Breastfeeding Intention	Skin-to-Skin Contact	EBF at Delivery	EBF at Discharge	EBF at 1–4 Weeks
	n (%)	**n (%)**	**n (%)**	**n (%)**	**n (%)**
Study outcomes					
Yes	21,232 (94.7)	16,022 (81.2)	19,355 (90.7)	22,555 (93.3)	19,244 (91.4)
No	629 (2.8)	3697 (18.8)	1973 (9.3)	1629 (6.7)	1809 (8.6)
Undecided	572 (2.5)	-	-	-	-
Socio-demographic factors					
Maternal age group					
20–34 years	21,048 (93.8)	18,651 (94.6)	20,023 (93.9)	22,690 (93.8)	1628 (90.0)
<20 years	103 (0.5)	113 (0.6)	112 (0.5)	1375 (5.7)	14 (9.2)
≥35 years	1282 (5.7)	955 (4.8)	1193 (5.6)	119 (0.5)	167 (0.8)
SES category					
High	10,304 (63.4)	9778 (52.9)	10,411 (52.1)	11,877 (52.5)	1109 (63.1)
Middle	7962 (32.8)	7268 (39.3)	7958 (39.8)	8922 (39.5)	588 (33.4)
Low	1598 (3.8)	1427 (7.7)	1612 (8.1)	1817 (8.0)	62 (3.5)
Smoking status					
No	21,860 (97.6)	17,937 (97.3)	19,520 (97.7)	22,207 (97.6)	1532 (92.9)
Yes	543 (2.4)	437 (2.4)	467 (2.3)	540 (2.4)	117 (7.1)
Supportive partner					
Yes	20,501 (97.2)	16,457 (97.2)	17,773 (97.2)	20,190 (97.3)	1454 (95.7)
No	585 (2.8)	481 (2.8)	508 (2.8)	569 (2.7)	66 (4.3)
Major nationality group					
Oceania	1237 (5.5)	1193 (6.1)	1247 (5.9)	1368 (5.7)	221 (12.2)
North-West Europe	360 (1.6)	326 (1.7)	343 (1.6)	373 (1.5)	18 (1.0)
Southern-Eastern Europe	1177 (5.3)	1028 (5.2)	1146 (5.4)	1262 (5.2)	128 (7.08)
North Africa and The Middle East	5100 (22.7)	4649 (23.6)	4901 (23.0)	5526 (22.8)	612 (33.8)
South-East Asia	5437 (24.2)	4958 (25.1)	5235 (24.6)	5868 (24.3)	487 (26.9)
North-East Asia	3150 (14.0)	2837 (14.4)	3048 (14.3)	3431 (14.2)	150 (8.3)

Table 2. *Cont.*

Variables	Breastfeeding Intention	Skin-to-Skin Contact	EBF at Delivery	EBF at Discharge	EBF at 1–4 Weeks
	n (%)	n (%)	n (%)	n (%)	n (%)
Southern and Central Asia	4636 (20.7)	3638 (18.5)	4158 (19.5)	4914 (20.3)	116 (6.4)
Americas	552 (2.5)	439 (2.2)	526 (2.5)	607 (2.5)	42 (2.3)
Sub-Saharan Africa	784 (3.5)	651 (3.3)	724 (3.4)	835 (3.5)	35 (1.9)
Health factors					
Antenatal health problems					
No	17,847 (82.4)	15,821 (83.0)	17,334 (83.7)	19,514 (83.3)	1496 (85.1)
Yes	3819 (17.6)	3245 (17.0)	3370 (16.3)	3916 (16.7)	263 (14.9)
Psychosocial intimate partner violence					
No	20,657 (98.4)	19,618 (98.4)	17,919 (98.4)	20,360 (98.5)	1517 (97.9)
Yes	335 (1.6)	273 (1.6)	290 (1.6)	316 (1.5)	33 (2.1)
Physical intimate partner violence					
No	20,663 (98.7)	16,616 (98.7)	17,911 (98.7)	20,356 (98.7)	1522 (98.1)
Yes	270 (1.3)	213 (1.3)	243 (1.3)	265 (1.3)	30 (1.9)
Type of delivery					
Normal vaginal	13,356 (59.6)	14,903 (75.7)	14,126 (66.3)	14,432 (59.7)	988 (54.7)
Assisted vaginal	2581 (11.5)	2878 (14.6)	2452 (11.5)	2759 (11.4)	163 (9.0)
Caesarean section	6473 (28.9)	1913 (9.7)	4730 (22.2)	6968 (28.8)	655 (36.3)
Antenatal depressive symptoms					
EPDS ≤ 9	16,543 (72.6)	13,406 (83.3)	14,392 (82.9)	16,259 (82.6)	1164 (79.6)
EPDS 10–12	2013 (10.1)	1577 (9.8)	1751 (10.1)	1992 (10.1)	146 (10.0)
EPDS ≥ 13	1465 (7.3)	1121 (6.9)	1222 (7.0)	1433 (7.3)	152 (10.4)
Postnatal depressive symptoms					
EPDS ≤ 9	15,451 (90.2)	13,538 (90.6)	14,739 (90.5)	16,628 (90.2)	1,489 (88.9)
EPDS 10–12	1055 (6.2)	880 (5.9)	973 (6.0)	1139 (6.2)	94 (5.6)
EPDS ≥ 13	633 (3.7)	523 (3.5)	579 (3.5)	677 (3.6)	92 (5.5)

n: cases; antenatal health problems included diabetes mellitus and/or hypertension; EBF at delivery was defined as infants who received only breast milk within the first 24 h post-delivery; EBF at discharge was measured as infants who received only breast milk in the 24 h preceding discharge from the maternity unit; EPDS: Edinburgh Postnatal Depression Scale; SES: Socioeconomic status.

In the antenatal period, almost all mothers intended to breastfeed their babies (94.7%). Approximately 81% of mothers practised skin-to-skin contact, while 91% and 93% exclusively breastfed at delivery and discharge, respectively. A sub-analysis of the data (i.e., the estimation of the confidence interval and p-value around the estimates, data not shown) suggested that there was no significant difference between EBF prevalence at delivery and discharge. In the early postnatal period, EBF remained high among CALD Australian mothers (91.4%; Table 2).

3.3. Determinants of Exclusive Breastfeeding Cessation in the Early Postnatal Period

The study showed that mothers who indicated no prenatal breastfeeding intention or who were undecided about breastfeeding during pregnancy were more likely to cease EBF in the early postnatal period compared to those who indicated prenatal breastfeeding intention in the complete case analyses (adjusted odds ratio (aOR) = 23.76, 95% CI 18.63–30.30, $p < 0.001$, for those with no prenatal breastfeeding intention and aOR = 6.15, 95% CI 4.74–7.98, $p < 0.001$, for those undecided) (Table 3).

Table 3. Determinants of exclusive breastfeeding cessation in the early postnatal period among CALD mothers in South Western Sydney and Sydney Local Health Districts, 2014–2016 (N = 25,407).

Study Factors	Complete Case Analysis				Multiple Imputation Analysis *			
	Unadjusted OR (95% CI)	*p* Value	Adjusted OR (95% CI) (a)	*p* Value	Unadjusted OR (95% CI)	*p* Value	Adjusted OR (95% CI) (a)	*p* Value
Antenatal breastfeeding intention								
Yes	1.00		1.00		1.00		1.00	
No	31.11 (25.41–38.10)	<0.001	23.76 (18.63–30.30)	<0.001	31.11 (29.90–32.37)	<0.001	27.13 (26.04–28.27)	<0.001
Undecided	7.01 (5.69–8.64)	<0.001	6.15 (4.74–7.98)	<0.001	7.00 (6.72–7.30)	<0.001	6.38 (6.11–6.66)	<0.001
Sociodemographic factors								
Supportive partner								
Yes	1.00		1.00		1.00		1.00	
No	1.81 (1.38–2.36)	<0.001	1.69 (1.20–2.38)	0.003	1.66 (1.58–1.74)	<0.001	1.60 (1.52–1.69)	<0.001
Socio-economic status								
Low	1.00		1.00					
Middle	0.67 (0.61–0.75)	<0.001	0.85 (0.72–0.99)	0.044	0.67 (0.65–0.68)	<0.001	0.84 (0.82–0.86)	<0.001
High	0.36 (0.28–0.47)	<0.001	0.48 (0.32–0.71)	<0.001	0.36 (0.34–0.38)	<0.001	0.59 (0.56–0.63)	<0.001
Maternal age group								
20–34 years	1.00		1.00		1.00		1.00	
<20 years	1.76 (1.48–2.08)	<0.001	1.72 (1.37–2.15)	<0.001	1.75 (1.69–1.81)	<0.001	1.75 (1.69–1.81)	<0.001
≥35 years	1.79 (1.02–3.15)	0.044	1.91 (0.93–3.93)	0.078	1.78 (1.60–1.99)	<0.001	1.61 (1.44–1.80)	<0.001
Smoking status								
No	1.00		1.00		1.00		1.00	
Yes	4.29 (3.45–5.33)	<0.001	3.39 (2.56–4.49)	<0.001	4.28 (4.10–4.47)	<0.001	3.81 (3.65–3.99)	<0.001
Major nationality group								
Oceania	1.00				1.00			
North-West Europe	0.25 (0.15–0.41)	<0.001	0.49 (0.25–0.97)	0.043	0.25 (0.23–0.28)	<0.001	0.47 (0.43–0.52)	<0.001
Southern-Eastern Europe	0.57 (0.45–0.73)	<0.001	0.73 (0.53–1.00)	0.051	0.57 (0.55–0.60)	<0.001	0.71 (0.68–0.74)	<0.001
North Africa and The Middle East	0.67 (0.56–0.79)	<0.001	0.65 (0.51–0.82)	<0.001	0.67 (0.65–0.69)	<0.001	0.64 (0.62–0.67)	<0.001
South-East Asia	0.45 (0.38–0.53)	<0.001	0.46 (0.36–0.58)	<0.001	0.45 (0.43–0.46)	<0.001	0.47 (0.45–0.49)	<0.001
North-East Asia	0.24 (0.19–0.31)	<0.001	0.41 (0.29–0.56)	<0.001	0.24 (0.23–0.26)	<0.001	0.43 (0.41–0.45)	<0.001
Southern and Central Asia	0.11 (0.09–0.14)	<0.001	0.18 (0.13–0.24)	<0.001	0.11 (0.11–0.12)	<0.001	0.14 (0.14–0.15)	<0.001
Americas	0.37 (0.26–0.53)	<0.001	0.40 (0.24–0.66)	<0.001	0.37 (0.35–0.40)	<0.001	0.41 (0.38–0.44)	<0.001
Sub-Saharan Africa	0.21 (0.14–0.31)	<0.001	0.25 (0.15–0.41)	<0.001	0.21 (0.20–0.23)	<0.001	0.24 (0.23–0.26)	<0.001
Health factors								
Antenatal depressive symptoms								
EPDS ≤ 9	1.00		1.00		1.00		1.00	
EPDS 10–12	1.03 (0.86–1.23)	0.783	1.10 (0.88–1.36)	0.398	1.02 (0.99–1.06)	0.161	1.00 (0.97–1.04)	<0.001
EPDS ≥ 13	1.59 (1.33–1.91)	<0.001	1.50 (1.20–1.89)	<0.001	1.59 (1.53–1.64)	<0.001	1.57 (1.51–1.62)	<0.001

Table 3. *Cont.*

Study Factors	Complete Case Analysis				Multiple Imputation Analysis *			
	Unadjusted OR (95% CI)	*p* Value	Adjusted OR (95% CI) (a)	*p* Value	Unadjusted OR (95% CI)	*p* Value	Adjusted OR (95% CI) (a)	*p* Value
Postnatal depressive symptoms								
EPDS ≤ 9	1.00		1.00		1.00		1.00	
EPDS 10–12	0.911 (0.73–1.13)	0.402	0.97 (0.73–1.30)	0.860	0.92 (0.88–0.96)	<0.001	1.00 (0.96–1.04)	0.885
EPDS ≥ 13	1.61 (1.28–2.01)	<0.001	2.07 (1.55–2.77)	<0.001	1.57 (1.50–1.63)	<0.001	1.66 (1.59–1.73)	<0.001
Psychosocial intimate partner violence								
No	1.00		1.00		1.00		1.00	
Yes	1.47 (1.02–2.12)	0.041	1.66 (1.10–2.53)	0.017	1.46 (1.36–1.57)	<0.001	1.50 (1.39–1.61)	<0.001
Physical intimate partner violence								
No	1.00		1.00		1.00		1.00	
Yes	1.57 (1.06–2.31)	0.023	1.49 (0.94–2.38)	0.093	1.56 (1.45–1.69)	<0.001	1.62 (1.50–1.75)	<0.001
Type of delivery								
Normal vaginal	1.00		1.00		1.00		1.00	
Assisted vaginal	0.79 (0.67–0.94)	0.008	0.90 (0.72–1.14)	0.386	0.79 (0.76–0.82)	<0.001	0.96 (0.88–0.92)	0.078
Caesarean section	1.36 (1.23–1.51)	<0.001	1.35 (1.18–1.55)	<0.001	1.36 (1.33–1.39)	<0.001	1.48 (1.45–1.52)	<0.001
Pre-existing maternal health problems								
No	1.00		1.00		1.00		1.00	
Yes	0.87 (0.76–1.00)	0.054	1.02 (0.83–1.07)	0.790	0.87 (0.85–0.89)	<0.001	0.95 (0.93–0.98)	0.004

(a): adjusted for maternal body mass index, gender of the baby, maternal alcohol intake, Aboriginality and birthing facility location, as well as socioeconomic and health factors.
* Sensitivity analyses following multiple imputations for missing values; pre-existing maternal health problems included diabetes mellitus and/or hypertension.

Mothers who reported not having a supportive partner during pregnancy were more likely to stop EBF in the early post-birth period compared to those who reported receiving support from their partner during pregnancy (aOR = 1.69, 95% CI: 1.20–2.38, $p = 0.003$). Mothers from higher SES groups were less likely to discontinue EBF in the early postnatal period compared to those from lower SES groups (aOR = 0.48, 95% CI: 0.32–0.71, $p < 0.001$ for high SES and aOR = 0.85, 95% CI: 0.85–0.99, $p = 0.044$ for middle). Low maternal age (<20 years) was associated with cessation of EBF in the early postnatal period compared to middle reproductive-aged mothers (20–34 years; aOR = 1.72, 95% CI: 1.37–2.15, $p < 0.001$). Mothers who reported tobacco smoking during pregnancy were more likely to stop EBF in the early postnatal period compared to their counterparts who reported not smoking (aOR = 3.39, 95% CI: 2.56–4.49, $p < 0.001$) (Table 3).

The odds of stopping EBF in the immediate postpartum period were higher among mothers who reported antenatal depressive symptoms (EPDS ≥ 13; aOR = 1.50, 95% CI: 1.20–1.89, $p < 0.001$), and those who reported postnatal depressive symptoms (EPDS ≥ 13; aOR = 2.07, 95% CI: 1.55–2.77, $p < 0.001$). The likelihood of discontinuing EBF in the immediate postnatal period was higher among mothers who reported a history of psychological intimate partner violence (aOR = 1.66, 95% CI: 1.10–2.53, $p = 0.017$), and those who had caesarean births (aOR = 1.35, 95% CI: 1.18–1.55, $p < 0.001$). The odds of ceasing EBF in the immediate postpartum period were lower among mothers from all major nationality groups compared to their counterparts in the reference group (Oceania) (Table 3). The effects of maternal age > 35 years, physical intimate partner violence, and having pre-existing maternal health problems on ceasing EBF in the immediate postnatal period were statistically significant in the imputation data compared to those in the complete case analysis. Furthermore, the 95% CI of the aOR for no maternal breastfeeding intention and major nationality group based on the imputation data is much narrower than the one obtained based on the original data set, possibly reflecting the effect of missing data or small sample size (Table 3).

4. Discussion

Our study indicates that most CALD Australian mothers had the intention to breastfeed (94.7%). Eighty-one percent of mothers practised skin-to-skin contact, while 91% and 93% exclusively breastfed at delivery and discharge, respectively. Notably, EBF remained high in the early postnatal period among CALD Australian mothers (91.4%). A lack of maternal prenatal breastfeeding intention (no prenatal breastfeeding intention or undecided) was the strongest risk factor for the cessation of EBF in the early postpartum period. Other significant factors associated with the cessation of EBF in the early postnatal period included a lack of partner support, antenatal and postnatal depressive symptoms, psychosocial IPV, caesarean birthing, low socioeconomic status, and young maternal age (<20 years).

Consistent with past reports from Australia [21] and internationally [38–40], the present study indicates that a mother's prenatal intention not to breastfeed or undecided were the strongest risk factors for the cessation of EBF in the early postnatal period among CALD Australian women. Studies suggest that a good personal attitude towards breastfeeding, encouraging social norms for breastfeeding at home and work and a personal dislike for formula feeding, were essential to a mother's decision to have a definite intention to breastfeed [38,41]. In addition, the level of social support for the mother at the time of breastfeeding from the partner, grandmothers/in-laws [42], or peers [43,44], and the mother's own attitude to breastfeeding were influential to a mother's breastfeeding behaviour [38]. Our study also suggests that the lack of a supportive partner was associated with cessation of EBF in the early postnatal period. While studies have indicated that partners are willing to provide the required support to improve breastfeeding outcomes for both the mother and baby, a lack of appropriate and/or conflicting information from health practitioners to fathers have been flagged as constraints to fathers' full participation in breastfeeding support [45,46]. The involvement of fathers (in addition to grandmothers/in-laws if present) in prenatal breastfeeding education sessions and postnatal support are key priority areas for improving breastfeeding among mothers [47].

In Australia, many epidemiological studies have indicated that higher maternal SES was associated with EBF [19,20]. Our study shows that CALD mothers from higher SES groups were less likely to cease EBF in the early postnatal period compared to those from lower SES groups. Similarly, evidence has shown that infants whose fathers were from high SES groups were more likely to be breastfed up to 6-weeks post-birth compared to infants with fathers of low SES [47]. Possible reasons for why higher SES mothers (CALD and non-CALD) engage in optimal breastfeeding may include increased uptake of breastfeeding-related information and better skills in negotiating flexible workplace hours, creating opportunities for breastfeeding [48,49]. Research shows that young maternal age (<20 years) was associated with increased risk of mental health issues, with subsequent impacts on employment and socioeconomic position in later life [50]. The present study shows that young maternal age (<20 years) is associated with cessation of EBF in the early postnatal period, in line with previously published studies [18,19]. In many Australian communities, charitable organisations provide parenting support, life support, and educational opportunities for young mothers and their babies to lead healthy and productive lives in their local communities [51]. Integration of these services with antenatal and postnatal breastfeeding services (where practicable) would be essential to improve breastfeeding outcomes among young mothers.

Our study demonstrates an association between self-reported maternal antenatal and postnatal depressive symptoms (EPDS $\geq$ 13) and cessation of EBF within 4-weeks postnatally. Past studies have indicated that perinatal depression is associated with suboptimal breastfeeding, including cessation of EBF in the early postnatal period [52–54]. Our finding highlights the importance of routine perinatal depression screening in Australia [55]. Detailed information on policy and research implications of Australian perinatal depression screening has been published elsewhere [13,31,55,56]. Furthermore, the present study shows that self-reported psychological intimate partner violence is associated with cessation of EBF in the early postnatal period, in line with previous studies [33,57,58]. In most Australian healthcare centres, routine screening of women in the antepartum and postpartum periods for depression [13,55] and IPV [33,59] is conducted in an effort to promptly identify at-risk mothers, ensure referral for clinical assessment, follow-up, and support. Our findings suggest that sustained advocacy is required for perinatal depression and IPV screening among Australian CALD women to improve EBF.

Past studies conducted in Australia and internationally, have shown that cigarette smoking is associated with suboptimal breastfeeding outcomes [18,60]. Similarly, the present study shows that cigarette smoking is associated with cessation of EBF in the early postnatal period among CALD mothers. Evidence suggests that while there is an association between cigarette smoking and suboptimal breastfeeding, the evidence for a plausible biological mechanism is weak [61]. Nevertheless, a recent review indicated that smoking reduces the protective effects of breast milk and also negatively modifies the infant's response to breastfeeding and breast milk [62]. A possible explanation for this association among smokers may stem from a lack of motivation to breastfeed (i.e., less likely to have breastfeeding intention or to initiate breastfeeding) and/or less desire to seek help with breastfeeding challenges compared to non-smokers [60,61,63]. Australia has legislated a range of anti-smoking strategies (including restrictions on advertising, incremental taxation and regulation) to reduce smoking in the community. These initiatives have been shown to be effective in reducing experimentation and uptake of smoking among young people and overall smoking rates across all socio-demographics in Australia [63]. Sustained implementation of these initiatives will have positive impacts on breastfeeding outcomes among CALD Australian mothers in the short- and long-term.

There is robust evidence in the literature which indicates that health facility birthing, mode of birthing, and professional assistance received during birthing are critical to a mother's breastfeeding initiation and continuation [18,64]. This possibly reflects the key role the Baby Friendly Hospital

Initiative (BFHI) plays in promoting, protecting, and supporting optimal breastfeeding in health facilities. Our study found that caesarean birthing was associated with cessation of EBF in the early postpartum period, which is similar to findings from previous studies [18,19]. Among Australian states and territories, evidence indicates that NSW has the lowest number of BFHI certified maternity centres, with implications for maternal breastfeeding experiences [18]. It is anticipated that the Australian National Breastfeeding Strategy 2019 and beyond will provide a roadmap for improving breastfeeding outcomes among CALD mothers in Australia, including increasing BFHI certified maternity centres in NSW [65]. The study showed that the odds of stopping EBF in the immediate postpartum period were lower among mothers from all major nationality groups compared to their counterparts in the reference group (Oceania). Future studies that focus on breastfeeding outcomes among sub-groups within the CALD populations may be warranted, as they would provide more insights for cultural care.

Limitations of this study are discussed. First, the cessation of breastfeeding in the early postnatal period was based on self-report, potentially leading a recall and/or measurement bias. The implication of this is that it may have resulted in an underestimation or overestimation of the relationship between the risk factors and the outcome. Second, the study was unable to assess or adjust for all potential determining factors (e.g., prematurity, level of support received postnatally, multi-parity, or partner education) as these may also affect the observed results. Third, we were unable to distinguish mothers who ceased EBF in the first, second, third, or fourth week postpartum. This analysis would have provided detailed information on early cessation of EBF postnatally among CALD Australian mothers. Fourth, the small sample size of mothers who indicated no prenatal breastfeeding intention or who were undecided may account for the large effect size. Fifth, the non-use of maternal and child health data from private healthcare and other local health districts in Sydney is a limitation in the present study. Finally, the unavailability of longitudinal data on EBF from 1 to 6 months postnatally and the use of secondary data were additional limitations in this study. Despite these limitations, the study provides breastfeeding data from CALD Australian women to inform population-level interventional strategies.

5. Conclusions

Our study suggests that many CALD mothers have definite intention to breastfeed, and most mothers practise skin-to-skin contact, EBF at delivery and at discharge from hospital post-birth. Notably, EBF remained high in the early postnatal period (within 4-weeks postpartum) among CALD Australian mothers. A lack of maternal prenatal breastfeeding intention and partner support, antenatal and postnatal depressive symptoms, psychosocial intimate partner violence, caesarean birthing, low socioeconomic status, and young maternal age (<20 years) were associated with the cessation of EBF in the early postnatal period among CALD Australian mothers. Our study provides insight into breastfeeding practices among CALD Australian mothers to inform targeted initiatives, especially those identified to be at risk of early cessation of EBF.

Author Contributions: Conceptualization, F.A.O.; data curation, F.A.O. and S.N.; formal analysis, F.A.O.; funding acquisition, F.A.O., J.U., J.P., B.B.A.M., and J.E.; investigation, F.A.O.; methodology, F.A.O.; project administration, F.A.O.; resources, F.A.O., A.M., A.P., and J.E.; software, F.A.O.; supervision, F.A.O.; validation, F.A.O., O.K.E., S.K., S.N., P.S., K.Y.A., A.M., O.O., K.A., A.P., B.B.A.M., and J.E.; visualization, F.A.O., O.K.E., S.N., P.S., K.Y.A., A.M., O.O., K.A., A.P., J.U., J.P., B.B.A.M., and J.E.; writing—original draft, F.A.O. and O.K.E.; writing—review and editing, F.A.O., O.K.E., S.K., S.N., P.S., K.Y.A., A.M., O.O., K.A., A.P., B.B.A.M., and J.E.

Acknowledgments: The authors are grateful to all the health professionals in South Western Sydney Local Health Districts and Sydney Local Health District who spent time entering the data, and also to personnel (particularly Leslie Cramer for data download) at the Information Management & Technology Division for the time spent in generating the data for the analysis. The authors are also grateful to the Early Years Research Group at the Ingham Institute, South Western Sydney Local Health District and the Healthy Home And Neighbourhood at the Sydney Local Health District for the initial funding. F.A.O. is also grateful to Melinda Wolfenden at THRI, Western Sydney University, for the time and effort in proofreading the grant application and excellent administrative support. The effort of Victoria Blight in securing the research grant is also acknowledged.

References

1. World Health Organization. Indicators for assessing infant and young child feeding practices: Part 1: Definitions. In Proceedings of the Consensus Meeting, Washington, DC, USA, 6–8 November 2007.
2. Gartner, L.M.; Morton, J.; Lawrence, R.A.; Naylor, A.J.; O'Hare, D.; Schanler, R.J.; Eidelman, A.I. American academy of pediatrics section on breastfeeding: Breastfeeding and the use of human milk. *Pediatrics* **2005**, *115*, 496–506. [PubMed]
3. Karlsson, O.; Rodosthenous, R.S.; Jara, C.; Brennan, K.J.; Wright, R.O.; Baccarelli, A.A.; Wright, R.J. Detection of long non-coding RNAs in human breastmilk extracellular vesicles: Implications for early child development. *Epigenetics* **2016**, *11*, 721–729. [CrossRef] [PubMed]
4. Fujita, M.; Lo, Y.J.; Brindle, E. Nutritional, inflammatory, and ecological correlates of maternal retinol allocation to breast milk in agro-pastoral Ariaal communities of northern Kenya. *Am. J. Hum. Biol.* **2017**, *29*, e22961. [CrossRef] [PubMed]
5. Verduci, E.; Banderali, G.; Barberi, S.; Radaelli, G.; Lops, A.; Betti, F.; Riva, E.; Giovannini, M. Epigenetic effects of human breast milk. *Nutrients* **2014**, *6*, 1711–1724. [CrossRef] [PubMed]
6. Mannan, H. Early Infant Feeding of Formula or Solid Foods and Risk of Childhood Overweight or Obesity in a Socioeconomically Disadvantaged Region of Australia: A Longitudinal Cohort Analysis. *Int. J. Environ. Res. Public Health* **2018**, *15*, 1685. [CrossRef] [PubMed]
7. Victora, C.G.; Horta, B.L.; de Mola, C.L.; Quevedo, L.; Pinheiro, R.T.; Gigante, D.P.; Gonçalves, H.; Barros, F.C. Association between breastfeeding and intelligence, educational attainment, and income at 30 years of age: A prospective birth cohort study from Brazil. *Lancet Glob. Health* **2015**, *3*, e199–e205. [CrossRef]
8. Victora, C.G.; Bahl, R.; Barros, A.J.; França, G.V.; Horton, S.; Krasevec, J.; Murch, S.; Sankar, M.J.; Walker, N.; Rollins, N.C. Breastfeeding in the 21st century: Epidemiology, mechanisms, and lifelong effect. *Lancet* **2016**, *387*, 475–490. [CrossRef]
9. León-Cava, N.; Lutter, C.; Ross, J.; Martin, L. *Quantifying the Benefits of Breastfeeding: A Summary of the Evidence*; Pan American Health Organization: Washington, DC, USA, 2002.
10. Australian Bureau of Statistics. Culturally and Linguistically Diversity (CALD) Characteristics. Available online: https://www.abs.gov.au/ausstats/abs@.nsf/Lookup/by%20Subject/4529.0.00.003~{}2014~{}Main%20Features~{}Cultural%20and%20Linguistic%20Diversity%20(CALD)%20Characteristics~{}13 (accessed on 18 January 2019).
11. Brewer, R. *Culturally and Linguistically Diverse Women in the Australian Capital Territory: Enablers and Barriers to Achieving Social Connectedness*; Women's Centre for Health Matters: Canberra, Australia, 2009.
12. Adily, A.; Ward, J. Improving health among culturally diverse subgroups: An exploration of trade-offs and viewpoints among a regional population health workforce. *Health Promot. J. Aust.* **2005**, *16*, 207–212. [CrossRef]
13. Ogbo, F.A.; Eastwood, J.; Hendry, A.; Jalaludin, B.; Agho, K.E.; Barnett, B.; Page, A. Determinants of antenatal depression and postnatal depression in Australia. *BMC Psychiatry* **2018**, *18*, 49. [CrossRef]
14. Aminisani, N.; Armstrong, B.K.; Canfell, K. Cervical cancer screening in Middle Eastern and Asian migrants to Australia: A record linkage study. *Cancer Epidemiol.* **2012**, *36*, e394–e400. [CrossRef]
15. Schmied, V.; Olley, H.; Burns, E.; Duff, M.; Dennis, C.-L.; Dahlen, H.G. Contradictions and conflict: A meta-ethnographic study of migrant women's experiences of breastfeeding in a new country. *BMC Pregnancy Childbirth* **2012**, *12*, 163. [CrossRef] [PubMed]
16. Gallegos, D.; Vicca, N.; Streiner, S. Breastfeeding beliefs and practices of African women living in Brisbane and Perth, Australia. *Mater. Child Nutr.* **2015**, *11*, 727–736. [CrossRef] [PubMed]
17. Joseph, J.; Brodribb, W.; Liamputtong, P. "Fitting-in Australia" as nurturers: Meta-synthesis on infant feeding experiences among immigrant women. *Women Birth* **2018**. [CrossRef] [PubMed]
18. Ogbo, F.A.; Eastwood, J.; Page, A.; Arora, A.; McKenzie, A.; Jalaludin, B.; Tennant, E.; Miller, E.; Kohlhoff, J.; Noble, J. Prevalence and determinants of cessation of exclusive breastfeeding in the early postnatal period in Sydney, Australia. *Int. Breastfeed. J.* **2017**, *12*, 16. [CrossRef] [PubMed]
19. Hauck, Y.L.; Fenwick, J.; Dhaliwal, S.S.; Butt, J. A Western Australian survey of breastfeeding initiation, prevalence and early cessation patterns. *Mater. Child Health J.* **2011**, *15*, 260–268. [CrossRef] [PubMed]
20. Amir, L.H.; Donath, S.M. Socioeconomic status and rates of breastfeeding in Australia: Evidence from three recent national health surveys. *Med. J. Aust.* **2008**, *189*, 254–256. [PubMed]

21. Forster, D.A.; McLachlan, H.L.; Lumley, J. Factors associated with breastfeeding at six months postpartum in a group of Australian women. *Int. Breastfeed. J.* **2006**, *1*, 18. [CrossRef] [PubMed]
22. Scott, J.; Landers, M.; Hughes, R.M.; Binns, C. Factors associated with breastfeeding at discharge and duration of breastfeeding. *J. Paediatr. Child Health* **2001**, *37*, 254–261. [CrossRef]
23. Craig, P.L.; Knight, J.; Comino, E.; Webster, V.; Pulver, L.J.; Harris, E. Initiation and duration of breastfeeding in an aboriginal community in south western Sydney. *J. Hum. Lact.* **2011**, *27*, 250–261. [CrossRef]
24. South Western Sydney Local Health District. *Research Strategy for South Western Sydney Local Health District 2012–2021*; South Western Sydney Local Health District: Sydney, Australia, 2012.
25. Sydney Local Health District. Planning. Available online: https://www.slhd.nsw.gov.au/planning/profiles.html (accessed on 22 June 2016).
26. National Health and Medical Research Council. *Infant Feeding Guidelines*; National Health and Medical Research Council: Canberra, Australia, 2012.
27. Bramson, L.; Lee, J.W.; Moore, E.; Montgomery, S.; Neish, C.; Bahjri, K.; Melcher, C.L. Effect of early skin-to-skin mother—Infant contact during the first 3 h following birth on exclusive breastfeeding during the maternity hospital stay. *J. Hum. Lact.* **2010**, *26*, 130–137. [CrossRef]
28. Crenshaw, J.T. Healthy birth practice# 6: Keep mother and baby together—It's best for mother, baby, and breastfeeding. *J. Perinat. Educ.* **2014**, *23*, 211–217. [PubMed]
29. Moore, E.R.; Bergman, N.; Anderson, G.C.; Medley, N. Early skin-to-skin contact for mothers and their healthy newborn infants. *Cochrane Database Syst. Rev.* **2016**. [CrossRef] [PubMed]
30. World Health Organization. *Guideline: Protecting, Promoting and Supporting Breastfeeding in Facilities Providing Maternity and Newborn Services*; CC BY-NC-SA 3.0 IGO; World Health Organization: Geneva, Switzerland, 2017.
31. Eastwood, J.; Ogbo, F.A.; Hendry, A.; Noble, J.; Page, A. Early Years Research Group. The impact of antenatal depression on perinatal outcomes in Australian women. *PLoS ONE* **2017**, *12*, e0169907. [CrossRef] [PubMed]
32. Australian Bureau of Statistics. *Technical Paper: Socio-Economic Indexes for Areas (SEIFA) 2011*; Commonwealth of Australia: Canberra, Australia, 2013.
33. New South Wales Health Department. *Unless They're Asked: Routine Screening for Domestic Violence in NSW Health: An Evaluation of the Pilot Project*; New South Wales Health: Sydney, Australia, 2001.
34. Binns, C.; Gilchrist, D.; Gracey, M.; Zhang, M.; Scott, J.; Lee, A. Factors associated with the initiation of breast-feeding by Aboriginal mothers in Perth. *Public Health Nutr.* **2004**, *7*, 857–861. [CrossRef] [PubMed]
35. Van Buuren, S.; Boshuizen, H.C.; Knook, D.L. Multiple imputation of missing blood pressure covariates in survival analysis. *Stat. Med.* **1999**, *18*, 681–694. [CrossRef]
36. Sterne, J.A.; White, I.R.; Carlin, J.B.; Spratt, M.; Royston, P.; Kenward, M.G.; Wood, A.M.; Carpenter, J.R. Multiple imputation for missing data in epidemiological and clinical research: Potential and pitfalls. *BMJ* **2009**, *338*, b2393. [CrossRef] [PubMed]
37. Spratt, M.; Carpenter, J.; Sterne, J.A.; Carlin, J.B.; Heron, J.; Henderson, J.; Tilling, K. Strategies for multiple imputation in longitudinal studies. *Am. J. Epidemiol.* **2010**, *172*, 478–487. [CrossRef]
38. Colaizy, T.T.; Saftlas, A.F.; Morriss, F.H. Maternal intention to breast-feed and breast-feeding outcomes in term and preterm infants: Pregnancy Risk Assessment Monitoring System (PRAMS), 2000–2003. *Public Health Nutr.* **2012**, *15*, 702–710. [CrossRef]
39. Wu, Y.; Ho, Y.; Han, J.; Chen, S. The influence of breastfeeding self-efficacy and breastfeeding intention on breastfeeding behavior in postpartum women. *J. Nurs.* **2018**, *65*, 42–50.
40. Stuebe, A.M.; Bonuck, K. What predicts intent to breastfeed exclusively? Breastfeeding knowledge, attitudes, and beliefs in a diverse urban population. *Breastfeed. Med.* **2011**, *6*, 413–420. [CrossRef]
41. Kools, E.J.; Thijs, C.; Vries, H.d. The behavioral determinants of breast-feeding in The Netherlands: Predictors for the initiation of breast-feeding. *Health Educ. Behav.* **2005**, *32*, 809–824. [CrossRef] [PubMed]
42. Negin, J.; Coffman, J.; Vizintin, P.; Raynes-Greenow, C. The influence of grandmothers on breastfeeding rates: A systematic review. *BMC Pregnancy Childbirth* **2016**, *16*, 91. [CrossRef] [PubMed]
43. Cameron, A.J.; Hesketh, K.; Ball, K.; Crawford, D.; Campbell, K.J. Influence of peers on breastfeeding discontinuation among new parents: The Melbourne InFANT Program. *Pediatrics* **2010**, *126*, e601–e607. [CrossRef] [PubMed]
44. Shakya, P.; Kunieda, M.K.; Koyama, M.; Rai, S.S.; Miyaguchi, M.; Dhakal, S.; Sandy, S.; Sunguya, B.F.; Jimba, M. Effectiveness of community-based peer support for mothers to improve their breastfeeding

practices: A systematic review and meta-analysis. *PLoS ONE* **2017**, *12*, e0177434. [CrossRef] [PubMed]
45. Susin, L.R.O.; Giugliani, E.R.J. Inclusion of fathers in an intervention to promote breastfeeding: Impact on breastfeeding rates. *J. Hum. Lact.* **2008**, *24*, 386–392. [CrossRef] [PubMed]
46. Tohotoa, J.; Maycock, B.; Hauck, Y.L.; Howat, P.; Burns, S.; Binns, C.W. Dads make a difference: An exploratory study of paternal support for breastfeeding in Perth, Western Australia. *Int. Breastfeed. J.* **2009**, *4*, 15. [CrossRef]
47. Maycock, B.; Binns, C.W.; Dhaliwal, S.; Tohotoa, J.; Hauck, Y.; Burns, S.; Howat, P. Education and support for fathers improves breastfeeding rates: A randomized controlled trial. *J. Hum. Lact.* **2013**, *29*, 484–490. [CrossRef]
48. Mitra, A.K.; Khoury, A.J.; Hinton, A.W.; Carothers, C. Predictors of breastfeeding intention among low-income women. *Mater. Child Health J.* **2004**, *8*, 65–70. [CrossRef]
49. McIntyre, E.; Hiller, J.E.; Turnbull, D. Determinants of infant feeding practices in a low socio-economic area: Identifying environmental barriers to breastfeeding. *Aust. N. Z. J. Public Health* **1999**, *23*, 207–209. [CrossRef]
50. Cooklin, A.R.; Canterford, L.; Strazdins, L.; Nicholson, J.M. Employment conditions and maternal postpartum mental health: Results from the Longitudinal Study of Australian Children. *Arch. Women's Ment. Health* **2011**, *14*, 217–225. [CrossRef]
51. New South Wales Health. Youth Health Resources and Contacts for Young People. Available online: https://www.health.nsw.gov.au/kidsfamilies/youth/Pages/yh-resources-for-young-people.aspx (accessed on 22 April 2019).
52. Grigoriadis, S.; VonderPorten, E.H.; Mamisashvili, L.; Tomlinson, G.; Dennis, C.-L.; Koren, G.; Steiner, M.; Mousmanis, P.; Cheung, A.; Radford, K. The impact of maternal depression during pregnancy on perinatal outcomes: A systematic review and meta-analysis. *J. Clin. Psychiatry* **2013**, *74*, 321–341. [CrossRef] [PubMed]
53. Dennis, C.-L.; McQueen, K. The relationship between infant-feeding outcomes and postpartum depression: A qualitative systematic review. *Pediatrics* **2009**, *123*, e736–e751. [CrossRef] [PubMed]
54. Rahman, A.; Hafeez, A.; Bilal, R.; Sikander, S.; Malik, A.; Minhas, F.; Tomenson, B.; Creed, F. The impact of perinatal depression on exclusive breastfeeding: A cohort study. *Mater. Child Nutr.* **2016**, *12*, 452–462. [CrossRef] [PubMed]
55. Beyondblue. Clinical practice guidelines for depression and related disorders—Anxiety, bipolar disorder and puerperal psychosis—In the perinatal period. In *A Guideline for Primary Care Health Professionals*; Beyondblue: Melbourne, Australia, 2011.
56. Buist, A.E.; Barnett, B.E.; Milgrom, J.; Pope, S.; Condon, J.T.; Ellwood, D.A.; Boyce, P.M.; Austin, M.-P.V.; Hayes, B.A. To screen or not to screen-that is the question in perinatal depression. *Med. J. Aust.* **2002**, *177*, S101–S105. [PubMed]
57. Kendall-Tackett, K.A. Violence against women and the perinatal period: The impact of lifetime violence and abuse on pregnancy, postpartum, and breastfeeding. *Trauma Violence Abus.* **2007**, *8*, 344–353. [CrossRef] [PubMed]
58. Martin-de-las-Heras, S.; Velasco, C.; Luna-del-Castillo, J.; Khan, K. Breastfeeding avoidance following psychological intimate partner violence during pregnancy: A cohort study and multivariate analysis. *BJOG Int. J. Obstet. Gynaecol.* **2018**, *126*, 778–783. [CrossRef] [PubMed]
59. Australian Institute of Health and Welfare. *Screening for Domestic Violence during Pregnancy: Options for Future Reporting in the National Perinatal Data Collection*; AIHW: Canberra, Australia, 2015.
60. Amir, L.H.; Donath, S.M. Does maternal smoking have a negative physiological effect on breastfeeding? The epidemiological evidence. *Birth* **2002**, *29*, 112–123. [CrossRef]
61. Amir, L.H. Maternal smoking and reduced duration of breastfeeding: A review of possible mechanisms. *Early Hum. Dev.* **2001**, *64*, 45–67. [CrossRef]
62. Napierala, M.; Mazela, J.; Merritt, T.A.; Florek, E. Tobacco smoking and breastfeeding: Effect on the lactation process, breast milk composition and infant development. A critical review. *Environ. Res.* **2016**, *151*, 321–338. [CrossRef]
63. Australian National Preventive Health Agency. *Smoking and Disadvantage*; Australian National Preventive Health Agency: Canberra, Australia, 2013.

64. Smith, J.; Cattaneo, A.; Iellamo, A.; Javanparast, S.; Atchan, M.; Gribble, K.; Hartmann, B.; Salmon, L.; Tawia, S.; Hull, N.; et al. *Review of Effective Strategies to Promote Breastfeeding: An. Evidence Check Rapid Review Brokered by the Sax Institute for the Department of Health*; Sax Institute: Sydney, Australia, 2018.
65. Australian Government Department of Health. Breastfeeding. Available online: http://www.health.gov.au/internet/main/publishing.nsf/Content/health-pubhlth-strateg-brfeed-index.htm (accessed on 22 April 2019).

5

Worldwide Variation in Human Milk Metabolome: Indicators of Breast Physiology and Maternal Lifestyle?

Melvin C. L. Gay [1,†], Petya T. Koleva [2,†], Carolyn M. Slupsky [3,†], Elloise du Toit [4,†], Merete Eggesbo [5,†], Christine C. Johnson [6,†], Ganesa Wegienka [6,†], Naoki Shimojo [7,†], Dianne E. Campbell [8,†], Susan L. Prescott [9,10,†], Daniel Munblit [11,12,†], Donna T. Geddes [1,†], Anita L. Kozyrskyj [13,*,†] and InVIVO LactoActive Study Investigators [†]

1 School of Molecular Sciences, University of Western Australia, Perth, WA 6009, Australia; melvin.gay@uwa.edu.au (M.C.L.G.); donna.geddes@uwa.edu.au (D.T.G.)
2 Department of Pediatrics, University of Alberta, Edmonton, Alberta, AB T6G 1C9, Canada; koleva@ualberta.ca
3 Departments of Nutrition/Food Science & Technology, University of California Davis, California, CA 95616-5270, USA; cslupsky@ucdavis.edu
4 Division of Medical Microbiology, University of Cape Town, Cape Town, Rondebosch 7701, South Africa; elloisedutoit@gmail.com
5 Department of Environmental Exposure and Epidemiology, Norwegian Institute of Public Health, Oslo N-0213, Norway; merete.eggesbo@fhi.no
6 Department of Public Health Sciences, Henry Ford Hospital, Detroit, MI 48208, USA; cjohnso1@hfhs.org (C.C.J.); gwegien1@hfhs.org (G.W.)
7 Department of Pediatrics, Chiba University, Chiba 260-8677, Japan; shimojo@faculty.chiba-u.jp
8 Department of Allergy and Immunology, Children's Hospital at Westmead, University of Sydney, Sydney, NSW 2145, Australia; dianne.campbell1@health.nsw.gov.au
9 School of Medicine, University of Western Australia, Nedlands, WA 6009, Australia; Susan.Prescott@telethonkids.org.au
10 ORIGINS Project, Telethon Kids Institute, Perth Children's Hospital, Perth, WA 6009, Australia
11 Department of Paediatrics, Imperial College London, London W2 1NY, UK; daniel.munblit08@imperial.ac.uk
12 Faculty of Pediatrics, Sechenov University, Moscow 119991, Russia
13 Departments of Pediatrics/Obstetrics & Gynecology, School of Public Health, University of Alberta, Edmonton, Alberta AB T6G 1C9, Canada
* Correspondence: kozyrsky@ualberta.ca
† InVIVO Planetary Health of the Worldwide Universities Network (WUN), West New York, NJ 10704, USA.

Abstract: Human milk provides essential substrates for the optimal growth and development of a breastfed infant. Besides providing nutrients to the infant, human milk also contains metabolites which form an intricate system between maternal lifestyle, such as the mother's diet and the gut microbiome, and infant outcomes. This study investigates the variation of these human milk metabolites from five different countries. Human milk samples (n = 109) were collected one month postpartum from Australia, Japan, the USA, Norway, and South Africa and were analyzed by nuclear magnetic resonance. The partial least squares discriminant analysis (PLS-DA) showed separation between either maternal countries of origin or ethnicities. Variation between countries in concentration of metabolites, such as 2-oxoglutarate, creatine, and glutamine, in human milk, between countries, could provide insights into problems, such as mastitis and/or impaired functions of the mammary glands. Several important markers of milk production, such as lactose, betaine, creatine, glutamate, and glutamine, showed good correlation between each metabolite. This work highlights the importance of milk metabolites with respect to maternal lifestyle and the environment, and also provides the framework for future breastfeeding and microbiome studies in a global context.

Keywords: human milk; milk metabolites; lactation; milk metabolomics

1. Introduction

Human milk provides all of the essential nutrients and bioactive substrates required for optimal growth and development of the nursing infant [1]. This includes not only large immunoglobulins and proteins, but also numerous low molecular weight substances, such as simple sugars and complex human milk oligosaccharides (HMOs), amino acids, short-chain fatty acids, and other energy metabolic pathway intermediates [2]. These nutrients work as part of a complex functional unit, operating in concert with intestinal enzymes to influence infant physiology. Many metabolites, such as HMOs, lactose, and other milk sugars, are also fermented by gut microbiota to generate additional metabolites. Variation in the human milk metabolome, namely with HMOs, is seen by maternal phenotype and diet [3]. Despite this, there are still only a few studies reporting on the determinants of small molecule concentrations in human milk or their role, and only limited studies on global regional differences in other milk components [4,5].

Patterns of infant growth are strong predictors of future cognitive performance and cardiometabolic health [6–8]. Breastfeeding may protect from rapid growth during infancy and the risk for overweight/obesity, diabetes, and high blood pressure [9]; however, this may vary with compositional factors in human milk [10]. Because human milk metabolites influence infant gut microbial composition, and gut microbial dysbiosis has been linked to future overweight [11,12], geographic variations in small milk molecules can conceivably predict regional differences in infant gut microbial development, infant growth, and future health. The activity of some milk metabolites directly reflects maternal diet, and hence would be a function of regional differences in dietary intake [13]. Taking as an example immune system activation of spillover lactose in the colon secondary to lactase deficiency in the small intestine [14], the activity of still other milk metabolites may be subject to regional differences in host genetics. With an aim to learn more about these less well-studied small molecular weight metabolites, we undertook a descriptive study of human milk metabolomics, comparing women from diverse geographical locations. Healthy women without atopic conditions were the focus of the comparison. We found regional differences in milk metabolites related to lactation performance that differentiated South African women from women from other countries.

2. Materials and Methods

With representation across ethnicity, maternal atopy status, and infant sex, 109 milk samples collected one month after birth were selected from six existing international cohorts: Perth, Australia (n = 29 from 2 cohorts which include 21 atopic mothers, i.e., Perth #1, [15] and 8 non-atopic mothers, i.e., Perth #2) [16]; Chiba, Japan (n = 12); Detroit, USA (n = 18) [17]; Oslo, Norway (n = 40) [18]; and Cape Town, South Africa (n = 10) [4]. The one-month postpartum time period was selected because human milk composition has stabilized by then [2]. Maternal atopy status was defined according to maternal report of asthma, eczema, allergies, or other atopic diseases, or at least one blood allergen-specific IgE level $\geq$ 35 kU/L for dust mite, dog, cat, Timothy grass, ragweed, *Alternaria alternate*, egg, or German cockroach. Research ethics approval was obtained from the Human Research Ethics Committee of The University of Western Australia, Human Research Ethics Committee of the Princess Margaret Hospital, Committee on Human Research of Chiba University, Institutional Review Board at Henry Ford Health System, Norwegian Regional Committees for Medical and Health Research Ethics, and University of Cape Town Human Research Ethical Committee.

Before sample collection, the mothers were given oral and written instructions for standardized collection of samples. Human milk samples were collected manually or with an electric breast pump into a sterile tube. Prior to collection, nipples and mammary areola were cleaned with soap and sterile water, and for the samples from South Africa, the area was additionally soaked with chlorhexidine to reduce contamination by skin microbes. All of the samples were kept frozen at −20 °C until delivery to the laboratory and then stored at −20 °C or −80 °C until further analysis. All the samples were shipped to Edmonton, Canada for storage, processing and Nuclear Magnetic Resonance (NMR) analysis at The Metabolomics Innovation Centre.

Milk metabolite levels were determined by NMR because of its high reproducibility and coverage of a large range of metabolites. Prior to NMR spectroscopy, milk samples were thawed on ice and mixed thoroughly. Approximately 500 μL of each sample was filtered to remove residual lipids and protein using Amicon Ultra 0.5 mL 3-kDa cutoff spin filter (Millipore Sigma, Burlington, MA, USA). The filtration was performed at 10,000× g for 15 min at 4 °C. Then, a 350 μL clear filtrate was placed in a 1.5-mL Eppendorf tube, followed by the addition of 70 μL of D_2O and 60 μL of standard buffer solution (585 mM $NaHPO_4$ (pH 7.0), 11.667 mM disodium-2,2-dimethyl-2-silapentane-5-sulfonate (DSS), and 0.47% NaN_3 in H_2O). The samples (460 μL) were then transferred to a regular NMR tube for subsequent NMR spectral analysis. All ^{1}H-NMR spectra were collected on a Varian 500 MHz Inova spectrometer equipped with a 5-mm HCN Z-gradient pulsed-field gradient cryogenic probe. ^{1}H-NMR spectra were acquired at 25 °C using the first transient of the Varian tnnoesy pulse sequence, which was chosen for its high degree of selective water suppression and quantitative accuracy of resonances around the solvent. Water suppression pulses were calibrated to achieve a bandwidth of 80 G. Spectra were collected with 128 transient and 8 steady-state scans using a 4-s acquisition time (48,000 complex points) and a 1-s recycle delay. Quality control (QC) mixtures which consisted of 4 metabolites at 1 mM were analyzed for every 20 to 25 samples, and a relative standard deviation of <2% was observed.

Before spectral analysis, all free induction decays were zero-filled to 64,000 data points and line broadened to 0.5 Hz. The methyl singlet produced by a known quantity of DSS was used as an internal standard for chemical shift referencing (set to 0 ppm) and for quantification. All ^{1}H-NMR spectra were processed and analyzed using the Chenomx NMR Suite Professional software package version 8.1 (Chenomx Inc., Edmonton, AB, Canada). The Chenomx NMR Suite software allows for qualitative and quantitative analysis of an NMR spectrum by manually fitting spectral signatures from an internal database to the spectrum. Typically, 90% of visible peaks were assigned to a compound, and more than 90% of the spectral area could be routinely fit using the Chenomx spectral analysis software. Most of the visible peaks were annotated with a compound name and expressed as μmol/L.

Statistical Analysis

Partial Least Square Discriminant Analysis (PLS-DA) was created using the Excel add-in Multibase 2015 package (Numerical Dynamics, Tokyo, Japan). PLS-DA was performed in order to maximize the separation between the different countries as well as the ethnicities of the mothers. Data preparation was made using the scaling method of standard deviations. Sample scatterplot and loading plots were compared where significant variables which contribute to sample distribution can be easily identified. Statistical analyses were carried out using R studio 1.1.414 (Rstudio Inc., Boston, MA, USA) with package nlme for linear mixed models to test for significant differences between the milk metabolites among different countries, and among ethnicities of the mothers. Milk metabolite levels were compared with each other using the Pearsons correlation across all the non-atopic mothers using Package corrplot [19]. Differences are considered to be significant if $p < 0.05$.

3. Results

Of the 109 participating women, 69% were Caucasian, 51% were nursing male infants, and 43% had a history of atopy; this comparison oversampled atopic women and their additional results are the subject of another paper. The majority of South African women were of mixed race and all were non-atopic; most of the comparator cohorts were of Caucasian ancestry. Of the women in the US cohort, 39% were African American (labelled as Black) and only one African-American woman was non-atopic. All women had delivered vaginally and did not receive intrapartum antibiotics.

3.1. Milk Metabolite Clusters by Country

A total of 28 metabolites were identified in the human milk of our descriptive study, including sugars (fucose, glucose, lactose), amino acids (alanine, glutamine, glutamate, glycine, isoleucine, leucine, valine), choline and its metabolites, and energy metabolites (acetone, citrate, creatine, creatine phosphate, creatinine, lactate, 2-oxoglutarate, pyruvate, succinate), as shown in Figure 1. Most of the measured metabolites were within the range of those reported in other studies at a comparable time postpartum [20,21].

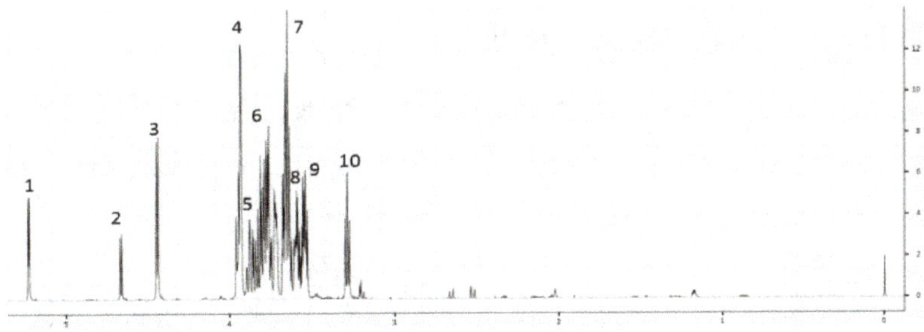

Figure 1. A representative ^{1}H nuclear magnetic resonance (NMR) spectrum of human milk. The ^{1}H chemical shifts for lactose are annotated 1 to 10.

The PLS plot in Figure 2 shows three main clusters of milk metabolites in women by country as follows: (1) South African, (2) Australian atopic and US, and (3) Australian non-atopic and Norwegian cohorts. Milk metabolites of Japanese women overlapped between those of Norwegian and South African women. Creatine and 2-oxoglutarate were the main drivers of milk metabolite differences between South Africa and other countries. Glutamine and phosphocholine differentiated the milk of Norwegian and US women.

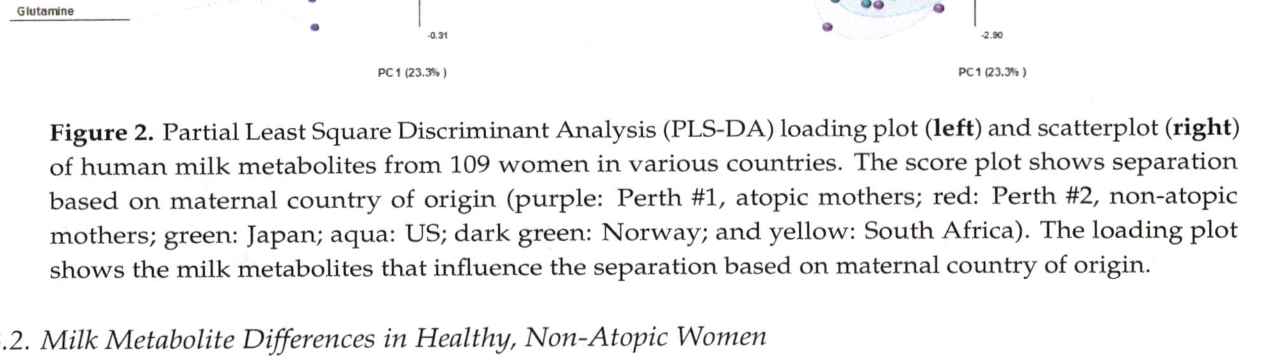

Figure 2. Partial Least Square Discriminant Analysis (PLS-DA) loading plot (**left**) and scatterplot (**right**) of human milk metabolites from 109 women in various countries. The score plot shows separation based on maternal country of origin (purple: Perth #1, atopic mothers; red: Perth #2, non-atopic mothers; green: Japan; aqua: US; dark green: Norway; and yellow: South Africa). The loading plot shows the milk metabolites that influence the separation based on maternal country of origin.

3.2. Milk Metabolite Differences in Healthy, Non-Atopic Women

Milk metabolite composition varied to the greatest extent between South African, and Norwegian or Australian women (Table 1). When compared to those of Norwegian women, the following milk metabolites were higher in concentration in South African women: lactose ($p = 0.02$), 2-oxoglutarate ($p < 0.001$), citrate (<0.001) and creatine ($p \leq 0.001$)/creatine-phosphate ($p = 0.02$) /creatinine ($p < 0.001$), as well as betaine ($p < 0.001$) and glycerol-phosphocholine ($p = 0.02$). Except for 2-oxoglurate and glycerol-phosphocholine, similar differences in these milk metabolites were observed between South African and Australian women. No country differences were observed in other milk sugars (glucose or fucose) or other energy metabolite (i.e., succinate) concentrations.

In addition, a statistical significance was also noted for lower milk levels of glutamine ($p < 0.001$) in Norwegian versus US women. Japanese women had significantly higher milk levels of pyruvate ($p < 0.01$) and lactate ($p < 0.01$) than Norwegian women. Milk levels of methanol were significantly lower ($p < 0.02$) in Norway versus all other countries.

Table 1. Comparison of milk metabolites concentrations (μmol/L) by country of origin.

MEAN (SD) Metabolites/Countries	South Africa	Japan	Norway	US	Perth #2
2-Oxoglutarate	79.6 (25.6)	79.1 (49.2) ##	30.5 (31.2) ***	39.0 (12.7) *	47.5 (19.9)
Acetone	13.2 (6.4)	19.8 (15.7)	10.8 (7.6)	11.4 (3.3)	13.3 (7.5)
Alanine	161.0 (93.5)	233.6 (96.8)	208.1 (84.5)	240.1 (91.9)	203.2 (48.4)
Betaine	668.1 (201.8)	355.3 (367.1)	180.4 (318.8) ***	408.4 (567.8)	58.8 (6.6) ***
Caprate	108.6 (124.7)	193.1 (216.3)	121.5 (120.3)	60.0 (90.6)	114.0 (42.9)
Caprylate	157.1 (137.2)	357.6 (497.0)	131.6 (207.1)	92.7 (132.5)	82.7 (47.1)
Choline	322.1 (194.9)	192.0 (128.3)	184.1 (163.7)	133.0 (77.0)	138.5 (71.1)
Citrate	5614 (3920)	2830 (1313) *	2718 (1361) ***	3642 (1272)	2856 (836.1) *
Creatine	274.7 (342.9)	60.3 (28.4) *	63.9 (26.9) ***	56.8 (23.4) *	66.5 (19.0) *
Creatine phosphate	49.6 (54.3)	45.2 (31.1)	20.6 (13.1) *	42.0 (12.7)	23.9 (7.6)
Creatinine	108.8 (82.7)	42.9 (15.4) **	43.7 (15.6) ***	57.3 (22.9) *	45.0 (5.7) **
Formate	83.4 (79.4)	112.2 (127.8)	902.0 (1695.2)	91.9 (55.7)	127.1 (24.9)
Fucose	278.5 (373.5)	570.9 (482.9)	330.5 (252.5)	344.4 (216.4)	382.3 (277.5)
Glucose	1347 (852.9)	1563 (1327)	926.4 (747.8)	1697 (413.5)	1699 (935.9)
Glutamate	858.9 (491.3)	1296 (565.8)	1467 (835.2)	1573 (830.2)	1554 (369.4)
Glutamine	282.0 (150.9)	103.0 (88.1)	101.9 (119.0)	514.2 (618.2) ###	207.6 (178.2)
Glycine	2796 (759.9)	3135 (1373)	2512 (1191)	1641 (1777)	1919 (949.5)
Guanidoacetate	4771 (1048)	3777 (1747)	3373 (2944)	3435 (1770)	1622 (286.5) *
Isoleucine	20.8 (12.2)	24.1 (25.9)	24.2 (21.1)	10.9 (2.6)	12.0 (4.0)
Lactate	213.7 (63.1)	3215 (5561) **##	443.5 (693.6)	137.8 (102.0)	125.7 (41.5)
Lactose	189,874 (34,234)	139,161 (83,333)	101,351 (84,404) *	161,160 (123,638)	83,524 (23,509) *
Leucine	33.7 (21.1)	49.9 (61.2)	66.2 (76.2)	30.9 (8.9)	34.0 (7.8)
Methanol	78.0 (17.6)	97.7 (49.2) ###	46.1 (19.3) ***	89.2 (6.7) ###	72.0 (6.8) #
Phosphocholine	636.9 (328.6)	784.7 (470.6)	463.7 (326.7)	698.3 (231.2)	488.4 (145.6)
Pyruvate	53.3 (29.5)	68.6 (69.8) ##	20.0 (26.3) *	31.7 (39.7)	6.3 (2.5) *
Succinate	48.3 (67.0)	47.9 (25.9)	210.8 (515.7)	21.2 (9.6)	49.3 (15.7)
Valine	35.3 (11.9)	63.9 (33.5)	65.6 (32.7) *	50.2 (21.1)	57.4 (17.6)
Glycerophosphocholine	797.6 (439.3)	645.0 (393.0)	414.9 (346.0) *	589.2 (239.7)	517.4 (118.5)
# metabolite differences with South Africa	na	4	11	3	7
# metabolite differences with Norway	-	4	na	2	1

* $p < 0.05$, ** $p < 0.01$, *** $p < 0.001$ when reference = South Africa; # $p < 0.05$, ## $p < 0.01$, ### $p < 0.001$ when reference = Norway; na: not applicable.

3.3. Milk Metabolite Correlations

Correlations between milk metabolites are reported in Figure 3. Both lactose and betaine were positively correlated with citrate, creatine, and the phosphocholines; milk lactose levels significantly rose with those of 2-oxoglutarate.

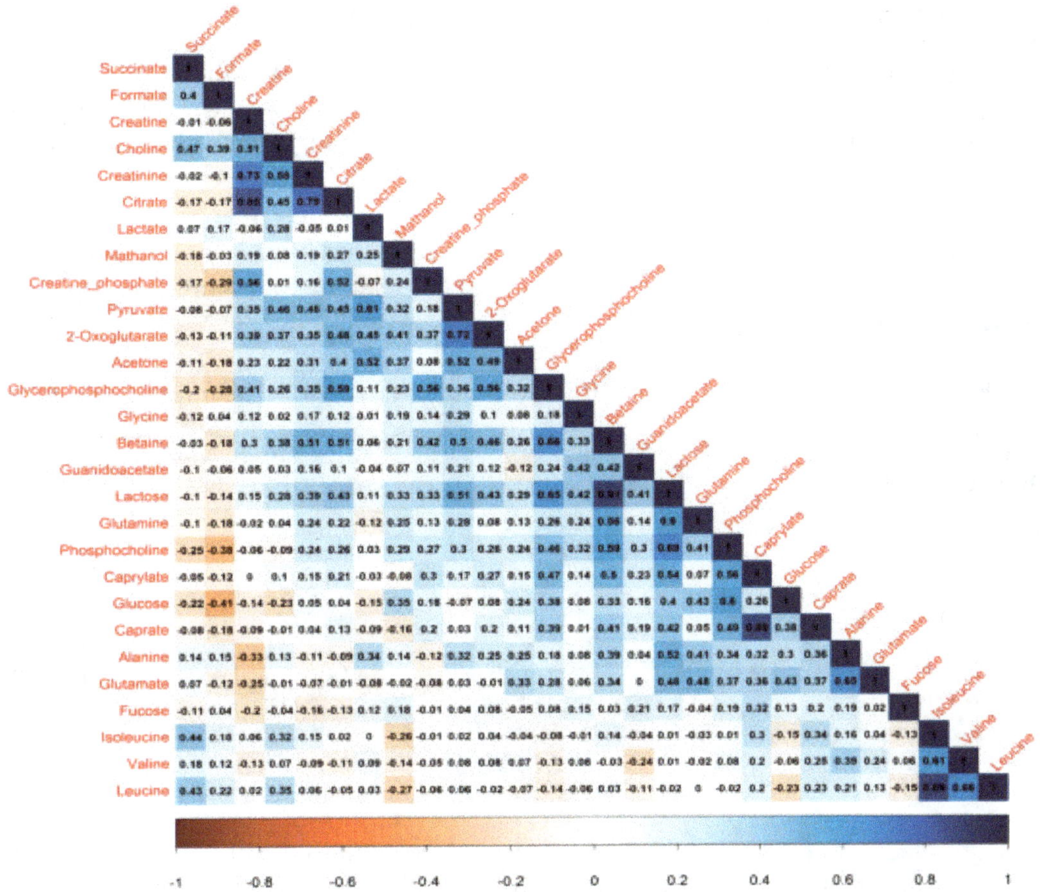

Figure 3. Correlation plot of 28 human milk metabolites from non-atopic mothers. Values shows Pearson correlation coefficients between pairs of metabolites. Positive correlation, zero correlation and negative correlation are represented by colors ranging from blue to white to red, respectively.

3.4. Milk Metabolite Clusters by Race/Ethnicity

Metabolite variation by ethnicity in the PLS plots was similar to country differences, showing three clusters of milk composition: Black, Caucasian and Asian (Figure 4). Milk lactate differentiated the Asian population from the rest. 2-Oxoglutarate and creatine were the main drivers of the milk cluster in the Black population, whereas the main milk metabolites in the Caucasian cluster were glutamate, glutamine, glucose, and phosphocholine.

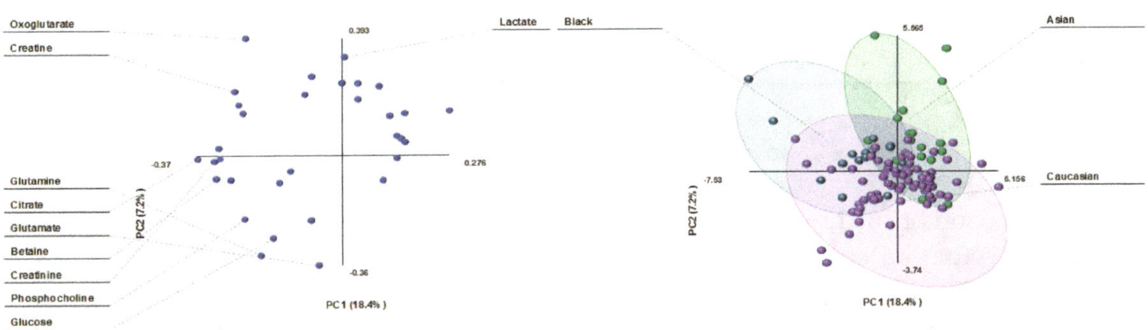

Figure 4. PLS-DA loading plot (**left**) and scatterplot (**right**) of human milk metabolites from women of different ethnic groups. The score plot shows separation based on maternal ethnicity (purple: Caucasian; green: Asian; and dark green: Black). The loading plot shows the milk metabolites that influence the separation based on maternal ethnicity.

3.5. Milk Metabolite Variation by Ethnicity in Healthy, Non-Atopic Women

2-Oxoglutarate (p = 0.008) and creatine (p = 0.02)/creatine phosphate (p = 0.008)/creatinine (p = 0.03), as well as betaine (p = 0.01) and glycerophosphocholine (p = 0.009) concentrations were higher in the milk of Black compared to Caucasian women (Table 2). Although lactose levels were also higher, this difference did not reach statistical significance (p = 0.07). In contrast, milk valine levels were lower in Black than in Caucasian women. In essence, these results compare mixed-race South African to Caucasian women, because only one US Black-race woman was a member of the Black race group. Compared to that of Asian women, the milk of Caucasians had significantly lower levels of lactate (p = 0.03) and fucose (p = 0.03).

Table 2. Comparison of milk metabolite concentrations (µmol/L) by maternal ethnicity.

MEAN (SD) Metabolites/Countries	Black	Caucasian	Asian
2-Oxoglutarate	75.4 (31.1)	37.6 (29.2) **	55.3 (47.1)
Acetone	12.9 (5.3)	11.9 (7.4)	14.2 (13.0)
Alanine	164.4 (87.9)	210.6 (82.1)	222.3 (90.9)
Betaine	581.1 (283.6)	204.9 (352.7) *	354.3 (390.1)
Caprate	77.2 (87.8)	109.8 (112.3)	185.1 (168.3)
Caprylate	134.7 (136.2)	118.1 (184.1)	266.9 (375.3)
Choline	285.1 (167.0)	170.2 (154.4)	218.7 (145.5)
Citrate	4892 (3687)	3123 (1833)	2776 (1061)
Creatine	229.4 (326.5)	77.6 (101.1) *	63.2 (28.5) *
Creatine phosphate	54.0 (56.2)	24.1 (13.7) **	35.9 (26.8)
Creatinine	89.7 (68.2)	51.6 (37.0) *	44.2 (15.0) *
Formate	86.5 (79.3)	582.6 (1363)	534.5 (1350)
Fucose	328.0 (376.9)	306.0 (236.6) #	556.4 (391.5)
Glucose	1264 (672.2)	1263 (866.0)	1148 (1083)
Glutamate	1021 (614.5)	1478 (791.6)	1272 (536.3)
Glutamine	252.4 (122.0)	204.7 (310.6)	89.5 (79.2)
Glycine	2646 (1051)	2360 (1307)	2596 (1169)
Guanidoacetate	4405 (1378)	2912 (2538)	4544 (1916)
Isoleucine	17.3 (11.5)	20.5 (18.4)	23.4 (21.8)
Lactate	198.2 (82.2)	339.5 (600.5) #	1918 (4213)
Lactose	178,365 (50,934)	110,060 (86,787)	131,284 (85,509)
Leucine	31.5 (14.8)	52.1 (56.4)	64.0 (87.0)
Methanol	80.4 (15.7)	59.3 (23.6)	71.0 (46.6)
Phosphocholine	584.6 (305.1)	521.9 (304.1)	642.5 (435.6)
Pyruvate	46.5 (25.3)	21.4 (29.6)	47.2 (58.8)
Succinate	36.1 (53.0)	152.7 (446.7)	100.8 (124.4)
Valine	34.6 (12.0)	61.1 (26.2) *	63.9 (40.5)
Glycerophosphocholine	846.4 (424.6)	467.7 (319.9) **	518.9 (327.7)
# metabolite differences with Black race	na	7	2
# metabolite differences with Asian race	3	na	2

* $p < 0.05$, ** $p < 0.01$, when reference = Black; # $p < 0.05$, when reference = Asian; na: not applicable.

4. Discussion

In this comparison of 109 human milk samples from five countries, clustering by country of origin was observed, such that milk metabolites in South African women differed substantially from those in Norwegian and US women, and women in either of the two Australian cohorts. Milk metabolites in Japanese women formed an overlapping cluster between Norway and South Africa. Creatine and 2-oxoglutarate were the milk metabolites mainly responsible for these regional differences; they were also the highest in South African women among the cohort. Differences in these milk metabolites were evident in a comparison of healthy, non-atopic women in all countries studied; lactose milk levels were also the highest in South African women. Since several low molecular weight metabolites levels are tightly controlled in human milk [3], identifying differences between maternal countries of origin are noteworthy. In the pursuant paragraphs, we summarize what is known about these metabolites, highlight other findings, and offer candidate explanations for the higher levels seen in South African women when compared to women living in Australia or the northern hemisphere.

After protein, lactose is the most plentiful component of human milk and often measured to reflect the carbohydrate energy content. Human milk lactose is found to be associated with infant growth in observational and simulation studies [22,23]. Since levels rise during the postpartum period in breastfeeding women [24], lactose has also been labelled as a marker for milk production. In our comparison, all human milk samples were obtained within one month of birth, removing timing of collection as an explanation for differences in milk lactose or other metabolite concentrations. In two to five months old infants, Gridneva et al. documented higher lactose milk levels in Australian women who breastfed more frequently [16]. Their results are congruent with a metabolomics study of sow milk, whereby Tan et al. reported higher milk lactose levels with higher rather than lower lactation performance [25]. Glucose and fucose, other sugars typically found in human milk, did not differ in their levels across country cohorts in our study. Lactose has also been found to have antimicrobial and innate immunity-inducing properties [2,26,27]. Hence, the much greater levels of milk lactose in South African women than in women living in more industrialized societies may reflect a greater breastfeeding frequency, or maternal programming to prevent infection.

Although milk sugars are the main substrates for energy generation and the production of oligosaccharides [28], little is known about these intermediate metabolites of the tricarboxylic acid energy cycle (TCA cycle), such as 2-oxoglutarate, citrate, or succinate. In our study, lactose levels were positively correlated with milk citrate and 2-oxoglutarate. Milk 2-oxoglutarate and citrate levels were also highest in South African women in our comparison; however, no differences were observed in milk succinate concentrations. As shown in a study of US women, the levels of milk 2-oxoglutarate in women feeding term infants typically decline within one month of birth [20]. Of note, lower 2-oxoglutarate levels have been detected in the milk of dairy cows with mastitis (breast duct infection), which is interpreted to be a function of greater consumption of this TCA cycle intermediate by resident microbiota or infecting microbes [3,29]. Mastitis and subclinical mastitis are common infections postpartum in industrialized countries [30], which offers another explanation for 2-oxoglutarate consumption and lower milk concentrations in US, Australian, and Norwegian women. Japanese women had higher milk levels of other energy-related intermediates such as lactate and pyruvate than Norwegian women; not much is known about the milk levels of these metabolites in humans. Compared to non-lactating cows, the TCA and related cycles, including pyruvate metabolism, were found to be most activated in the mammary glands of lactating cows [31]; pyruvate and lactate were among the 118 metabolites shared between the mammary gland and milk.

Lactose is produced by mammary cells, but other low-weight molecules are speculated to diffuse into human milk and serve as indicators of maternal plasma levels [2]. Methanol is found in human milk and can originate from maternal circulation following the consumption of fruits, vegetables, alcohol, and artificial sweeteners, and from exposure to environmental tobacco smoke [32]. Other examples are betaine, a choline metabolite whose levels increase with dietary intake of choline [33]. Consistently, milk betaine and the phosphocholines were positively correlated in our study. We also found milk methanol to be lowest in Norwegian women, whereas betaine levels were lowered in Australian milk. Milk creatinine (derived from creatine, an energy metabolite) levels are also related to circulating blood levels [34]; urinary creatinine also reportedly rises postpartum during breastfeeding [24]. In lactating cows, creatine and lactose are the two metabolites found in the stomach, serum, milk, and urine, denoting their importance in the lactation process [31]. Of note, betaine is an osmolytic and its supplementation can increase milk yield in cows [35]. Together with the higher levels of milk lactose and betaine, elevated levels of milk creatine or its metabolite, creatinine, may indicate higher milk production in South African women.

In Tan et al.'s study of sow milk [25], glutamate and glutamine were additional markers of high milk production. Glutamate is produced when 2-oxoglutarate combines with glutamine. Glutamine and glutamate are the most abundant amino acids in human milk, increasing with each stage of lactation, and are largely derived during lactation from muscle protein breakdown of glutamine [21,36]. Higher levels of the amino acid valine have also been found to be associated with higher bovine milk yield [37]. It is then noteworthy that glutamate was the metabolite which distinguished US human milk composition from that of Norwegian and Japanese women. Milk glutamine levels were significantly lower in Norwegian and Japanese than in US women, which is consistent with the general observation that glutamine levels are higher in North America than in Asia [21]. Both glutamine and glutamate are important energy sources for intestinal cells and are needed for infant growth. When Dangat et al. compared healthy women in India to women with maternal conditions such as pre-eclampsia, which are associated with growth retardation in offspring, they found healthy women to have higher glutamine and glutamate levels in their milk, as well as higher lactose concentrations [38].

Ethnic differences between the same milk metabolome of mixed Black and Caucasian women were consistent with the country variation we observed, and further indicated a similarity among Caucasian women in Norway, Australia, and the US, potentially in terms of breastfeeding practices and/or maternal diet, health status, or genetics. Maternal diet has a reported influence on some human milk constituents, such as fatty acids, vitamins, and minerals; maternal intake of carbohydrates or fat is unrelated to milk lactose levels, but little is known about other low molecular weight substrates [13]. Since several low molecular metabolites detected in milk can be consumed or produced by resident microbiota, ethnic differences in these milk metabolites may also be a function of variation in human milk microbiota. As shown by Kumar et al., human milk microbial composition can vary according to the degree of societal industrialization, whereby the abundance of Proteobacteria is observed to be higher in milk samples of South African women [4]. In this regard, human milk lactose levels have been reported by others to vary inversely with milk Enterobacteria [26]. Further, maternal intake of lactose has been inversely correlated with milk concentrations within the Firmicutes phylum [39]. Unfortunately, data on maternal diet was not collected at the time that human milk samples were obtained in our study. Additionally, no women of Asian ethnicity were present in the Australian or US cohorts, and too few non-atopic women of Black race were recruited in the US cohort to speculate on genetic versus environmental origins of the milk metabolite variation.

The strengths of this international comparative study are that all human milk samples were selected at the same stage of lactation with similar maternal characteristics, and processed with NMR spectroscopy in one center. As has been reported for other milk constituents [40], despite not following an identical protocol for milk collection, the individual country samples were similar across several milk metabolites whose levels have been reported to be tightly controlled [20].

5. Conclusions

Human milk composition is optimal for infant growth and development. As we and others seek to determine how societal factors impact on the infant gut microbiome, immune development and subsequent health, understanding population differences in early nutrition is essential. This present work should be considered a first step in helping to frame breastfeeding/microbiome studies in a global context. It reminds us that regional maternal diet and breastfeeding practices have the capacity to influence milk composition. In addition to trying to understand this variation, we must also leverage study findings to inform policy, especially in times of change. In our study, the milk composition of South African women had higher levels of lactose, creatine and energy metabolites. How will South African infants fare against the rising trends of not being fed colostrum, receiving short exclusive breastfeeding and being introduced to solids at an early stage [41] in a country historically known for lower infant growth failure rates than it neighbors [42]? Understanding people and their place and purpose on this planet is essential to understanding the complexity we face in harnessing the health of the microbiome.

Author Contributions: Formal analysis, M.C.L.G.; Funding acquisition, E.d.T., M.E., C.C.J., G.W., N.S., D.E.C., S.L.P., D.M., D.T.G., and A.L.K.; Investigation, P.T.K.; Supervision, E.d.T., M.E., C.C.J., G.W., N.S., D.E.C., S.L.P., D.M., D.T.G., and A.L.K.; Visualization, M.C.L.G.; Writing—review & editing, M.C.L.G., P.T.K., C.M.S., E.d.T., M.E., C.C.J., G.W., N.S., D.E.C., S.L.P., D.M., D.T.G., and A.L.K.

Acknowledgments: We are grateful to the mothers who provided their valuable data in the individual study cohorts and the research assistants who collected it. We would also like to acknowledge the contributions of Sarah Bridgman and Jennifer Petrie in formatting the manuscript. inVIVO LactoActive study investigators: Anita L. Kozyrskyj (lead), University of Alberta; Dianne E. Campbell, Children's Hospital at Westmead & University of Sydney; Cecilie Dahl, Norwegian Institute of Public Health; Elloise du Toit, University of Cape Town; Merete Eggesbo, Norwegian Institute of Public Health; Melvin C. L. Gay, University of Western Australia; Donna T. Geddes, University of Western Australia; Aveni Haynes, University of Western Australia; Peter Hsu, Children's Hospital at Westmead & University of Sydney; Petya T. Koleva, University of Alberta; Christine C. Johnson, Henry Ford Hospital; Charles Mackay, Monash University; Daniel Munblit, Imperial College London & Sechenov University; John Penders, Maastricht University; Harald Renz, University of Marburg; Susan L. Prescott, Perth Children's Hospital & University of Western Australia; Naoki Shimojo, Chiba University; Carolyn M. Slupsky, University of California Davis; Carel Thijs, Maastricht University; Ganesa Wegienka, Henry Ford Hospital; Christina West, Umea University.

References

1. Hennet, T.; Borsig, L. Breastfed at tiffany's. *Trends Biochem. Sci.* **2016**, *41*, 508–518. [CrossRef] [PubMed]
2. Demmelmair, H.; Koletzko, B. Variation of metabolite and hormone contents in human milk. *Clin. Perinatol.* **2017**, *44*, 151–164. [CrossRef] [PubMed]
3. Smilowitz, J.T.; O'Sullivan, A.; Barile, D.; German, J.B.; Lonnerdal, B.; Slupsky, C.M. The human milk metabolome reveals diverse oligosaccharide profiles. *J. Nutr.* **2013**, *143*, 1709–1718. [CrossRef] [PubMed]
4. Kumar, H.; du Toit, E.; Kulkarni, A.; Aakko, J.; Linderborg, K.M.; Zhang, Y.; Nicol, M.P.; Isolauri, E.; Yang, B.; Collado, M.C.; et al. Distinct patterns in human milk microbiota and fatty acid profiles across specific geographic locations. *Front. Microbiol.* **2016**, *7*, 1619. [CrossRef] [PubMed]
5. Fu, Y.; Liu, X.; Zhou, B.; Jiang, A.C.; Chai, L. An updated review of worldwide levels of docosahexaenoic and arachidonic acid in human breast milk by region. *Public Health Nutr.* **2016**, *19*, 2675–2687. [CrossRef] [PubMed]
6. Victora, C.G.; Adair, L.; Fall, C.; Hallal, P.C.; Martorell, R.; Richter, L.; Sachdev, H.S. Maternal and child undernutrition: Consequences for adult health and human capital. *Lancet* **2008**, *371*, 340–357. [CrossRef]
7. Adair, L.S.; Fall, C.H.; Osmond, C.; Stein, A.D.; Martorell, R.; Ramirez-Zea, M.; Sachdev, H.S.; Dahly, D.L.; Bas, I.; Norris, S.A.; et al. Associations of linear growth and relative weight gain during early life with adult health and human capital in countries of low and middle income: Findings from five birth cohort studies. *Lancet* **2013**, *382*, 525–534. [CrossRef]
8. Garza, C.; Borghi, E.; Onyango, A.W.; de Onis, M. Parental height and child growth from birth to 2 years in the WHO multicentre growth reference study. *Matern. Child Nutr.* **2013**, *9*, 58–68. [CrossRef] [PubMed]
9. Victora, C.G.; Bahl, R.; Barros, A.J.; Franca, G.V.; Horton, S.; Krasevec, J.; Murch, S.; Sankar, M.J.; Walker, N.; Rollins, N.C. Breastfeeding in the 21st century: Epidemiology, mechanisms, and lifelong effect. *Lancet* **2016**, *387*, 475–490. [CrossRef]
10. Munblit, D.; Peroni, D.G.; Boix-Amoros, A.; Hsu, P.S.; Van't Land, B.; Gay, M.C.L.; Kolotilina, A.; Skevaki, C.; Boyle, R.J.; Collado, M.C.; et al. Human milk and allergic diseases: An unsolved puzzle. *Nutrients* **2017**, *9*, 894. [CrossRef] [PubMed]
11. Davis, J.C.; Totten, S.M.; Huang, J.O.; Nagshbandi, S.; Kirmiz, N.; Garrido, D.A.; Lewis, Z.T.; Wu, L.D.; Smilowitz, J.T.; German, J.B.; et al. Identification of oligosaccharides in feces of breast-fed infants and their correlation with the gut microbial community. *Mol. Cell Proteomics* **2016**, *15*, 2987–3002. [CrossRef] [PubMed]
12. Koleva, P.T.; Bridgman, S.L.; Kozyrskyj, A.L. The infant gut microbiome: Evidence for obesity risk and dietary intervention. *Nutrients* **2015**, *7*, 2237–2260. [CrossRef] [PubMed]
13. Bravi, F.; Wiens, F.; Decarli, A.; Dal Pont, A.; Agostoni, C.; Ferraroni, M. Impact of maternal nutrition on breast-milk composition: A systematic review. *Am. J. Clin. Nutr.* **2016**, *104*, 646–662. [CrossRef] [PubMed]
14. Wahlqvist, M.L. Lactose nutrition in lactase nonpersisters. *Asia Pac. J. Clin. Nutr.* **2015**, *24*, S21–S25. [PubMed]

15. Taylor, A.L.; Dunstan, J.A.; Prescott, S.L. Probiotic supplementation for the first 6 months of life fails to reduce the risk of atopic dermatitis and increases the risk of allergen sensitization in high-risk children: A randomized controlled trial. *J. Allergy Clin. Immunol.* **2007**, *119*, 184–191. [CrossRef] [PubMed]
16. Gridneva, Z.; Kugananthan, S.; Hepworth, A.R.; Tie, W.J.; Lai, C.T.; Ward, L.C.; Hartmann, P.E.; Geddes, D.T. Effect of human milk appetite hormones, macronutrients, and infant characteristics on gastric emptying and breastfeeding patterns of term fully breastfed infants. *Nutrients* **2016**, *9*, 15. [CrossRef] [PubMed]
17. Wegienka, G.; Havstad, S.; Joseph, C.L.; Zoratti, E.; Ownby, D.; Woodcroft, K.; Johnson, C.C. Racial disparities in allergic outcomes in african americans emerge as early as age 2 years. *Clin. Exp. Allergy* **2012**, *42*, 909–917. [CrossRef] [PubMed]
18. Eggesbo, M.; Thomsen, C.; Jorgensen, J.V.; Becher, G.; Odland, J.O.; Longnecker, M.P. Associations between brominated flame retardants in human milk and thyroid-stimulating hormone (TSH) in neonates. *Environ. Res.* **2011**, *111*, 737–743. [CrossRef] [PubMed]
19. Package "Corrplot". Available online: https://cran.r-project.org/web/packages/corrplot/corrplot.pdf. (accessed on 23 August 2018).
20. Spevacek, A.R.; Smilowitz, J.T.; Chin, E.L.; Underwood, M.A.; German, J.B.; Slupsky, C.M. Infant maturity at birth reveals minor differences in the maternal milk metabolome in the first month of lactation. *J. Nutr.* **2015**, *145*, 1698–1708. [CrossRef] [PubMed]
21. Zhang, Z.; Adelman, A.S.; Rai, D.; Boettcher, J.; Lonnerdal, B. Amino acid profiles in term and preterm human milk through lactation: A systematic review. *Nutrients* **2013**, *5*, 4800–4821. [CrossRef] [PubMed]
22. Prentice, P.; Ong, K.K.; Schoemaker, M.H.; van Tol, E.A.; Vervoort, J.; Hughes, I.A.; Acerini, C.L.; Dunger, D.B. Breast milk nutrient content and infancy growth. *Acta Paediatr.* **2016**, *105*, 641–647. [CrossRef] [PubMed]
23. Nilsson, A.; Mardinoglu, A.; Nielsen, J. Predicting growth of the healthy infant using a genome scale metabolic model. *NPJ Syst. Biol. Appl.* **2017**, *3*, 3. [CrossRef] [PubMed]
24. Sachse, D.; Baerug, A.; Sletner, L.; Birkeland, K.I.; Nakstad, B.; Jenum, A.K.; Berg, J.P. Urine nmr metabolomics analysis of breastfeeding biomarkers during and after pregnancy in a large prospective cohort study. *Scand. J. Clin. Lab. Investig.* **2014**, *74*, 264–272. [CrossRef] [PubMed]
25. Tan, C.; Zhai, Z.; Ni, X.; Wang, H.; Ji, Y.; Tang, T.; Ren, W.; Long, H.; Deng, B.; Deng, J.; et al. Metabolomic profiles reveal potential factors that correlate with lactation performance in sow milk. *Sci. Rep.* **2018**, *8*, 10712. [CrossRef] [PubMed]
26. Boix-Amoros, A.; Collado, M.C.; Mira, A. Relationship between milk microbiota, bacterial load, macronutrients, and human cells during lactation. *Front. Microbiol.* **2016**, *7*, 492. [CrossRef] [PubMed]
27. Cederlund, A.; Kai-Larsen, Y.; Printz, G.; Yoshio, H.; Alvelius, G.; Lagercrantz, H.; Stromberg, R.; Jornvall, H.; Gudmundsson, G.H.; Agerberth, B. Lactose in human breast milk an inducer of innate immunity with implications for a role in intestinal homeostasis. *PLoS ONE* **2013**, *8*, e53876. [CrossRef] [PubMed]
28. Cocinero, E.J.; Carcabal, P. Carbohydrates. *Top. Curr. Chem.* **2015**, *364*, 299–333. [PubMed]
29. Xi, X.; Kwok, L.Y.; Wang, Y.; Ma, C.; Mi, Z.; Zhang, H. Ultra-performance liquid chromatography-quadrupole-time of flight mass spectrometry ms(e)-based untargeted milk metabolomics in dairy cows with subclinical or clinical mastitis. *J. Dairy Sci.* **2017**, *100*, 4884–4896. [CrossRef] [PubMed]
30. Axelsson, D.; Blomberg, M. Prevalence of postpartum infections: A population-based observational study. *Acta. Obstet. Gynecol. Scand.* **2014**, *93*, 1065–1068. [CrossRef] [PubMed]
31. Sun, H.Z.; Shi, K.; Wu, X.H.; Xue, M.Y.; Wei, Z.H.; Liu, J.X.; Liu, H.Y. Lactation-related metabolic mechanism investigated based on mammary gland metabolomics and 4 biofluids' metabolomics relationships in dairy cows. *BMC Genom.* **2017**, *18*, 936. [CrossRef] [PubMed]
32. Dorokhov, Y.L.; Shindyapina, A.V.; Sheshukova, E.V.; Komarova, T.V. Metabolic methanol: Molecular pathways and physiological roles. *Physiol. Rev.* **2015**, *95*, 603–644. [CrossRef] [PubMed]
33. Fischer, L.M.; da Costa, K.A.; Galanko, J.; Sha, W.; Stephenson, B.; Vick, J.; Zeisel, S.H. Choline intake and genetic polymorphisms influence choline metabolite concentrations in human breast milk and plasma. *Am. J. Clin. Nutr.* **2010**, *92*, 336–346. [CrossRef] [PubMed]
34. Balzer, M.S.; Gross, M.M.; Lichtinghagen, R.; Haller, H.; Schmitt, R. Got milk? Breastfeeding and milk analysis of a mother on chronic hemodialysis. *PLoS ONE* **2015**, *10*, e0143340. [CrossRef] [PubMed]
35. Peterson, S.E.; Rezamand, P.; Williams, J.E.; Price, W.; Chahine, M.; McGuire, M.A. Effects of dietary betaine on milk yield and milk composition of mid-lactation holstein dairy cows. *J. Dairy Sci.* **2012**, *95*, 6557–6562. [CrossRef] [PubMed]

36. Manso, H.E.; Filho, H.C.; de Carvalho, L.E.; Kutschenko, M.; Nogueira, E.T.; Watford, M. Glutamine and glutamate supplementation raise milk glutamine concentrations in lactating gilts. *J. Anim. Sci. Biotechnol.* **2012**, *3*, 2. [CrossRef] [PubMed]
37. Wu, X.; Sun, H.; Xue, M.; Wang, D.; Guan, L.L.; Liu, J. Serum metabolome profiling revealed potential biomarkers for milk protein yield in dairy cows. *J. Proteomics* **2018**, *184*, 54–61. [CrossRef] [PubMed]
38. Dangat, K.; Upadhyay, D.; Kilari, A.; Sharma, U.; Kemse, N.; Mehendale, S.; Lalwani, S.; Wagh, G.; Joshi, S.; Jagannathan, N.R. Altered breast milk components in preeclampsia; an in-vitro proton nmr spectroscopy study. *Clin. Chim. Acta* **2016**, *463*, 75–83. [CrossRef] [PubMed]
39. Williams, J.E.; Carrothers, J.M.; Lackey, K.A.; Beatty, N.F.; York, M.A.; Brooker, S.L.; Shafii, B.; Price, W.J.; Settles, M.L.; McGuire, M.A.; et al. Human milk microbial community structure is relatively stable and related to variations in macronutrient and micronutrient intakes in healthy lactating women. *J. Nutr.* **2017**, *147*, 1739–1748. [PubMed]
40. Munblit, D.; Treneva, M.; Peroni, D.G.; Colicino, S.; Chow, L.; Dissanayeke, S.; Abrol, P.; Sheth, S.; Pampura, A.; Boner, A.L.; et al. Colostrum and mature human milk of women from London, Moscow, and Verona: Determinants of immune composition. *Nutrients* **2016**, *8*, e695. [CrossRef] [PubMed]
41. Budree, S.; Goddard, E.; Brittain, K.; Cader, S.; Myer, L.; Zar, H.J. Infant feeding practices in a south African birth cohort-a longitudinal study. *Matern. Child Nutr.* **2017**, *13*, 13. [CrossRef] [PubMed]
42. Osgood-Zimmerman, A.; Millear, A.I.; Stubbs, R.W.; Shields, C.; Pickering, B.V.; Earl, L.; Graetz, N.; Kinyoki, D.K.; Ray, S.E.; Bhatt, S.; et al. Mapping child growth failure in Africa between 2000 and 2015. *Nature* **2018**, *555*, 41–47. [CrossRef] [PubMed]

6

Hormones in Breast Milk and Effect on Infants' Growth

Alessandra Mazzocchi [1], Maria Lorella Giannì [1,2], Daniela Morniroli [1,2], Ludovica Leone [1], Paola Roggero [1,2], Carlo Agostoni [1,3,*], Valentina De Cosmi [3] and Fabio Mosca [1,2]

1 Department of Clinical Sciences and Community Health, University of Milan, 20122 Milan, Italy
2 Fondazione IRCCS Ca' Granda Ospedale Maggiore Policlinico, NICU, 20122 Milan, Italy
3 Fondazione IRCCS Ca' Granda Ospedale Maggiore Policlinico, Pediatric Intermediate Care Unit, 20122 Milan, Italy
* Correspondence: carlo.agostoni@unimi.it

Abstract: Breast milk is characterized by a dynamic and complex composition which includes hormones and other bioactive components that could influence infant growth, development, and optimize health. Among the several beneficial effects associated with prolonged breastfeeding, a 13% decrease in the risk of overweight and obesity has been reported. Recent research has focused on breast milk hormones contributing to the appetite and energy balance regulation and adiposity. Accordingly, we conducted a literature systematic review with the aim to provide an update on the effect of leptin, ghrelin, Insulin Growth Factor 1, adiponectin, and insulin on infants' and children's growth and body composition. The revised literature reveals contrasting findings concerning the potential role of all these hormones on modeling growth and fat mass apposition and health outcomes later in life. Further studies are needed to gain further insight into the specific role of these bioactive components in metabolic pathways related to body composition. This could help gain a further insight on infants' growth, both in physiological and pathological settings.

Keywords: hormones; adipokines; breast milk; growth; body composition; term infant

1. Introduction

Breast milk (BM) is the only species-specific human food tailored to meet infants' needs through the adaptation of its micro and macronutrient content and bioactive components, depending upon the mother–infant dyad characteristics (i.e., gestational age at birth, birth weight, etc.) [1,2].

Furthermore, the dynamic composition of BM also allows mother–infant signaling over lactation [3,4]. As a result, the infant is guided in the developmental and physiological processes through breastfeeding, whose crucial role in promoting healthy growth and optimal cognitive development is widely acknowledged [2,5]. Breastfeeding is beneficial through an epigenetic effect that is demonstrated to be dose-dependent [6]. However, although our understanding of the bioactive, non-nutritional compounds of BM and their dynamic changes over time has improved, the complexity of BM composition and the synergistic mechanisms responsible for its life-long biological effects have not yet been unraveled [7]. Among the several beneficial health effects associated with prolonged breastfeeding, a 13% decrease in the risk of overweight and obesity development has been reported [8]. In light of the well-known different growth trajectory and body composition development that characterize breastfed infants in comparison to formula-fed ones [9,10], gaining further insight into the factors that contribute to infants' appetite regulation and metabolic programming in the long run is, therefore, crucial for developing adequate strategies aimed at obesity prevention [11,12]. Accordingly, recent research has focused on BM hormones involved in the regulation of appetite and energy balance and adiposity, with the aim of identifying the factors that modulate their concentration throughout lactation and elucidating their potential biological relevance within this context [13,14]. We conducted a literature review with the aim of providing an update on the effects of BM leptin, ghrelin, Insulin Growth Factor 1 (IGF-1), adiponectin, and insulin found within BM on infants' and children's growth and body composition.

2. Methods

We performed a review using PUBMED, searching for all trails published in English from 2009 up to July 2019. The following key words were used: "Leptin" OR "Ghrelin" OR "IGF-1" OR "Adiponectin" OR "Insulin" OR "Adipokines" AND "BM" OR "donor milk" OR "banked milk" AND "weight gain" OR "body composition" OR "obesity" OR "adiposity" OR "growth" AND "infant" OR "children". In this review, observational studies examining the effects of these BM hormones on infants' and children's anthropometry and growth were selected. A total of 344 articles were initially identified and, among them, 30 studies were retrieved and evaluated for inclusion as relevant studies for the analysis by reviewing the abstract, and, when necessary, the full text. A manual bibliographic cross-referencing was also performed. We also reviewed the reference lists of relevant studies in order to detect other relevant primary sources.

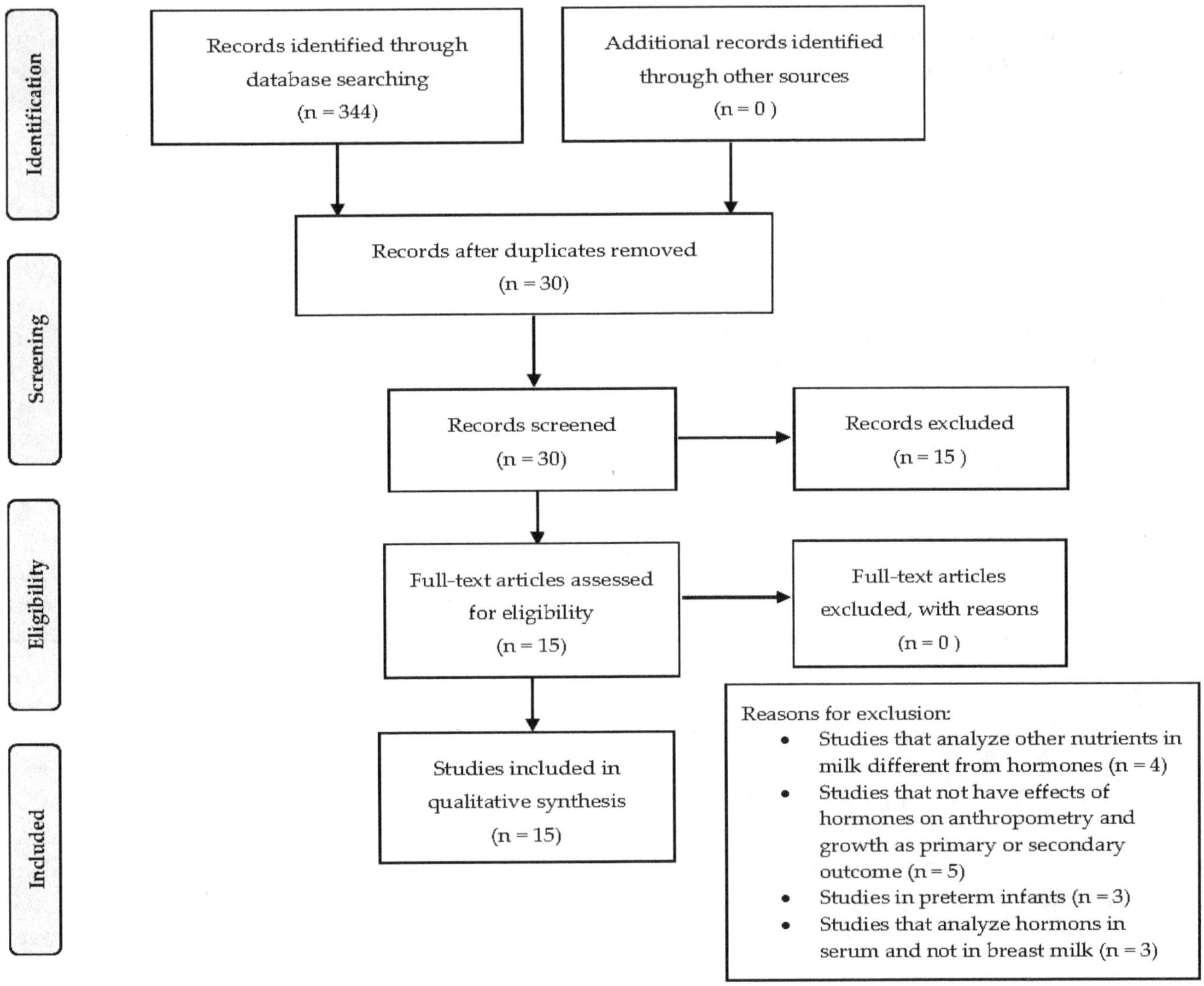

Figure 1. PRISMA diagram of search strategy.

Articles were considered as relevant and included in the analysis if (a) they reported the effect of milk hormones on infant growth; (b) included weight gain, body composition, obesity, adiposity as outcome measures; and (c) enrolled human participants. The selection procedure used for identifying and including the studies is summarized in Figure 1. Finally, we included 15 observational studies for the review. Three researchers independently searched, screened, and identified studies and abstracted and tabulated data. Discrepancies were addressed and sorted out by discussion.

3. Results

Young et al. [15] performed a prospective study of 41 healthy, term, breastfed infants, with the aim of assessing components in BM that are related with infant growth and may affect fat-free mass (FFM) or fat mass (FM) deposition thorughout the first four months of life. A significant association between the trajectory of weight for length Z-scores (WLZ) and BM insulin was detected. However, the effect differed by maternal body mass index (BMI), being the association negative among infants of normal weight mothers. In the multivariable model, mean BM insulin quintiles were significantly associated with infant fat gain rate, suggesting the role of this hormone in regulating fat-mass accretion. On the contrary, an inverse association among BM adiponectin content and rate of fat gain was found.

Kon et al. [16] assessed 103 mother–infant pairs during the first three months of lactation and reported higher BM concentration of IGF-1 in the mothers of infants with high weight gain than in the mothers of those with low and normal weight gain at all study points. BM leptin and ghrelin content tended to show a similar behavior at two and three months of lactation and at one and two months of lactation, respectively. These results suggest that both leptin and ghrelin contribute to infants' weight gain. On the contrary, in another prospective study, Yis et al. [17] found that neither BM ghrelin nor BM leptin was correlated with anthropometric data in breastfed infants. They only observed positive correlations when they analyzed hormones sampled in infants' serum, in particular between ghrelin and triceps skinfold thickness (TSF), and leptin and weight, TSF and weight gain at three months of age. Gridneva and colleagues [18] showed a different effect of BM leptin and adiponectin content on infant FFM and FM deposition through the first 12 months of life: Specifically, they saw an inverse association between the daily intake of adiponectin and the infant fat-free mass but a positive relationship with infant fat mass. At one year, higher intake of BM leptin was associated with higher fat mass deposition. Interestingly, contrasting data were found in this study by Fields et al. [19], where authors observed that milk leptin concentration reduces through lactation and it was higher in obese mothers; furthermore, this hormone shows a negative association with infant length, FM percentage, total FM, and trunk fat at six months of age. In a previous pilot study on 19 exclusively breastfeeding mother–infant dyads [20], Fields observed that greater BM leptin was associated with lower BMI-for-age z-score (BMIZ), and higher content of BM insulin was associated with lower infant weight, BMIZ, and FFM. All these results concerning leptin suggest that this hormone may have a role both with regard to FM and FFM deposition. The relationship between BM adiponectin, leptin, and insulin with infant body composition was assessed in 430 mother–infant dyads taking part into the Canadian Healthy Infant Longitudinal Development (CHILD) Study [21]. Data showed an inverse correlation between BM leptin and insulin content and infant WLZ and BMIZ at four months of age, whereas no significant association was found between BM adiponectin concentrations and infant body composition. Meyer et al. [22] longitudinally investigated the correlation among BM leptin and adiponectin with body composition in children aged three to five years. The authors previously reported a positive association between BM adiponectin concentration and FM and weight gain in infants in the first two years of age. However, the findings of this analysis failed to demonstrate a significant relationship of BM leptin and adiponectin levels, assessed at six weeks and four months after delivery, with later body composition characteristics. Brunner and colleagues [23] investigated the association of leptin and adiponectin in BM with infant weight gain and body composition using skinfold thickness assessment in the first 24 months of life. Although BM leptin assessed at four months was negatively associated with concurrent infant weight, BMI, and FFM, no relationship with infant growth and body composition at later ages was reported. On the contrary, there was a tendency for BM adiponectin to be negatively associated with infant growth parameters in the first four months of age, but afterwards, it was positively associated with infant weight gain and FM up to the first 24 months of life. Mohamad et al. [24], assessed the relationship of maternal serum and BM adipokines with infant adiposity development. A higher BM adiponectin concentration at two months after delivery was associated with reduced infant body weight, BMIZ, and abdominal circumference at two months of age. After adjusting for confounders, BM adiponectin at two months postpartum was the only factor that remained independently associated with infant adiposity at two months of age. This result indicates that BM adiponectin may be protective on infant adiposity development in the early postnatal period. Cesur et al. [25] investigated the relationship between ghrelin and adiponectin content in BM and serum samples of 25 mother–infant pairs with the anthropometry of newborn infants at one and four months of life. BM ghrelin content was significantly higher than the infant and maternal serum ghrelin at both study points. Moreover, the level of the fourth month BM ghrelin level positively correlated with infants' weight gain throughout the study. Larsson et al. [26] aimed to identify the determinants of early growth by comparing two groups of exclusively breastfed infants, one with excessive weight gain and the second one with a normal growth pattern during the first five months. The lack of difference in the BM intake at the age of five months between the groups suggests that the high weight gain could be driven by factors related to milk composition. Accordingly, the leptin content was significantly decreased in the BM of the group characterized by high weight gain, thus stimulating appetite and milk intake in this group of infants. Anyhow, it has to be considered that, in this study, measurement of BM was carried out only at five months of age and not earlier, when growth velocity was considerably higher. Ucar and colleagues [27] investigated whether leptin may exert an effect on satiety by comparing the formilk and hindmilk leptin concentrations in 18 lactating women. However, no differences were found between the leptin levels of BM samples assessed during the two different phases of feeding at breast. Additionally, no association between leptin concentrations in both BM and maternal plasma and infants' body weight, BMI, TSF, and left upper arm circumference measurements was found. Concerning the role of adiponectin in BM, a longitudinal observational study of two cohorts of 45 mother–infant pairs was carried out to determine an association between milk adiponectin and infant growth. No significant difference was detected among the two cohorts at the beginning of the study. However, higher BM adiponectin was associated, through the first six months, with lower infant adiposity—in particular, with weight-for-age z-score (WAZ) and WLZ, but not length for age z-score (LAZ), after adjusting for confounders and irrespective of the cohort [28]. Similarly, a negative association between adiponectin and infant growth (i.e., weight-for-height z-score (WHZ) and head circumference) in two cohorts of infants from 48 healthy mothers and from 48 mothers with gestational diabetes mellitus was found [12]. No associations between BM insulin, leptin, and ghrelin concentrations and infant WHZ and head circumference resulted [12]. In Table 1 the main findings of the studies meeting the inclusion criteria are shown.

Table 1. Observational studies on hormones' dosage in breast milk and infants' growth and anthropometry.

Study	Sample Size	Growth and Anthropometric Outcomes	Hormones in Breast Milk	Major Findings
[12]	96 BF infants	Infant body weight (kg), length (cm), WLZ, head circumference (cm).	Adiponectin, leptin, insulin and ghrelin	Adiponectin inversely associated with WLZ and head circumference ($p \leq 0.003$). Association between adiponectin and insulin and head circumference ($p \leq 0.007$ and $p \leq 0.049$, respectively).
[15]	41 BF infants	WLZ, % body fat from skinfolds from 0 to 4 mo.	Leptin, adiponectin, ghrelin, insulin	Negative association between HM insulin and WLZ trajectory in infants of normal weight mothers ($p = 0.028$)
[16]	103 BF infants	Weight gain (g/mo).	Leptin, adiponectin, ghrelin, IGF-1	Correlation between breast milk IGF-1 and infant weight gain (r = 0.294, $p = 0.043$). Higher ghrelin levels at 1 and 2 mo and higher leptin levels at 2 and 3 mo of lactation ($p < 0.05$) in infants with high weight gain (>1000 g/mo).
[17]	24 BF infants	Infant's body weight (g), length (cm), triceps skinfold thickness (mm), postnatal weight gain (g) at 3 and 6 mo of age.	Ghrelin, leptin	No correlation between breast-milk ghrelin or breast-milk leptin with anthropometric data.
[18]	20 BF infants	Infant's body weight (g), length (cm), BMI (kg/m^2), ultrasound skinfolds, bioimpedance spectroscopy and FMI (FM (kg)/length (m)^2), FFMI (FFM (kg)/length (m)^2).	Adiponectin, leptin	Higher intake of adiponectin associated with lower infant FFM ($p = 0.005$) and FFM index ($p = 0.009$) and higher FM ($p < 0.001$), FM index (FMI; $p < 0.001$), and %FM ($p < 0.001$). Higher intake of leptin associated with larger increases in infant adiposity (2–12 month): FM, $p = 0.0006$; %FM, $p = 0.0004$.
[19]	37 BF infants	Infant's body weight (g), length (cm), FM (g and %), FFM (g), trunk fat mass (g).	Insulin, leptin	Inverse association between leptin levels at 1 mo and infant length ($p = 0.0257$), FM % ($p = 0.0223$), FM (g) ($p = 0.0226$), and trunk fat mass ($p = 0.0111$) at 6 mo.

Table 1. *Cont.*

Study	Sample Size	Growth and Anthropometric Outcomes	Hormones in Breast Milk	Major Findings
[20]	19 BF infants	Infant's body weight (g), length (cm), WLZ, BMIZ, FM (g and %), FFM (g), trunk fat mass (g) at 1 mo of age	Leptin, insulin	Leptin associated with lower BMIZ (r = −0.54, $p = 0.03$). Higher concentrations of insulin associated with lower infant weight, relative weight, and FFM (r = −0.49–0.58, $p < 0.06$).
[21]	430 BF infants	Infant's body weight (g), length (cm), WFL, BMIZ at 4 mo and 1 yrs of age.	Adiponectin, leptin, insulin	Higher leptin associated with lower infant WLZ at 4 mo (β − 0.67, 95% confidence interval (CI): −1.17, −0.17 for highest vs lowest quintile) and 1 yrs (β − 0.58, 95% CI: −1.02, −0.14). Insulin showed a U-shaped association, with intermediate concentrations predicting the lowest infant WLZ at 4 mo (β − 0.51, 95% CI: −0.87, −0.15 for third vs lowest quintile) and 1 yrs (β − 0.35, 95% CI: −0.66, −0.04). Adiponectin not associated with infant body composition.
[22]	147 BF infants	Infant's body weight (kg), BMI percentiles, sum of four skinfolds (mm), FM (kg and %), FFM (kg) at 3, 4, and 5 yrs of age.	Adiponectin, leptin	No association between leptin or total adiponectin levels assessed at 6 weeks post-delivery with children's body weight, BMI percentiles, sum of four skinfolds, measurements, FM (kg and %), or FFM (kg).
[23]	188 BF infants	The relationship of BM leptin and adiponectin with infant weight gain and body composition up to the age of 2 yrs.	Adiponectin, leptin	Milk leptin at 4 mo negatively associated with infant weight ([95%CI]: −604.96 g [−1166.19; −43.72], $p = 0.037$) and FFM (−400.95 g [−777.64; −24.25], $p = 0.039$) at the age of 4 mo. Adiponectin tended to be negatively associated with infant FFM ($p = 0.015$) and weight ($p = 0.054$) in the first 4 mo, but afterwards was positively related to weight gain ($p = 0.027$) and the sum of skinfolds ($p = 0.047$) up to 2 years.

Table 1. *Cont.*

Study	Sample Size	Growth and Anthropometric Outcomes	Hormones in Breast Milk	Major Findings
[24]	155 BF infants	Infant's body weight (kg) and BMIZ, abdominal circumference (cm).	Leptin, adiponectin	The higher level of adiponectin at 2 mo postpartum associated with reduced infant body weight ($\beta = -0.54$ $p = 0.003$), BMIZ ($\beta = -0.79$, $p = 0.008$) and abdominal circumference at 2 mo of age ($\beta = -2.34$, $p = 0.003$). No association between adiponectin at birth and 2 mo with infant adiposity at 6 and 12 mo of age. An increased maternal ALR was related to reduced infant BMIZ at birth.
[25]	25 BF infants	Infant's body weight (g), length (cm), BMI (kg/m^2).	Ghrelin, adiponectin	Positive correlation between the level of the 4th mo ghrelin level and infants' weight gain ($r = 0.51$, $p = 0.025$).
[26]	30 BF infants	Infant's body weight (g), length (cm), WAZ, LAZ, BAZ, TSFZ, SSFZ.	Leptin, adiponectin	A 40% reduction of median leptin content at 5 mo in the high weight gain group ($p = 0.045$). At 5 mo, no significant associations between milk concentrations of hormones and infants' WAZ, BAZ or LAZ, or energy and hormones and infant's anthropometry (WAZ, BAZ, or LAZ) or change in these z-scores from birth to the 5 mo visit (all $p > 0.11$).
[27]	18 BF infants	Infant's body weight (kg), BMI (kg/m^2), triceps skinfold thickness (mm), left upper arm circumference (mm).	Leptin	No correlation between Log leptin concentrations and infants' body weight, BMI, triceps skinfold thickness, and left upper arm circumference measurements ($p > 0.05$).
[22]	322 BF infants	Infant's body weight (kg), length (cm), WAZ, BMI (kg/m^2), LAZ, WLZ.	Adiponectin	During the first 6 months, higher adiponectin associated with lower infant WAZ ($\beta = 0.20 \pm$ standard error (SE) 0.04, $p = 0.0001$) and WLZ ($\beta = 0.29 \pm 0.08$, $p = 0.0002$) Adiponectin not associated with infant length.

Mo = months; yrs = years; BF = breastfed; FM = fat mass; FFM = fat-free mass; FMI = FM index; FFMI = FFM index; BMI = body mass index; WAZ = weight for age z-score; WLZ = weight-for-length/height z-score; LAZ = length-for-age z-score; BMIZ = BMI z-score; TSFZ = triceps skinfold-for-age z-score; SSFZ = subscapular skinfold-for-age; ALR = maternal adiponectin to leptin ratio; β = beta regression coefficient.

4. Discussion

In this systematic review, we explored updated evidences on five hormones (leptin, ghrelin, IGF-1, adiponectin, insulin) described in BM that are also related with hunger, fat deposition, and adipose tissue metabolism in all stages of life. Leptin is an hormone synthetized by adipose cells and mucosal cells in the small intestine; it regulates energy homeostasis by interacting with its receptors in the hypothalamus, inhibiting hunger [29]. As a result, fat storage in adipocytes is decreased [30]. In newborns, Chaoimh et al. [31] found a negative relationship between cord leptin content and weight gain, demonstrating that a low weight gain is accompanied by a reduced fat mass deposition in the early postnatal period. Accordingly, BM leptin has been reported to be inversely associated with infant global adiposity and trunk fat at six months of age [19]. Moreover, a higher content of BM leptin was associated with lower WLZ and BMIZ in infants [20,21]. However, this effect appears to be temporary, as indicated by the lack of effect of leptin levels in BM on body composition in the first years of age [22,23]. Interestingly, despite this well-known anti-adiposity effect, BM leptin content has also been positively correlated with higher weight gain in infants in the early postnatal period, and increased adiposity as far as 12 months of lactation [16,18]. Consistently with these results, a possible relationship of BM leptin with body fat stores and infant adiposity has been suggested by Savino and colleagues, who determined leptin values in serum and in the mothers' BM. The authors found positive correlations between BM leptin and infant serum leptin, and between infant serum leptin and both infants' BMI and weight [32]. Yis et al. also found a positive correlation with leptin serum level in infants, but failed to demonstrate a significant correlation with BM leptin levels [17]. These inconstistent results may pose a doubt on BM leptin's hormonal role during lactation, which could differ from what is known to be its primary role in human body, as hypothesized by Ucar and colleagues who failed to demonstrate a role played by leptin BM levels as a satiety factor, and also showed no correlation with infants' weight and adiposity [27]. Opposite to leptin, ghrelin is considered to be the "hunger hormone". It is a neuropetide secreted by specific gastrointestinal cells when the stomach is empty, that acts on the hypothalamus to stimulate appetite, increase gastric acid secretion, and improve gastrointestinal motility [33]. A different relationship between the serum content of hormones involved in satiety and appetite regulation, including ghrelin, has been found by Vásquez-Garibay et al. [34]. Specifically, the authors demonstrated a more significant association in breastfeeding mother–infant pairs than in formula-fed ones. Moreover, Cesur et al. found that ghrelin in BM is significantly higher than serum ghrelin, both in the infants' and the mothers' samples through first months of lactation [25]. However, although there is agreement regarding the role of breastfeeding in modulating the mechanisms underlying satiety and appetite regulation, studies available in the literature on BM ghrelin and infants' weight gain have shown inconsistent results. While Kon and colleagues [16] reported a positive correlation between BM ghrelin in the first two months of lactation with higher weight gain in infants, the results were not confirmed by Yis et al., despite again finding a positive correlation with infants' serum ghrelin levels and TSF [17]. Equally to ghrelin, adiponectin is a peptide with hormonal functions that stimulate hunger, acting on the hypothalamus. It is produced specifically by the adipose tissue, and its serum levels are inversely correlated with the FM percentage of the body in the adult population [35]. Its levels in BM and association with infants' FM and growth have been explored by many studies included in this review, with inconsistent results. Young et al. inversely correlated BM adiponectin levels with FM gain in healthy term infants, consistent with its hormonal function [12], whereas Gridneva and colleagues found a correlation with a higher adiposity in the first year of life [18]. Similar results, both with a positive or negative correlation, were obtained in all other studies explored, whereas the largest cohort CHILD study failed to find any association between adiponectin BM levels and infants' body composition [21]. IGF-1 is part of countless metabolic pathways of cells' signaling with their environment, often referred as IGF "axis" that plays a primary role in cell proliferation and inhibition of cell death (apoptosis) in both physiological and pathological states [36]. IGF-1 expression is also required for achieving maximal growth in developing organisms [37]. In this review, we found only one study that explored IGF-1 BM levels and infants' growth. Kon et al. reported a higher BM level of IGF-1 in those mothers whose infants showed a higher weight gain [16]. Insulin is a peptide that acts as a hormone, produced by specific endocrine cells located in the pancreatic tissue. It is considered to be the most important anabolic hormone and promotes cellular intake glucose in muscle and adipose tissue [38]. According to these functions, its levels in BM have been demonstrated to positively correlate with infant WLZ trajectory in the first months of life [12]. However, similarly to other hormones listed above, these findings were not confirmed by other studies considered in this review. However, limitations should be noted when interpreting the results. First of all, more longitudinal investigations are needed, especially during the early lactation period, to clarify the effects of breast milk hormones on growth and regulation of nutrition in infancy and childhood. The use of different outcomes to measure the child's growth was a further limitation of the review. The duration of the studies was until different ages and in some studies, it was not possible to arrange clinical visits before the age of five to six months. Finally, infant growth was evaluated using anthropometric measurements: More accurate measurements of body composition will help accurately evaluate the mediation effect of hormones in BM.

5. Conclusions

The inconsistent findings of the studies considered in this review could be explained with the concomitant action of countless factors interfering with infants' body composition during the first years of life. While some of these, including basic subject characteristics, could be identified and controlled, other factors such as synergetic or antagonist functions of many other bioactive components of BM, that could play a role in modeling growth and FM apposition, are difficult—if not impossible—to take into account. Although further studies are needed to determine the specific role of hormones and adipokines in BM, undoubtedly, these bioactive components participate in metabolic pathways related to body composition. The understanding of these pathways could help gain further insight on infants' growth, both in physiological and pathological settings.

Author Contributions: A.M., V.D.C., M.L.G., and D.M. drafted the manuscript; proof read, ordered the references, made determinations and gave technical support in data interpretation, and final revision of the draft. C.A. and F.M. critically reviewed the paper. All the others authors contributed significantly to the paper and agreed to the manuscript in its current form.

Acknowledgments: Supported by a contribution from the Italian Ministry of Health (IRCCS grant).

References

1. Kramer, M.S.; Guo, T.; Platt, R.W.; Shapiro, S.; Collet, J.P.; Chalmers, B.; Hodnett, E.; Sevkovskaya, Z.; Dzikovich, I.; Vanilovich, I. PROBIT Study Group. Breastfeeding and infant growth: Biology or bias? *Pediatrics* **2002**, *110*, 343–347. [CrossRef] [PubMed]
2. Mosca, F.; Giannì, M.L. Human milk: Composition and health benefits. *Pediatr. Med. Chir.* **2017**. [CrossRef] [PubMed]
3. Sharp, J.A.; Modepalli, V.; Enjapoori, A.K.; Bisana, S.; Abud, H.E.; Lefevre, C.; Nicholas, K.R. Bioactive Functions of Milk Proteins: A Comparative Genomics Approach. *J. Mammary Gland Biol. Neoplasia* **2014**, *19*, 289–302. [CrossRef] [PubMed]
4. Andreas, N.J.; Kampmann, B.; Mehring Le-Doare, K. Human breast milk: A review on its composition and bioactivity. *Early Hum. Dev.* **2015**, *91*, 629–635. [CrossRef] [PubMed]
5. Verduci, E.; Banderali, G.; Barberi, S.; Radaelli, G.; Lops, A.; Betti, F.; Riva, E.; Giovannini, M. Epigenetic effects of human breast milk. *Nutrients* **2014**, *6*, 1711–1724. [CrossRef] [PubMed]
6. Pauwels, S.; Symons, L.; Vanautgaerden, E.L.; Ghosh, M.; Duca, R.C.; Bekaert, B.; Freson, K.; Huybrechts, I.; Langie, S.A.S.; Koppen, G.; et al. The Influence of the Duration of Breastfeeding on the Infant's Metabolic Epigenome. *Nutrients* **2019**, *11*, 1408. [CrossRef] [PubMed]

7. Fields, D.A.; Schneider, C.R.; Pavela, G. A narrative review of the associations between six bioactive components in breast milk and infant adiposity. *Obesity* **2016**, *24*, 1213–1221. [CrossRef] [PubMed]
8. Victora, C.G.; Bahl, R.; Barros, A.J.; França, G.V.; Horton, S.; Krasevec, J.; Murch, S.; Sankar, M.J.; Walker, N.; Rollins, N.C. Lancet Breastfeeding Series Group. Breastfeeding in the 21st century: Epidemiology, mechanisms, and lifelong effect. *Lancet* **2016**, *387*, 475–490. [CrossRef]
9. Lind, M.V.; Larnkjær, A.; Mølgaard, C.; Michaelsen, K.F. Breastfeeding, Breast Milk Composition, and Growth Outcomes. In *Recent Research in Nutrition and Growth*; Karger Publishers: Basel, Switzerland, 2018; Volume 89, pp. 63–77.
10. Kugananthan, S.; Gridneva, Z.; Lai, C.T.; Hepworth, A.R.; Mark, P.J.; Kakulas, F.; Geddes, D.T. Associations between Maternal Body Composition and Appetite Hormones and Macronutrients in Human Milk. *Nutrients* **2017**, *9*, 252. [CrossRef] [PubMed]
11. Rito, A.I.; Buoncristiano, M.; Spinelli, A.; Salanave, B.; Kunešová, M.; Hejgaard, T.; Solano, M.G.; Fijałkowska, A.; Sturua, L.; Hyska, J.; et al. Association between Characteristics at Birth, Breastfeeding and Obesity in 22 Countries: The WHO European Childhood Obesity Surveillance Initiative—COSI 2015/2017. *Obes. Facts* **2019**, *12*, 226–243. [CrossRef]
12. Yu, X.; Rong, S.S.; Sun, X.; Ding, G.; Wan, W.; Zou, L.; Wu, S.; Li, M.; Wang, D. Associations of breast milk adiponectin, leptin, insulin and ghrelin with maternal characteristics and early infant growth: A longitudinal study. *Br. J. Nutr.* **2018**, *120*, 1380–1387. [CrossRef] [PubMed]
13. Neville, M.C.; Anderson, S.M.; McManaman, J.L.; Badger, T.M.; Bunik, M.; Contractor, N.; Crume, T.; Dabelea, D.; Donovan, S.M.; Forman, N.; et al. Lactation and neonatal nutrition: Defining and refining the critical questions. *J. Mammary Gland Biol. Neoplasia* **2012**, *17*, 167–188. [CrossRef] [PubMed]
14. Badillo-Suárez, P.A.; Rodríguez-Cruz, M.; Nieves-Morales, X. Impact of Metabolic Hormones Secreted in Human Breast Milk on Nutritional Programming in Childhood Obesity. *J. Mammary Gland Biol. Neoplasia* **2017**, *22*, 171–191. [CrossRef] [PubMed]
15. Young, B.E.; Levek, C.; Reynolds, R.M.; Rudolph, M.C.; MacLean, P.; Hernandez, T.L.; Friedman, J.E.; Krebs, N.F. Bioactive components in human milk are differentially associated with rates of lean and fat mass deposition in infants of mothers with normal vs. elevated BMI. *Pediatric Obes.* **2018**, *13*, 598–606. [CrossRef] [PubMed]
16. Kon, I.Y.; Shilina, N.M.; Gmoshinskaya, M.V.; Ivanushkina, T.A. The study of breast milk IGF-1, leptin, ghrelin and adiponectin levels as possible reasons of high weight gain in breast-fed infants. *Ann. Nutr. Metab.* **2014**, *65*, 317–323. [CrossRef] [PubMed]
17. Yiş, U.; Oztürk, Y.; Sişman, A.R.; Uysal, S.; Soylu, O.B.; Büyükgebiz, B. The relation of serum ghrelin, leptin and insulin levels to the growth patterns and feeding characteristics in breast-fed versus formula-fed infants. *Turk. J. Pediatrics* **2010**, *52*, 35–41.
18. Gridneva, Z.; Kugananthan, S.; Rea, A.; Lai, C.T.; Ward, L.C.; Murray, K.; Hartmann, P.E.; Geddes, D.T. Human Milk Adiponectin and Leptin and Infant Body Composition over the First 12 Months of Lactation. *Nutrients* **2018**, *10*, 1125. [CrossRef] [PubMed]
19. Fields, D.A.; George, B.; Williams, M.; Whitaker, K.; Allison, D.B.; Teague, A.; Demerath, E.W. Associations between human breast milk hormones and adipocytokines and infant growth and body composition in the first 6 months of life. *Pediatric Obes.* **2017**, *12*, 78–85. [CrossRef] [PubMed]
20. Fields, D.A.; Demerath, E.W. Relationship of insulin, glucose, leptin, IL-6 and TNF-α in human breast milk with infant growth and body composition. *Pediatric Obes.* **2012**, *7*, 304–312. [CrossRef]
21. Chan, D.; Goruk, S.; Becker, A.B.; Subbarao, P.; Mandhane, P.J.; Turvey, S.E.; Lefebvre, D.; Sears, M.R.; Field, C.J.; Azad, M.B. Adiponectin, leptin and insulin in breast milk: Associations with maternal characteristics and infant body composition in the first year of life. *Int. J. Obes.* **2018**, *42*, 36–43. [CrossRef]
22. Meyer, D.M.; Brei, C.; Stecher, L.; Much, D.; Brunner, S.; Hauner, H. The relationship between breast milk leptin and adiponectin with child body composition from 3 to 5 years: A follow-up study. *Pediatric Obes.* **2017**, *12*, 125–129. [CrossRef] [PubMed]
23. Brunner, S.; Schmid, D.; Zang, K.; Much, D.; Knoeferl, B.; Kratzsch, J.; Amann-Gassner, U.; Bader, B.L.; Hauner, H. Breast milk leptin and adiponectin in relation to infant body composition up to 2 years. *Pediatric Obes.* **2015**, *10*, 67–73. [CrossRef] [PubMed]

24. Mohamad, M.; Lim, P.; Wang, Y.; Soo, K.; Mohamed, H. Maternal Serum and Breast Milk Adiponectin: The Association with Infant Adiposity Development. *Int. J. Environ. Res. Public Health* **2018**, *15*, 1250. [CrossRef] [PubMed]
25. Cesur, G.; Ozguner, F.; Yilmaz, N.; Dundar, B. The relationship between ghrelin and adiponectin levels in breast milk and infant serum and growth of infants during early postnatal life. *J. Physiol. Sci.* **2012**, *62*, 185–190. [CrossRef] [PubMed]
26. Larsson, M.; Lind, M.; Larnkjær, A.; Due, A.; Blom, I.; Wells, J.; Michaelsen, K. Excessive weight gain followed by catch-down in exclusively breastfed infants: An exploratory study. *Nutrients* **2018**, *10*, 1290. [CrossRef] [PubMed]
27. Ucar, B.; Kırel, B.; Bör, Ö.; Kılıç, F.S.; Doğruel, N.; Aydoğdu, S.D.; Tekin, N. Breast milk leptin concentrations in initial and terminal milk samples: Relationships to maternal and infant plasma leptin concentrations, adiposity, serum glucose, insulin, lipid and lipoprotein levels. *J. Pediatric Endocrinol. Metab.* **2000**, *13*, 149–156. [CrossRef]
28. Woo, J.G.; Guerrero, M.L.; Altaye, M.; Ruiz-Palacios, G.M.; Martin, L.J.; Dubert-Ferrandon, A.; Newburg, D.S.; Morrow, A.L. Human milk adiponectin is associated with infant growth in two independent cohorts. *Breastfeed. Med.* **2009**, *4*, 101–109. [CrossRef] [PubMed]
29. Flier, J.S.; Maratos-Flier, E. Leptin's Physiologic Role: Does the Emperor of Energy Balance Have No Clothes? *Cell Metab.* **2017**, *26*, 24–26. [CrossRef] [PubMed]
30. Brennan, A.M.; Mantzoros, C.S. Drug Insight: The role of leptin in human physiology and pathophysiology—Emerging clinical applications. *Nat. Clin. Pract. Endocrinol. Metab.* **2006**, *2*, 318–327. [CrossRef]
31. Chaoimh, C.N.; Murray, D.M.; Kenny, L.C.; Irvine, A.D.; Hourihane, J.O.; Kiely, M. Cord blood leptin and gains in body weight and fat mass during infancy. *Eur. J. Endocrinol.* **2016**, *175*, 403–410. [CrossRef]
32. Savino, F.; Sardo, A.; Rossi, L.; Benetti, S.; Savino, A.; Silvestro, L. Mother and Infant Body Mass Index, Breast Milk Leptin and Their Serum Leptin Values. *Nutrients* **2016**, *8*, 383. [CrossRef] [PubMed]
33. Schwartz, M.W.; Woods, S.C.; Porte, D., Jr.; Seeley, R.J.; Baskin, D.G. Central nervous system control of food intake. *Nature* **2000**, *404*, 661–671. [CrossRef] [PubMed]
34. Vásquez-Garibay, E.M.; Larrosa-Haro, A.; Guzmán-Mercado, E.; Muñoz-Esparza, N.; García-Arellano, S.; Muñoz-Valle, F.; Romero-Velarde, E. Serum concentration of appetite-regulating hormones of mother-infant dyad according to the type of feeding. *Food Sci. Nutr.* **2019**, *7*, 869–874. [CrossRef] [PubMed]
35. Ukkola, O.; Santaniemi, M. Adiponectin: A link between excess adiposity and associated comorbidities? *J. Mol. Med.* **2002**, *80*, 696–702. [CrossRef] [PubMed]
36. Nemet, D.; Cooper, D.M. Exercise, diet, and chilhood obesity: The GH-IGF-I connection. *J. Pediatric Endocrinol. Metab.* **2002**, *15*, 751–757. [CrossRef]
37. De Jong, M.; Cranendonk, A.; Twisk, J.W.; van Weissenbruch, M.M. IGF-I and relation to growth in infancy and early childhood in very-low-birth-weight infants and term born infants. *PLoS ONE* **2017**, *12*, e0171650. [CrossRef] [PubMed]
38. Dimitriadis, G.; Mitrou, P.; Lambadiari, V.; Maratou, E.; Raptis, S.A. Insulin effects in muscle and adipose tissue. *Diabetes Res. Clin. Pract.* **2011**, *93*, S52–S59. [CrossRef]

7

What Evidence do we have for Pharmaceutical Galactagogues in the Treatment of Lactation Insufficiency?

Luke E. Grzeskowiak [1,2,*], Mary E. Wlodek [3] and Donna T. Geddes [4]

1 Adelaide Medical School, Robinson Research Institute, The University of Adelaide, Adelaide, SA 5005, Australia
2 SA Pharmacy, Flinders Medical Centre, SA Health, Bedford Park, Adelaide, SA 5042, Australia
3 Department of Physiology, The University of Melbourne, Melbourne, VIC 3010, Australia; m.wlodek@unimelb.edu.au
4 School of Molecular Sciences, The University of Western Australia, Crawley, Perth, WA 6009, Australia; donna.geddes@uwa.edu.au
* Correspondence: luke.Grzeskowiak@adelaide.edu.au

Abstract: Inadequate breast milk supply is a frequently reported reason for early discontinuation of breastfeeding and represents a critical opportunity for intervening to improve breastfeeding outcomes. For women who continue to experience insufficient milk supply despite the utilisation of non-pharmacological lactation support strategies, pharmacological intervention with medications used to augment lactation, commonly referred to as galactagogues, is common. Galactagogues exert their pharmacological effects through altering the complex hormonal milieu regulating lactation, particularly prolactin and oxytocin. This narrative review provides an appraisal of the existing evidence regarding the efficacy and safety of pharmaceutical treatments for lactation insufficiency to guide their use in clinical practice. The greatest body of evidence surrounds the use of domperidone, with studies demonstrating moderate short-term improvements in breast milk supply. Evidence regarding the efficacy and safety of metoclopramide is less robust, but given that it shares the same mechanism of action as domperidone it may represent a potential treatment alternative where domperidone is unsuitable. Data on remaining interventions such as oxytocin, prolactin and metformin is too limited to support their use in clinical practice. The review provides an overview of key evidence gaps and areas of future research, including the impacts of pharmaceutical galactagogues on breast milk composition and understanding factors contributing to individual treatment response to pharmaceutical galactagogues.

Keywords: galactagogues; low milk supply; lactation; breast milk; breast feeding

---

1. Mothers' Own Breast Milk is Best

Breast milk is considered the optimal source of enteral nutrition to support the growth and development of all infants [1]. Exclusive breastfeeding is advocated for the first six months, with the continuation of breastfeeding supported until the age of two years or longer [2]. Infants who are not breastfed or are breastfed for shorter durations are at an increased risk of early and later-life morbidities and mortality [1–3]. Specifically, the reduced provision of breast milk is associated with increased risks of gastrointestinal, urinary, respiratory and middle-ear infections, together with a range of non-communicable diseases such as asthma, allergies, obesity and diabetes, and some childhood cancers [4]. Breastfeeding also confers a range of maternal benefits, which include reduced risks of breast, endometrial and ovarian cancer, together with faster return to pre-pregnancy weight and improvements in the psychological wellbeing [4,5].

The provision of mothers' own breast milk is particularly important in the feeding of vulnerable preterm infants, where superiority of mothers' own milk to donor human milk and infant formula with respect to the composition and bioactivity are critically important [3]. The use of mothers' own breast milk during hospitalisation reduces the incidence and severity of preventable morbidities, including necrotizing enterocolitis (NEC), late onset sepsis, chronic lung disease, retinopathy of prematurity, rehospitalisation after discharge, and neurodevelopmental problems in infancy and childhood [3]. For example, a recent Cochrane review showed that preterm infants receiving infant formula are three times more likely to develop NEC, which has a mortality rate of 20–40% [6]. The benefits are further exemplified by evidence from a cohort of very low birth weight infants where for every 10 mL/kg/day increase in the ingestion of mothers' own breast milk, the odds of rehospitalisation up to 30 months of age decreased by 5% [7]. These benefits extend long-term, with predominant breast milk feeding in the first 28-days of life is associated with better IQ, academic achievement, working memory, and motor function at seven years of age in very preterm infants [8]. In addition, the ability for a mother to provide her own breast milk provides psychological benefits including greater feelings of attachment, empowerment, and confidence [9].

The reality, however, is that many mothers face challenges related to initiating and sustaining breastfeeding. One of the key challenges related to breast milk production, with perceived inadequate breast milk supply is a frequently reported reason for early discontinuation of breastfeeding or decreased exclusivity in women who have initiated breastfeeding [10]. As an example of the potential magnitude of the problem, a large survey of 1323 mothers in the US highlighted that 50% of women stopped breastfeeding earlier than they had intended due to insufficient breast milk supply [11]. These surveys however, suffer a lack of objective evidence to confirm whether the low milk supply is real or perceived. Further, they often do not include information about early breastfeeding practices during the establishment of lactation such as the frequent emptying of the breast. Nevertheless, even if true lactation insufficiency is a fraction of previously reported figures, a significant opportunity exists for the development and implementation of strategies targeting improvements in breast milk supply to improve breastfeeding outcomes and subsequent maternal and infant health. In light of this, there continues to be widespread interest in and use of medications to augment lactation, commonly referred to as galactagogues. Prior to appraising the evidence regarding the role of pharmaceutical galactagogues in the treatment of lactation insufficiency, it is necessary to consider the physiology of lactation.

2. Physiology of Lactation

The development of functional lactation is a multi-stage event and is regulated by a complex hormonal milieu that includes numerous reproductive hormones (e.g., oestrogen, progesterone, prolactin, oxytocin) and metabolic hormones (e.g., glucocorticoids, insulin, insulin-like growth factor 1 (IGF-I), growth hormone, and thyroid hormone) [12]. Secretory differentiation occurs in mid- to late pregnancy when the differentiation of mammary epithelial cells into lactocytes occurs, conferring the ability to synthesize and secrete key components of human milk. This process is largely driven by circulating levels of oestrogen and progesterone that not only stimulate milk duct development, but also suppress prolactin's action on milk production during pregnancy. Secretory activation is triggered by the sudden drop in progesterone following delivery of the placenta, accompanied by high levels of circulating prolactin. Secretory activation is confirmed by the onset of copious milk secretion and typically occurs between 24–102 h (average 60 h) after birth. This is often described as the milk 'coming in'. Milk ejection is primarily regulated by oxytocin, which stimulates the contraction of myoepithelial cells around the alveoli and facilitates milk release [13]. Once lactation is established, an autocrine control (local feedback) mechanism regulates ongoing milk production, meaning supply is largely based on the effective removal of milk from the breast and is less sensitive to circulating levels of prolactin [13].

Given the important roles of prolactin and oxytocin in regulating milk secretion and milk ejection, these hormones have become common pharmacological targets for influencing breast milk supply. Figure 1 provides an overview of endogenous and exogenous factors influencing prolactin and oxytocin, while also highlighting mechanisms of action of common pharmaceutical galactagogues. A more detailed review of the neuroendocrine regulation of prolactin and oxytocin secretion and function can be found elsewhere and is beyond the scope of this review [14]. In brief, the production of prolactin in the anterior pituitary is regulated by the presence of prolactin inhibiting factors (PIF) and prolactin releasing factors (PRF), which are controlled by the hypothalamus. The concentrations of these inhibitory and stimulatory factors is influenced by a variety of external stimuli such as infant suckling, sounds of the infant crying, and stress. The key PIF is dopamine, which exerts an inhibitory effect on prolactin production. Positive external stimuli lead to an inhibitory effect on dopamine release and a resultant increase in prolactin levels. Similarly, medications that block dopamine, such as the dopamine antagonists domperidone and metoclopramide, block its inhibitory effects and result in an increase in prolactin secretion. In contrast, a range of hormones act to stimulate prolactin production, including thyrotropin releasing hormone, cortisol, and oxytocin. Other hormones that exert direct or indirect effects on the mammary gland to influence milk synthesis include the growth hormone, prolactin and insulin. Milk contains a small whey protein called the feedback inhibitor of lactation (FIL). The accumulation of milk in the breast leads to milk stasis and an increased concentration of FIL, which provides a negative feedback to slow milk production by inhibiting the action of prolactin on lactocytes.

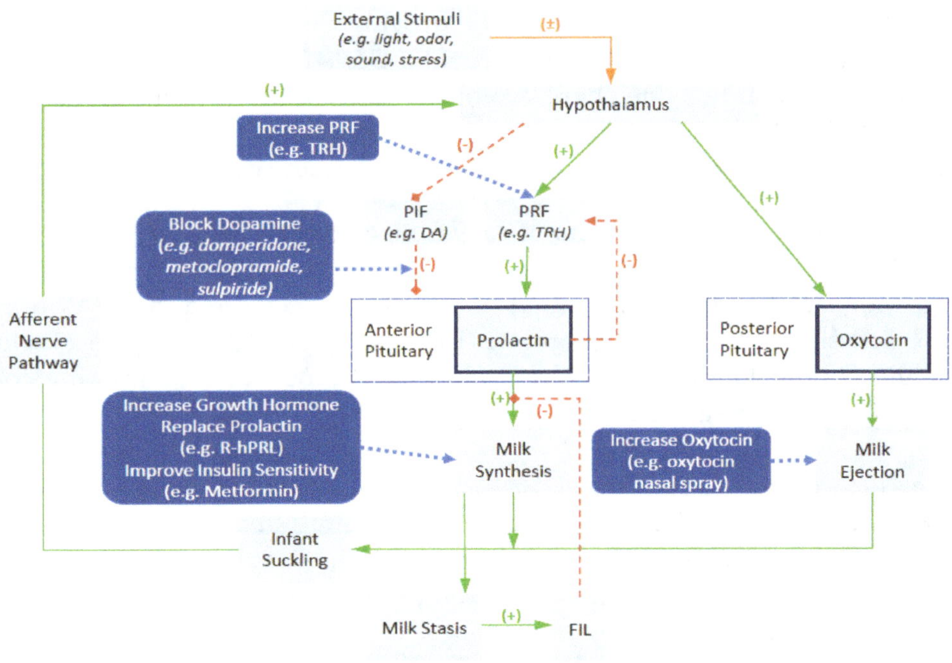

Figure 1. Physiology of lactation and mechanisms of action of various pharmaceutical galactagogues (Adapted from [14–16]). Abbreviations: TRH, thyrotrophin releasing hormone; PIF, prolactin inhibitory factor; PRF, prolactin releasing factor; DA, dopamine; R-hPRL, recombinant human prolactin; FIL, feedback inhibitor of lactation.

3. Risk Factors for Lactation Insufficiency

Three key aspects are required for establishing an adequate breast milk supply including sufficient mammary tissue, normal hormone levels, and regular effective removal of milk [17]. Insufficient mammary tissue can be the result of hypoplastic breasts, breast surgery such as mastectomy or breast reduction, or cyst removal [18]. Numerous maternal factors can influence hormone levels including retained placenta, severe postpartum haemorrhage, hypothyroidism, high levels of stress or anxiety, certain medications, anaemia, diabetes, obesity, polycystic ovary syndrome, cigarette smoking, or alcohol consumption [17,18]. Lastly, the effective and regular removal of milk can be influenced by the method and frequency of expressing if indirectly feeding the infant, or the inability for infants to effectively remove milk from the breast if feeding directly as a result of issues such as poor attachment, low infant intraoral vacuums and delivery complications. Factors such as the use of infant formula, early introduction of solids, infant sedation, or infant medical problems (e.g., low birth weight, congenital abnormalities, illness) may also exacerbate poor feeding and ineffective removal of breast milk [18].

In particular, mothers of preterm infants face many challenges in establishing and maintaining an adequate supply of breast milk during their infant's prolonged hospitalisation. This is driven by multiple factors including; physiological immaturity of the breast associated with preterm birth, maternal morbidities, inability for the preterm infant to breastfeed directly from the breast, and the stress of having an infant admitted to the Neonatal Intensive Care Unit (NICU). Each of these factors has the ability to interfere with the establishment of normal milk supply, with one previous study demonstrating that 82% of women birthing preterm experienced delayed secretory activation [19]. While longer-term breastfeeding outcomes were not collected for this cohort, other studies in mothers of term infants have demonstrated that delayed secretory activation is associated with an increased risk of early cessation of breastfeeding [20].

4. Use of Galactagogues in Clinical Practice

Relatively little evidence exists regarding the prevalence of pharmaceutical galactagogue use. A recent clinical practice survey of Australian Neonatal Units (NNUs) identified that 100% of NNUs reported domperidone as their first line pharmacological agent of choice in the management of lactation insufficiency [21]. While 75% of NNUs reported having a clinical guideline on domperidone, significant variability was evident across these guidelines with respect to the dose and duration of treatment.

The preference towards the use of domperidone for lactation insufficiency is supported by a recent audit of phone calls to an Australian pregnancy and lactation counselling service regarding the use of galactagogues during lactation highlighted that domperidone accounted for >90% of phone calls [22]. In contrast, the discussion of herbal galactagogues increased from 0% in 2001 to 23% in 2014. Overall, these findings highlight the popularity of domperidone use in the Australian setting, together with the increasing popularity of herbal galactagogues.

Three studies have examined patterns of domperidone use over the past 10–15 years. An Australian study undertaken at a single tertiary level maternity hospital identified the increasing prevalence of use from 0.1% of all deliveries in 2000 to 5% in 2010 [23]. A recognised limitation of this study lies in the fact that it likely underestimates total domperidone use, as it could not take into account domperidone dispensed from community pharmacies. In comparison, a Canadian study investigated the number of women that dispensed domperidone in the first six months postpartum among 320,351 live births occurring between 2002 and 2011 [24]. Over this time period the prevalence of domperidone use increased from 7% to 18% in women delivering at term and 17% to 32% in women delivering preterm. The most recent study used data from the Clinical Practice Research Datalink in England and demonstrated a 3.8-fold increase in postpartum domperidone prescribed from 0.56 per 100 person-years in 2002–2004 to 2.1 per 100 person-years in 2011–2013, with overall use much lower than that reported in previous studies [25]. Risk factors commonly associated with domperidone use in these studies included preterm birth, delivery by caesarean section, maternal obesity, diabetes or gestational diabetes, and primiparity [24–26].

5. Efficacy and Safety of Galactagogues

In order to evaluate the efficacy and safety of galactagogues we searched four electronic databases from inception to January 2019: Ovid Medline, EMBASE, Web of Science, and SCOPUS. Medical subject headings (e.g., MeSH headings) and free word combinations using Boolean logic of the following search items were used: 'galactagogues' OR individual medication names (e.g., 'domperidone') AND 'lactation' OR 'low milk supply'. Previous reviews, bibliographies of published trials and cross references were also searched. No language restrictions were applied. For the evaluation of galactagogue efficacy, studies were restricted to those investigating the use of galactagogues in the treatment of established lactation insufficiency and using controlled study designs. Studies investigating herbal galactagogues were excluded from this review.

An overview of controlled intervention trials evaluating the efficacy of various galactagogues is provided in Table 1. Domperidone [27–37] and metoclopramide [28,29,38–40] appear to be the most commonly studied galactagogues in the setting of established lactation insufficiency, with limited studies evaluating the effects of other galactagogues including sulpiride [41,42], growth hormone [43,44], human recombinant prolactin [45], thyrotropin releasing hormone [46,47], and metformin [48]. No studies have evaluated the use of oxytocin in the treatment of lactation insufficiency. The focus of this review is on the use of galactagogues in the treatment of lactation insufficiency, studies that included women without an established diagnosis of lactation insufficiency were not considered [49–59].

5.1. Domperidone

Domperidone is a dopamine antagonist and is thought to act as a galactagogue by increasing serum prolactin (Figure 1). The majority of studies evaluating the effects of domperidone have been undertaken among mothers of preterm infants. Treatment durations (five to 28 days) and treatment initiation (>1 to >3 weeks post-partum) varied widely between studies. The most commonly used interventional dose consisted of 10 mg three times daily, with two studies evaluating a higher dose of 20 mg three times daily [27,34].

All placebo-controlled studies demonstrate treatment effects in favor of domperidone. Five studies involving mothers of preterm infants have recently been combined in a meta-analysis, demonstrating that the administration of 30 mg/day led to a modest increase in maternal breast milk volume of 88 mL daily [60]. Missing from this meta-analysis was the recent study by Fazilla et al., which demonstrated a similar improvement to the previous pooled estimate of 109 mL/day (95%CI 69 to 149 mL/day) [32]. Effects of domperidone on mothers of term infants is limited to two studies [33,35], with both demonstrating treatment effects in favor of domperidone compared with placebo. Inam et al. utilised a treatment target of 50 mL per single expression episode (both breasts) with 36 of 50 (72%) women in the domperidone arm achieving this target compared with 11 of 40 (22%) women in the placebo arm ($p = 0.002$) [33]. Petraglia et al. evaluated changes in breast milk supply by weighing infants before and after breast feeding, demonstrating greater improvement in daily breast milk supply among women receiving domperidone (347 ± 36 to 673 ± 44 mL/day), compared with placebo (335 ± 30 to 398 ± 45 mL/day; $p < 0.01$) [35].

Table 1. Overview of controlled studies evaluating the efficacy of pharmaceutical galactagogues for the treatment of lactation insufficiency.

Study (Country)	Intervention (n/N) and Dose	Duration (Days)	Delivery Gestation (Weeks)	Infant Age (Weeks)	Effect on Milk Production
Domperidone					
Asztalos 2017 (Canada) [37]	*Domperidone* (45): 10 mg TDS *Placebo* (40/45)	14	<30	>1 to ≤3	Change in milk supply: *Domperidone*: 121 (±96) to 267 (±189) mL/day; *Placebo*: 115 (±95) to 217 (±168) mL/day; $p = 0.20$
Campbell-Yeo 2010 (Canada) [30]	*Domperidone* (21/22): 10 mg TDS *Placebo* (24)	14	<31	≥3	Change in milk supply: *Domperidone*: 184 (±167) to 380 (±202) mL/day; *Placebo*: 218 (±155) to 251 (±172) mL/day
da Silva 2001 (Canada) [31]	*Domperidone* (6/11): 10 mg TDS *Placebo* (8/9)	7	<37 †	Any	Difference from baseline: *Domperidone*: 49.5 (±29.4) mL/day; *Placebo*: 8.0 (±39.5) mL/day; $p < 0.05$
Fazilla 2017 (Indonesia) [32]	*Domperidone* (25): 10 mg TDS *Placebo* (25):	7	<37	>1	Difference from baseline: *Domperidone*: 181.6 (±80.2) mL/day; *Placebo*: 72.4 (±57.8) mL/day; $p = 0.0001$
Inam 2013 (Pakistan) [33]	*Domperidone* (50): 10 mg TDS *Placebo* (50)	7	Term	1	Number reaching target of ≥ 50 mL per single expression: *Domperidone*: 36/50 (76%); *Placebo*: 11/50 (22%); $p = 0.002$
Knoppert 2013 (Canada) [34]	*Domperidone* (5/8): 10 mg TDS *Domperidone* (6/7): 20 mg TDS	28	<33	≥2 to ≤3	Change in milk supply: 10 mg TDS: 150 to 420 mL/day; 20 mg TDS: 300 to 720 mL/day
Petraglia 1985 (Italy) [35]	*Domperidone* (9): 10 mg TDS *Placebo* (8)	10	Term	>2	Change in milk supply: *Domperidone*: 347 (±36) to 673 (±44) mL/day; *Placebo*: 335 (±30) to 398 (±45) mL/day; $p < 0.01$
Rai 2016 (India) [36]	*Domperidone* (14/16): 10 mg TDS *Placebo* (16)	7	<37†	≥1 to ≤2	Difference from baseline: Domperidone: Median 186.0 (IQR 126.5 to 240) mL/day; Placebo: Median 70 (IQR 49.5 to 97); $p = 0.004$
Wan 2008 (Australia) [27]	*Domperidone* (4/7): 10 mg TDS & 20 mg TDS	7–14	<37	>2	Change in milk supply: Baseline: 208.8 (±182.3) mL/day; 30 mg: 566.4 (±229.3) mL/day; 60 mg: 705.6 (±388.1) mL/day
Metoclopramide					
Kauppila 1981 (Finland) [39]	*Metoclopramide* (37/45): 5 mg TDS, 10 mg TDS, 15 mg TDS & *placebo*	14	Term	>1	Difference from baseline (single feed): 5 mg TDS: 11.2 ± 28.1 mL; 10 mg TDS: 42.5 ± 34.7 mL; 15 mg TDS: 50.0 ± 35.9 mL; *Placebo*: 4.0 ± 27.5 mL
Kauppila 1985 (Finland) [38]	*Metoclopramide* (8): 10 mg TDS *Placebo* (5)	21	Term	≥4 to ≤20	Change in milk supply: *Metoclopramide*: 285 (±75) to 530 (±162) mL/day ($p < 0.01$); *Placebo*: individual results not stated
Sakha 2008 (Iran) [40]	*Metoclopramide* (10): 10 mg TDS *Placebo* (10)	15	Term	NR	Infant weight gain: *Metoclopramide*: 328.5 g; *Placebo*: 351.5 g ($p = 0.68$)
Domperidone/Metoclopramide					
Blank 2000 (Australia) [28]	*Domperidone* (9): 10 mg TDS *Metoclopramide* (11): 10 mg TDS *Placebo* (9)	5	<34	≥1	Change in milk supply: *Domperidone*: 120 (±81) to 239 (±105) mL/day; *Metoclopramide*: 100 (±53) to 184 (±100) mL/day; *Placebo*: 143 (±57) to 172 (±117) mL/day
Ingram 2012 (Canada) [29]	*Domperidone* (31/38): 10 mg TDS *Metoclopramide* (34/42): 10 mg TDS	10	<37†	NR	Change in milk supply: *Domperidone*: 174 (±126) to 285 (±158) mL/day; *Metoclopramide*: 133 (±115) to 212 (±154) mL/day; *Difference*: 31.0 (−5.67 to 67.6) mL/day
Sulpiride					
Ylikorkala 1982 (Finland) [41]	*Sulpiride* (14): 50 mg TDS *Placebo* (12/14)	28	NS	≤16	Difference from baseline: *Sulpiride*: 265 mL/day; *Placebo*: −50 mL/day
Ylikorkala 1984 (Finland) [42]	*Sulpiride* (13/14): 50 mg TDS *Placebo* (11/14)	14	NS	≤16	Difference from baseline: *Sulpiride*: 646 (±67) mL/day; *Placebo*: 428 (±71) mL/day ($p < 0.05$)

Table 1. *Cont.*

Study (Country)	Intervention (n/N) and Dose	Duration (Days)	Delivery Gestation (Weeks)	Infant Age (Weeks)	Effect on Milk Production
Human Growth Hormone (hGH)					
Gunn 1996 (New Zealand) [43]	*hGH* (9/10): 0.2 IU/kg/day SC (max 16 IU/kg/day) *Placebo* (9/10)	7	26–34	NR	Change from baseline: *hGH*: 139 (±49) to 175 (±46) mL/day; $p < 0.01$ *Placebo*: 93 (±50) to 102 (±69) mL/day; p = NS
Milsom 1998 (New Zealand) [44]	*hGH* (5): 0.05 IU/kg/day SC *hGH* (5): 0.1 IU/kg/day SC *hGH* (6): 0.2 IU/kg/day SC	7	Term	<16	Percentage increase in breast milk volume: High dose group (0.2 IU): 36 ± 12.6 Low/Mid dose group (0.05/0.1 IU): 4.7 ± 9.7; $p < 0.04$
Recombinant Human Prolactin (R-hPRL)					
Powe 2010 (USA) [45]	*R-hPRL* (3): 60 mcg/kg SC BD *R-hPRL* (3): 60 mcg/kg SC daily *Placebo* (4)	7	24–32	≥1 to ≤4	Percentage change in milk supply: *R-hPRL* (Twice Daily): 429 (±338%); *R-hPRL* (Once Daily): 44 (±28%); *Placebo*: −12 (±27%)
Thyrotrophin-Releasing Hormone (TRH)					
Zarate 1975 (Mexico) [46]	*TRH* (5): 20 mg TDS PO *Placebo* (4)	7	NR	NR	No change in milk production (actual volume not reported)
Peters 1991 (Germany) [47]	*TRH* (10): 1 mg QID IN *Placebo* (9)	10	Term	Day 6	Change from baseline: *TRH*: 142.0 (±33.9) to 253.0 (±105.3) g/day ($p = 0.014$); *Placebo*: 150.0 (±46.2) to 140.6 (±57.7) g/day ($p = 0.87$)
Metformin					
Nommsen-Rivers 2019 (USA) [48]	*Metformin* (10): Day 1–7 – 750 mg/day; Day 8–14 – 1500 mg/day; Day 14–28 – 2000 mg/day *Placebo* (5)	28	Term	1–8	Difference from baseline: *Metformin*: Median 8 (IQR −23 to 33) mL/day; *Placebo*: Median −58 (IQR −62 to −1) mL/day

Abbreviations: TDS, three times daily; BD, twice daily; SC, subcutaneous; IN, intranasal; QID, four times daily; NR, not reported. † denotes infants admitted to neonatal unit.

Two underpowered studies have compared the effects of different doses of domperidone [27,34]. One of these was a small case-crossover study where women were randomised to receive an initial dose of 30 mg/day or 60 mg/day, then crossover to the other arm of the study after 7–14 days of treatment. Daily milk volume production was only reported for four of six women who were considered treatment responders, with daily breast milk volume increasing from 208.8 ± 182.3 mL/day at baseline to 566.4 ± 229.3 mL/day at a dose of 30 mg/day and 705.6 ± 388.1 mL/day at a dose of 60 mg/day [27]. The reported increases were statistically significantly higher compared with baseline values, but the small sample size of four women prohibited the identification of statistically significant differences between the two different doses. In contrast, Knoppert et al. randomised 15 women to either receive 30 mg/day or 60 mg/day for four weeks [34]. Daily breast milk volume increased from a median of 150 to 420 mL/day among those receiving the 30 mg/day dose, and 300 to 720 mL/day among those receiving the 60 mg/day dose, but the differences between the groups were not statistically significant [34]. Collectively, while these two studies provide promising evidence of potential further improvements in daily breast milk volume with the use of a higher dose of domperidone (i.e., 60 mg/day compared to 30 mg/day), further research is required to determine if a higher dose can be considered superior.

Maternal adverse events most commonly associated with the use of domperidone in clinical trials include headache, dry mouth, and gastrointestinal disturbances. That said, compared to placebo, no increased risk of maternal adverse events (RR 1.05; 95%CI 0.65–1.71) has been identified in clinical trials. Similarly, no trials have reported an increased risk of adverse neonatal events [58,59]. Indeed the concentrations of domperidone in breast milk are low with the absolute infant dose only 0.04 (95%CI 0.03–0.07) micrograms/kg/day for a maternal dose of 30 mg/day, and 0.07 (95%CI 0.05–0.11) micrograms/kg/day for a maternal dose of 60 mg/day [27]. One small case-crossover study demonstrated a higher prevalence of adverse events with a higher dose of domperidone [27]. Among the seven study participants, there were a total of five adverse events reported at 30 mg/day (abdominal cramping [$n = 1$], dry mouth [$n = 3$], headache [$n = 1$]), and 12 adverse events reported at 60 mg/day (abdominal cramping [$n = 2$], constipation [$n = 1$], dry mouth [$n = 5$], depressed mood [$n = 1$], headache [$n = 3$]) [27]. Also, one woman withdrew from the study as a result of experiencing severe abdominal cramps while receiving 60 mg/day [27]. In contrast, a more recent double blind randomised controlled trial comparing 30 mg/day to 60 mg/day identified no adverse events in either group [34]. Therefore, while it currently remains unclear, it is possible that a higher dose of domperidone may be associated with a greater risk of maternal adverse events.

The use of domperidone in lactation has been the subject of controversy due to an increased risk of ventricular arrhythmia (VA) and sudden cardiac death of approximately four per 1000 person-years observed among non-lactating adults, including males and females [61,62]. This increased risk relates to the potential of domperidone to prolong the QT interval [63], but the relevance to lactating women has been questioned [64–68]. Domperidone was initially developed as an antiemetic and prokinetic, with previous recommended doses ranging from 30 mg/day to 60 mg/day or greater [66]. Some observational studies suggested that the risk of VA or sudden cardiac death may be increased if daily doses were greater than 30 mg or if patients were male or greater than 60 years old [61,62]. More detail regarding domperidone and QT interval effects among non-lactating adults can be found elsewhere [61,62].

Numerous studies provide reassuring evidence as to the safety of domperidone use in lactating women. A recent randomised double-blind, placebo- and positive-controlled safety study identified that among healthy female volunteers, domperidone at doses up to 80 mg/day did not cause clinically relevant QTc-interval prolongation [69]. Further, all women participating in the trial by Asztalos et al. had an ECG at baseline and at the end of the study. They observed no evidence of prolongation of the QTc-interval with any mother participating in the trial [62]. Perhaps the strongest evidence to guide the clinical practice comes from a recent Canadian population-based cohort study of 320,351 women, of which 45,163 were prescribed domperidone within six months postpartum [70]. The primary outcome consisted of ventricular arrhythmia and data were obtained on whether or not women had a previous history of ventricular arrhythmia. No cases of ventricular arrhythmia were identified among those women with no prior history [71]. All cases of ventricular arrhythmia were observed among women with a previous history. Taken together, these results provide supporting evidence for the limited increased risk of ventricular arrhythmia among women with no previous medical history, and strengthens the support that domperidone should be avoided in those women with a previous history. Notably, among this cohort 90% of women received a dose of domperidone greater than 30 mg/day, suggesting limited impact of dose on ventricular arrhythmia risk. In light of such evidence it appears that domperidone can be used safely, but should be avoided or used with extreme caution in women with established risk factors for QTc-prolongation. This includes women taking medications that inhibit the metabolism of domperidone and/or also prolong the QTc-interval (e.g., fluconazole, erythromycin), and women with a personal or family history of cardiac arrhythmia or family history of unexplained sudden death. Clinical protocols regarding the use of domperidone in clinical practice have been developed and serve to facilitate safer prescribing practices and minimize potential adverse reactions in mothers and their hospitalized premature infants [72].

5.2. *Metoclopramide*

Similar to domperidone, metoclopramide is a dopamine antagonist and is thought to act as a galactagogue by increasing serum prolactin (Figure 1). In contrast to domperidone, the majority of clinical studies have evaluated the use of metoclopramide among mothers of term infants. Four studies have evaluated a standard dose of 10 mg three times daily, with the treatment duration varying from five to 21 days. One study evaluated three difference metoclopramide doses [39]. Three studies directly measured changes in breast milk volume, one study indirectly evaluated breast milk volume based on infant weight measures before and after a single feed, while the last study evaluated infant weight gain. A dose-response case-cross-over study identified a significant increase from baseline in breast milk yield during a single feed following use of 30 mg/day (42.5 ± 34.7 mL) and 45 mg/day (50.0 ± 35.9 mL) doses, but not 15 mg/day (11.2 ± 28.1 mL) or placebo (4.0 ± 27.5 mL) [39]. Blank et al. identified a greater increase in breast milk volume in those receiving metoclopramide compared with placebo (84 mL/day compared to 29 mL/day, but the difference between the groups was not statistically significantly different [28]. Kauppila et al. identified a significant increase in breast milk supply during the study among those receiving metoclopramide (285 ± 75 mL /day to 530 ± 162 mL /day ($p < 0.01$)), but change in breast milk supply was not reported for those in the placebo arm [38].

Adverse events associated with metoclopramide have been incompletely described. Kauppila et al. reported adverse events occurring among six of eight women, which included tiredness ($n = 6$), headache ($n = 1$), and nausea ($n = 1$) [38]. In the dose-response study by Kauppila et al. seven women complained of side-effects including tiredness ($n = 1$), headache ($n = 1$), anxiety ($n = 1$), hair loss ($n = 1$) and intestinal disorders ($n = 1$), but the relationship between the adverse events and dose were not described [39]. While greater amounts of metoclopramide are secreted into the breast milk compared with domperidone, the reported absolute infant dose ranging from six to 24 micrograms/kg/day is still well below the recommended pediatric dose of 500 micrograms/kg/day [73]. Notably, metoclopramide was detected in the plasma of one infant and while no short-term neonatal adverse events have been identified, whether infants are more susceptible to potential longer-term adverse events of metoclopramide is unknown. This is of concern given the ease with which metoclopramide crosses the blood-brain barrier and therefore the potential to interrupt dopamine signaling in the newborn.

Similar to domperidone, metoclopramide also has the potential to cause serious maternal adverse events. Given that metoclopramide has the ability to cross the blood-brain barrier, it is more likely to cause central nervous system side effects than domperidone. Of particular concern is the increased risk of depression, which is already increased in the postpartum period. In the study by Ingram et al., two of 29 (7%) women receiving open-label metoclopramide after the initial 10-day trial reported experiencing depression [29]. Metoclopramide also has the ability to cause serious and potentially permanent extrapyramidal side effects such as tardive dyskinesia, for which it carries a black box warning in the product information. As such, it is recommended that metoclopramide not be used for longer than five days and that the maximum dose be limited to 10 mg three times daily. A large international internet survey of women who took metoclopramide to increase breast milk supply found that 4.8% of women had either palpitations or racing heart rate, 12% reported depression, and 1 to 7% reported other central nervous system side effects ranging from dizziness and headache to involuntary grimacing and tremors [74]. The overall adverse event profile of metoclopramide makes it less desirable than domperidone to use as a galactagogue, with evidence directly comparing the two outlined below.

5.3. Domperidone Compared To Metoclopramide

While domperidone and metoclopramide are both dopamine antagonists and increase serum prolactin concentrations, they do differ with respect to some pharmacodynamic properties. One of these key properties relates to the ability to cross the blood-brain barrier, with only metoclopramide able to do so in appreciable quantities. This has led to questions regarding potential differences in the efficacy and safety of these two medications. Two studies have directly compared outcomes among women taking domperidone and metoclopramide. Blank et al. identified a slightly greater increase in the daily breast milk volume among nine women receiving domperidone (120 ± 81 mL/day to 239 ± 105 mL/day) than among eleven women receiving metoclopramide (100 ± 53 mL/day to 184 ± 100 mL /day) [28]. The 35 mL/day difference between those receiving domperidone and metoclopramide, however, was not statistically significant. Ingram et al. demonstrated a similar difference in breast milk volume for those receiving domperidone compared with metoclopramide (31.0 mL/day; 95%CI −5.67 to 67.6 mL/day), among a total sample of 65 women [29].

When it comes to maternal adverse events, Blank et al. reported that minor neurobehavioral symptoms of either drowsiness, sleep disturbance, restlessness or dizziness were experienced by two of nine women taking domperidone and two of 11 women taking metoclopramide [28]. In contrast, Ingram et al. reported that seven (20%) of women taking metoclopramide reported experiencing adverse events compared with just three (10%) of women taking domperidone. Notably, one woman taking metoclopramide withdrew from the study due to experiencing bad headaches and dry mouth [29]. Greater incidence of adverse events with metoclopramide is also evident from observational studies, with a 2010 Internet survey of 1990 mothers identifying a 7-fold increased risk of depression, and 4 to 19-fold increased risk of symptoms commonly associated with tardive dyskinesia (e.g., tremors, involuntary grimaces, and jerking) among women taking metoclopramide compared with domperidone [75].

5.4. Sulpiride

Sulpiride is a dopamine antagonist, traditionally used as an antipsychotic, and is thought to act as a galactagogue by increasing serum prolactin (Figure 1). The effects of sulpiride in increasing breast milk supply have been evaluated in two placebo-controlled studies [41,42]. Both utilised a dose of 50 mg three times daily compared with placebo, with the treatment duration ranging from 14 to 28 days. It is unclear from both studies as to the infant gestational age. Both studies demonstrated a greater increase in breast milk volume among those receiving sulpiride, with improvements of 218 mL/day and 315 mL/day and associated reductions in the requirement for supplemental feeds. However, both studies experienced greater than 20% loss to follow-up in the placebo group which was reported to be due to insufficient treatment response, indicating significant potential for bias. While previous clinical trials in lactation have reported few adverse events associated with the use of sulpiride and the doses used in these trials are lower than those thought to produce significant neuroleptic effects in adults, data are still limited and there remains concerns regarding potential maternal or infant effects. Common adverse events include sedation and weight gain, while sulpiride may also cause extrapyramidal side effects similar to metoclopramide. Of greater concern is that the relative infant exposure to sulpiride through breast milk is up to 20% of the maternal weight-adjusted dose [49], which is much greater than that for other galactagogues.

5.5. Growth Hormone

The exact mechanisms of action of growth hormone in lactation remain unclear. The growth hormone is released by the anterior pituitary gland and acts synergistically to prolactin [12]. Administration of the growth hormone has been demonstrated to increase secretion of the insulin-like growth factor, providing evidence that the galactopoietic response to the growth hormone occurs as a result of indirect effects on mammary glands [44]. Two studies have evaluated the administration of the human growth hormone [43,44]. The first placebo-controlled study enrolled mothers of preterm infants (<34 week's gestation) and involved a subcutaneous administration of 0.2 international units/kg/day for seven days. Those receiving growth hormone experienced an increase in breast milk volume (139 ± 49 to 175 ± 46 mL/day; $p < 0.01$), but no difference was evident among those receiving placebo (93 ± 50 to 102 ± 69 mL/day; p = not stated). The second study, by the same authors, enrolled mothers of term infants and investigated three doses ranging from 0.05 to 0.2 international units/kg/day for seven days [44]. Women in the high dose arm (0.2 IU) experienced a greater percentage increase in breast milk volume than those in the low- (0.05 IU) and mid- (0.1 IU) dose arms (36 ± 12.6% compared to. 4.7 ± 9.7%; $p < 0.04$) [44]. Absolute differences in milk volume identified in the two previously reported studies were 25 and 86 mL/day, respectively. No maternal or infant adverse events were reported within either study. Overall, the relatively modest improvements in breast milk supply observed with growth hormone do not seem to justify the high costs and administration challenges associated with the treatment, particularly in comparison to alternative galactagogues such as domperidone or metoclopramide.

5.6. Recombinant Human Prolactin

Given that prolactin is a critical component of establishing lactation, the direct administration of prolactin is viewed as an approach for treating lactation insufficiency that is the result of prolactin deficiency (Figure 1). One study that involved the administration of recombinant human prolactin (r-hPRL) was identified [45]. The placebo-controlled study enrolled mothers of preterm infants (<32 weeks gestation) with prolactin deficiency, and involved subcutaneous administration of either 60 micrograms/kg twice daily or 60 micrograms/kg once daily for seven days. The subgroup analysis revealed that milk volumes were higher in the group treated with twice daily r-hPRL (429 ± 338%) than in the group receiving only placebo (−12 ± 27%; $p < 0.05$). No significant differences were observed with respect to maternal or infant adverse events. While data are limited, this study demonstrates that r-hPRL may be a viable option for the treatment of lactation insufficiency among women with established prolactin deficiency. Given the high costs and administration challenges associated with the treatment, this remains a treatment for rare situations where alternative prolactin stimulating medications such as domperidone are unsuitable, as is the case with the Sheehan syndrome or congenital prolactin deficiency where lactotrophs are absent or reduced in number.

5.7. Thyrotrophin Releasing Hormone

The thyrotrophin-releasing hormone (TRH) acts on the anterior pituitary to increase serum prolactin concentrations (Figure 1). Two studies were identified that involved the administration of TRH, producing mixed results [46,47]. One study randomised women to receive either TRH ($n = 5$) or placebo ($n = 4$) orally [47]. Among women treated with TRH, only one woman experienced an increase in serum prolactin. Actual breast milk volumes were not described, with the effect on milk production reported as 'no change' for all women among the treatment and placebo arms of the study. The second study enrolled mothers of term infants and involved the intranasal administration of 1 mg four times daily for 10 days. Those receiving TRH experienced an increase in breast milk volume (142.0 ± 33.9 g/day to 253.0 ± 105.3 g/day; $p = 0.014$), but no difference was evident among those receiving placebo (150.0 ± 46.2 g/day to 140.6 ± 57.7 g/day; $p = 0.87$). The increase in breast milk volume was accompanied by an observed increase in basal prolactin levels from a mean of 117 (± 45) micrograms/L to 173 (± 56) micrograms/L among women receiving TRH, whereas those receiving placebo experienced a decrease in basal prolactin levels (137 ± 70 micrograms/L to 82 ± 38 micrograms/L). No maternal or infant adverse events were reported in these two studies. However, reported effects on thyroid function have been mixed based on open-label non-controlled studies, with one demonstrating no changes in maternal or infant thyroid function [47], while one study identified two cases of maternal hyperthyroidism among 13 women treated with TRH which required treatment discontinuation [59]. Given the potential severity of adverse events and mixed findings of previous studies, more research on the use of TRH is necessary before its consideration in clinical practice.

5.8. Oxytocin

Despite the important role of oxytocin in regulating milk ejection, no studies have evaluated the use of oxytocin in the setting of established lactation insufficiency. Existing literature is restricted to studies enrolling women soon after delivery, with treatment undertaken in an effort to augment early milk supply and prevent the development of lactation insufficiency [53,54,56–58]. These studies have produced conflicting findings and their relevance to the treatment of women with established lactation insufficiency is uncertain. As it currently stands, there is insufficient evidence whether oxytocin may be an effective treatment for lactation insufficiency. However, given evidence that acute or chronic stress can interfere with oxytocin secretion, inhibiting both milk transfer and mother-infant bonding [20], further research on the potential usefulness of oxytocin in the setting of established lactation insufficiency is warranted, particularly among mothers of preterm infants where high levels of anxiety and depressive symptoms are common.

5.9. Metformin

Metformin is commonly used in the management of type 2 diabetes and is thought to act as a galactagogue through its role as an insulin-sensitising medication (Figure 1). The effects of metformin in increasing breast milk supply have been evaluated in one placebo controlled study [48]. The pilot study enrolled mothers of term infants who were experiencing low breast milk production and who had at least one sign of insulin resistance (e.g., elevated fasting plasma glucose). Women were randomised to either metformin ($n = 10$) or placebo ($n = 5$) with metformin dose increasing from 750 mg/day to 2000 mg/day over a 28-day treatment period. Peak median change in the milk output did not differ between those receiving metformin (+8; IQR –23 to 33 mL/day) or placebo (–58; IQR –62 to –1 mL/day) ($p = 0.31$). Notably, a greater increase in milk output was evident among those who managed to continue taking metformin for the entire treatment period, but only 20% of women assigned to the metformin arm experienced any actual improvement in milk output to day 28. Gastrointestinal adverse events were commonly reported, including diarrhoea (56%), nausea/vomiting (44%), and abdominal pain or cramping (56%), but were mostly of mild or moderate severity. One woman discontinued metformin due to the severity of abdominal cramping. No infant adverse events were reported. Given evidence on metformin is restricted to a small pilot study, its potential role as a galactagogue remains uncertain.

5.10. Summary of Galactagogue Efficacy and Safety

The largest and strongest body of evidence supports the use of domperidone as the first-line medication for the pharmacological management of lactation insufficiency. Domperidone represents a low cost treatment that is well tolerated, with moderate quality evidence that it produces a modest increase in breast milk supply in mothers of preterm infants. Whether results are translatable to mothers of term infants remain unclear as there are a limited number of high quality studies that include this patient population. Domperidone has been associated with serious adverse events and therefore is not suitable for all women, however, following appropriate screening prior to prescribing the risk of serious adverse events appear negligible. There is weak evidence that domperidone may be slightly more effective than metoclopramide and that adverse events are more likely to occur with metoclopramide than domperidone. Metoclopramide may be an appropriate alternative for use in women where domperidone is unsuitable. Antipsychotics do not reflect a viable therapeutic option for the management of lactation insufficiency, largely owing to their side effects such as extrapyramidal reactions and weight gain. Limited evidence and difficulties with respect to access to and administration of medications such as growth hormone, recombinant human prolactin and thyrotrophin-releasing hormone make these less desirable treatment options. Lastly, while an initially promising therapy for improving breast milk supply among women with signs of insulin resistance, initial findings from a pilot study evaluating metformin do not provide compelling evidence to support its use as a therapeutic treatment of lactation insufficiency.

6. Methodological Challenges and Evidence Gaps Regarding Galactagogues

6.1. Previous Study Limitations

Clinical studies evaluating the use of pharmaceutical galactagogues suffer from a number of important methodological limitations. Highlighting these limitations is not only important in considering the quality of existing evidence, but also in informing future research endeavors. The major limitation of the existing evidence lies in the small number of women included in clinical trials, limiting the potential to comprehensively evaluate both the efficacy and safety of these medications. Studies ranged from 7 to 100 participants, with a median of only 24. Many studies were therefore underpowered to detect statistically or clinically significant differences in breast milk supply or adverse events. Further, smaller studies face greater challenges in achieving balance in the distribution of baseline covariates across study groups. For example, in the study by Nommsen-Rivers et al., six out of 10 (60%) women receiving metformin were also taking the herbal galactagogue fenugreek, compared with one out of five (20%) women in the placebo arm [48]. In the study by Knoppert et al., five out of seven (71%) women in the high dose domperidone arm were primiparous, compared with three out of eight (38%) in the low dose domperidone arm [34], whereas in the study by da Silva et al. six out of nine (67%) women in the placebo arm were primiparous, compared with six out of seven (86%) in the domperidone arm [31]. Such differences in the baseline distribution of factors potentially related to breast milk volume or treatment response to galactagogue can significantly bias study findings and highlights the importance of large, appropriately controlled trials.

Many studies suffer from potential selection bias due to the high loss to follow-up in one or both treatment arms. This is particularly important where the loss to follow-up is related to the treatment response and only including data on those successfully completing the study potentially biases the results towards those with more favorable treatment response. Greater than 10% loss to follow-up in one or both intervention arms was evident among nine studies [28,29,31,34,36,37,39,41,42].

Non-pharmacological breastfeeding strategies are the mainstay of treatment for lactation insufficiency, but their implementation and utilisation across clinical trials of galactagogues is often incompletely described. This makes it unclear what strategies have been utilised and whether these have been applied equally across treatment groups.

Two studies reported the encouragement of skin-to-skin contact between the mother and infant [29,37], while some provided advice regarding the minimum number of times women expressed each day, ranging from four to eight however the frequency of pumping was not accounted for despite strong relationships with the milk volume [28,29,34,37,43,48]. All studies where mothers were expressing breast milk reported the use of electric pumps, which have been shown to be more effective in the establishment of milk production than hand expression [75].

Definitions for lactation insufficiency varied widely across studies and involved the use of an absolute volume measure (e.g., <500 mL/day) [27,28,33,34,38,44,45], relative volume measure (e.g.,

< 250 mL/kg/day) [29,35,37,39,41,42,46], requirement for supplemental feeds [30–32,43], insufficient infant weight gain [39], or certain reduction in supply based on previous milk production [14,23,37]. Given that there is no universally accepted definition of lactation insufficiency in the literature, it is unsurprising that definitions used across studies vary greatly. It is uncertain, however, whether the baseline milk volume has any impact on the treatment response to pharmaceutical galactagogues and this could possibly explain some heterogeneity across clinical studies. Linked with this concept is the complete absence of any noted targets regarding the optimal breast milk volume in previously published clinical trials. This is particularly important for mothers of preterm infants where the inclusion of an optimal treatment target could have an impact on the treatment response. For example, if the target is simply defined as meeting the infants' daily feed requirements and the infant is only 1 kg, the target is approximately 150 mL. As the infant grows, however, that target will shift and women whose daily breast milk production remains at 150 mL/day will find it difficult to keep up with their infants' demands and this may lead to eventual cessation of breastfeeding. As an example, Meier and Engstrom have suggested that for mothers of very low birth weight infants a desirable milk volume target is at least 350 mL/day by the end of the second postnatal week [76]. Higher volumes (e.g., 600 to 800 mL/day) are considered even more desirable and are more likely to sustain long-term breastfeeding outcomes [76]. Among the studies included in this review, the median breast milk volume increased from 146 mL/day to 276 mL/day, with only five studies reporting a final mean volume above the proposed target of 350 mL/day [27,30,34,35,38], with all involving the use of either domperidone or metoclopramide. This indicates that the hormonal manipulation utilising existing therapeutic approaches may not be adequate to reverse the poor development of the mammary gland during pregnancy and milk synthesis after it is has been established.

While galactagogues may provide short-term improvements in breast milk supply, their relationship to longer-term breastfeeding outcomes is unknown. Long-term outcomes are particularly challenging to assess among placebo controlled trials as once the trial has completed many women are often able to take the intervention medication off-label. This means long-term outcomes become confounded by maternal behaviors following completion of the trial. With that in mind, few studies have reported long-term breastfeeding outcomes. Asztalos et al. provided the most comprehensive evaluation, with 60% of women still breastfeeding once their infants reached the term gestation corrected age, with 70% requiring additional supplementation [37]. Notably, 67% of women were still using lactation-inducting compounds following completion of the study. A major criticism of previous studies is that the majority only compare differences in supply between groups, not adjusting for baseline milk production. Adjusting for baseline values has been demonstrated to significantly improve statistical power, particularly where there is a strong correlation between baseline and final value [77].

Lastly, while no specific methodological limitation of the studies were included in this review, it is worthwhile to comment on the large number of studies that have investigated the use of pharmaceutical galactagogues in the setting where lactation insufficiency has not been diagnosed [49–58]. We do not feel that one can accurately draw evidence on the efficacy or safety of galactagogues where they are utilised in the absence of a clear established clinical indication. There is currently no evidence to support the prophylactic administration of galactagogues in the absence of the diagnosis of lactation insufficiency, while an associated concern with the use of galactagogues is that they may come at the cost of appropriate utilisation of non-pharmacological treatment strategies.

6.2. *Impact of Galactagogues on Breast Milk Composition*

Prolactin is thought to mediate changes in breast milk composition occurring during normal lactogenesis [78]. In vitro and animal studies provide evidence that in early lactation prolactin promotes the closure of epithelial tight junctions between alveolar cells and increases the synthesis of α-lactalbumin, which in turn increases breast milk volume [78]. Prolactin has also been demonstrated to influence secretion of immunomodulatory factors in breast milk, with the decreasing concentrations of these factors occurring over the course of lactation mirroring reductions in serum prolactin concentrations also occurring over time [78]. Whether galactagogues, particularly those altering prolactin concentrations, alter the macronutrient composition of the human milk has been examined in just two studies, one involving domperidone [30], and the other recombinant human prolactin [78]. These studies evaluated changes in a number of breast milk constituents including sodium, calcium, lactose, citrate, protein, fat, alpha-lactalbumin, IgA, and oligosaccharides. Such changes in breast milk composition are particularly important for preterm infants, who have higher protein, energy, mineral, and electrolyte requirements than term infants and are at risk of cumulative nutritional deficits and postnatal growth restriction during early life [79]. As such, multi-component breast milk fortifiers (including protein) are routinely added to expressed breast milk to assist preterm infants in meeting their nutrition and growth requirements.

Powe et al. investigated the composition of breast milk among 11 women receiving recombinant human prolactin. The mean time following birth was 12 weeks and ranged from 3.5 to 39 weeks). Overall compositional changes mirrored those in women undergoing normal lactogenesis, with an observed increase in lactose and calcium concentrations, and decreased sodium concentrations that all fell within normal ranges [78]. The observed 200 mL/day increase in breast milk production was thought to be related to the increasing synthesis of alpha-lactalbumin and a corresponding increase in lactose levels, which acts as an osmotic agent to draw additional fluid into milk secretory vesicles [78]. Further, greater maturity was reflected by a decrease in milk sodium concentration, consistent with the closure of tight junctions between the mammary epithelial cells. Lastly, recombinant human prolactin administration led to an increase in overall oligosaccharide concentrations [78]. Oligosaccharide concentrations traditionally decrease during lactogenesis, but observed increases in both neutral and acidic oligosaccharide levels could indicate immunological benefits for the infants. In contrast, no statistically significant differences were observed with respect to changes in milk fat, protein or citrate levels.

In comparison to Powe et al., Campbell-Yeo et al. investigated changes in breast milk composition among a cohort of 45 women randomised to either domperidone or placebo. The mean time following birth was not reported, but 75% of women were randomised prior to four weeks. Compared to those receiving placebo, women administered domperidone experienced a greater improvement in breast milk volume of 163 mL/day, with significant increases in breast milk carbohydrate and calcium, but not sodium. While not statistically significant, mean breast milk protein declined by 9.6% in the domperidone group and increased by 3.6% in the placebo group ($p = 0.16$) [30]. The mechanisms contributing to a possible decrease in the protein concentration are unclear, but are comparable to the 15% reduction in protein observed by Powe et al. following the administration of recombinant human prolactin. It is well known that the milk produced by mothers of preterm infants is higher in protein and this becomes comparable to the breast milk produced by mothers of term infants by 10–12 weeks postpartum [80]. It is possible that the administration of galactagogues altering prolactin levels results in a more rapid transition towards mature breast milk with a resultant reduction in the protein concentration occurring as a natural result of increasing breast milk volume. However, given the limited evidence available, future studies evaluating whether galactagogues alter human breast milk composition are required before a more definitive conclusion can be reached. In order to evaluate this effectively, a comparison of breast milk composition must be made to mothers unaffected by lactation insufficiency in order to determine whether any changes in composition are just reflective of improvements in breast milk supply, or the direct effect of galactagogues. Therefore, a key evidence gap relates to the need for a more comprehensive evaluation of breast milk composition that takes into account postnatal age and breast milk volume.

6.3. Predicting Treatment Response to Galactagogues

There are many factors associated with breastfeeding success, with non-pharmacological treatment strategies clearly first-line in the management of lactation insufficiency. Despite adherence to such strategies (e.g., expressing technique, expressing frequency), the treatment response to galactagogues is noted to be variable in clinical practice. Despite this anecdotal experience, we are unaware of any prospective studies that have examined predictors of treatment response to galactagogues such as domperidone. Most clinical studies simply report the average treatment effect of the galactagogue used, but a small number of studies have reported the individual level data with significant variability in treatment response evident. Wan et al. examined changes in daily breast milk volume in response to treatment with either 30 mg or 60 mg daily doses of domperidone. Among the six women studied, two demonstrated no improvement at all in the daily breast milk volume, representing a non-response rate of 33% [27]. A similar treatment response was identified by Da Silva et al. with two of seven women experiencing less than 10% improvement in daily breast milk volume following the treatment with domperidone, representing a non-response rate of 30% [31].

Given these findings, understanding factors that contribute towards the response to domperidone is important in identifying groups of women most likely to benefit from treatment, while also enabling the potential identification of other important targets for improving breast milk volume. One such factor may be maternal BMI, where it has already been previously reported that overweight/obese mothers of term infants experience a lower prolactin response to infant suckling [81]. The possible impacts of maternal obesity on treatment response to domperidone have been investigated in a recent retrospective cohort study of mothers of preterm infants. In this study, a significant treatment interaction was observed between domperidone and obesity, with obese women less likely to still be breastfeeding their infants at discharge from the Neonatal Unit than non-obese women, despite both receiving domperidone [82]. Obese women were also noted to be more likely to require a prolonged course of domperidone [82]. This may be due to hormonal or inflammatory differences associated with obesity and warrants further investigation. Of particular interest is the role of the toll-like receptor 4 (TLR4) immune signalling pathway, which plays an important role in obesity and the metabolic syndrome [83]. Further, the TLR4 pathway, regardless of whether it is activated by an infection or a sterile inflammatory pathway, is recognised as a key mediator of preterm labor [84]. This is important as TLR4 signalling may be a key factor involved in the delayed secretory activation and development of low milk supply, commonly experienced by many mothers of preterm infants. When exposed to a bacterial by-product in a mouse model of mastitis [85], it is the TLR4 signalling that is responsible for low milk supply, not the bacterium itself [86]. This surprising finding has led to a new paradigm for lactation insufficiency, whereby TLR4 signalling leads to lactocyte cell death and consequently a reduced capacity to produce milk [87]. The presence of asymptomatic breast inflammation could result in unresponsiveness to domperidone (or other galactagogues) whereby the prolactin-mediated signal to stimulate lactocytes to produce more milk is negated by the inflammatory signal. No studies have prospectively evaluated the role of such inflammatory factors in the development of low milk supply or the response to treatment with galactagogues such as domperidone.

In addition to previously described factors, serum prolactin levels could determine the treatment response to galactagogues that alter prolactin concentrations. Kauppila et al. demonstrated that three of five mothers who did not respond to the metoclopramide treatment had the highest basal prolactin levels [72]. Further, while the effects of parity on changes in breast milk supply following treatment with domperidone or metoclopramide have not been previously investigated, there is evidence that nulliparous women are more sensitive to the prolactin stimulatory effects of domperidone/metoclopramide than parous women [88]. This could necessitate the need for different doses or treatment approaches based on parity, but requires further investigation.

Other factors that could influence the treatment response to galactagogues include gestational age at birth and timing of the treatment initiation following birth. Both of these were explored in the recent EMPOWER study, which evaluated the use of domperidone compared to placebo over 14 days [37]. Following the end of the initial treatment period women who received placebo went on to receive domperidone for 14 days. This enabled investigation of the potential effects of delaying the treatment with domperidone for 14 days. At the end of 28 days, the mean daily milk volume was similar between those who immediately started on domperidone compared with those who had treatment with domperidone delayed by 14 days (290 ± 211 mL/day vs. 302 ± 230 mL/day; $p = 0.88$) [37]. Additionally, they observed no significant difference between the number of women who had delivered between 23–26 weeks gestation or 27–29 weeks gestation and achieved a 50% increase in breast milk volume (72.9% compared to 64.2%; $p = 0.38$) [89].

7. Conclusions

The largest and strongest body of evidence supports the use of domperidone as the first-line medication for the pharmacological management of lactation insufficiency but the observed treatment effects are modest at best. There is currently insufficient evidence to determine whether the use of galactagogues has any negative impacts on the micro- and macro-nutrient composition of breast milk and this requires further research. There is emerging evidence of potential differences in the treatment response to galactagogues and further research in this space is critical for improving the therapeutic management of lactation insufficiency. There is a critical need for studies identifying underlying mechanisms contributing towards the development of lactation insufficiency and how these impact the treatment response to various pharmaceutical galactagogues. Such knowledge would facilitate the development and evaluation of novel pharmaceutical treatments for lactation insufficiency while also improve our understanding of individual variability in treatment response to improve utilisation and outcomes of existing treatments.

Author Contributions: Conceptualization, L.E.G.; Writing—Original Draft Preparation, L.E.G.; Writing—Review and Editing, M.E.W., D.T.G.

Acknowledgments: L.E.G. acknowledges the salary support provided by an Australia National Health and Medical Research Council (NHMRC) Early Career Fellowship (GNT 1070421), Robinson Research Institute Career Development Fellowship and Lloyd Cox Research Fellowship. D.T.G. acknowledges the salary support provided by an unrestricted research grant from Medela AG (Switzerland).

References

1. Gartner, L.M.; Morton, J.; Lawrence, R.A.; Naylor, A.J.; O'Hare, D.; Schanler, R.J.; Eidelman, A.I. Breastfeeding and the use of human milk. *Pediatrics* **2005**, *115*, 496–506.
2. Kramer, M.S.; Kakuma, R. Optimal duration of exclusive breastfeeding. *Cochrane Database Syst. Rev.* **2012**, *8*, CD003517. [CrossRef]
3. Meier, P.; Patel, A.; Esquerra-Zwiers, A. Donor human milk update: Evidence, mechanisms, and priorities for research and practice. *J. Pediatr.* **2017**, *180*, 15–21. [CrossRef]
4. Chung, M.; Raman, G.; Chew, P.; Magula, N.; Trikalinos, T.; Lau, J. Breastfeeding and maternal and infant health outcomes in developed countries. *Evid. Technol. Asses. (Full Rep.)* **2007**, *153*, 1–186.
5. Victora, C.G.; Bahl, R.; Barros, A.J.; França, G.V.; Horton, S.; Krasevec, J.; Murch, S.; Sankar, M.J.; Walker, N.; Rollins, N.C. Breastfeeding in the 21st century: Epidemiology, mechanisms, and lifelong effect. *Lancet* **2016**, *387*, 475–490. [CrossRef]
6. Quigley, M.; Embleton, N.; McGuire, W. Formula versus donor breast milk for feeding preterm or low birth weight infants. *Cochrane Database Syst. Rev.* **2018**, *6*, CD002971. [CrossRef]
7. Vohr, B.R.; Poindexter, B.B.; Dusick, A.M.; McKinley, L.T.; Higgins, R.D.; Langer, J.C.; Poole, W.K. Persistent beneficial effects of breast milk ingested in the neonatal intensive care unit on outcomes of extremely low birth weight infants at 30 months of age. *Pediatrics* **2007**, *120*, e953–e959. [CrossRef]
8. Belfort, M.B.; Anderson, P.J.; Nowak, V.A.; Lee, K.J.; Molesworth, C.; Thompson, D.K.; Doyle, L.W.; Inder, T.E. Breast milk feeding, brain development, and neurocognitive outcomes: A 7-year longitudinal study in infants born at less than 30 weeks' gestation. *J. Pediatr.* **2016**, *177*, 133–139. [CrossRef] [PubMed]
9. Bell, E.H.; Geyer, J.; Jones, L. A structured intervention improves breastfeeding success for ill or preterm infants. *MCN Am. J. Matern. Child. Nurs.* **1995**, *20*, 309–314. [CrossRef] [PubMed]

10. Amir, L.H. Breastfeeding: Managing 'supply' difficulties. *Aust. Fam. Physician* **2006**, *35*, 686–689.
11. Li, R.; Fein, S.B.; Chen, J.; Grummer-Strawn, L.M. Why mothers stop breastfeeding: Mothers' self-reported reasons for stopping during the first year. *Pediatrics* **2008**, *122*, S69–S76. [CrossRef] [PubMed]
12. Lee, S.; Kelleher, S.L. Biological underpinnings of breastfeeding challenges: The role of genetics, diet and environment on lactation physiology. *Am. J. Physiol. Heart Circ. Physiol.* **2016**, *311*, E405–E422. [CrossRef] [PubMed]
13. Neville, M.C. Anatomy and physiology of lactation. *Pediatr. Clin. North. Am.* **2001**, *48*, 13–34. [CrossRef]
14. Crowley, W.R. Neuroendocrine regulation of lactation and milk production. *Compr. Physiol.* **2015**, *5*, 255–291.
15. Forinash, A.B.; Yancey, A.M.; Barnes, K.N.; Myles, T.D. The use of galactogogues in the breastfeeding mother. *Ann. Pharmacother.* **2012**, *46*, 1392–1404. [CrossRef]
16. Stuebe, A.M.; Grewen, K.; Pedersen, C.A.; Propper, C.; Meltzer-Brody, S. Failed lactation and perinatal depression: Common problems with shared neuroendocrine mechanisms? *J. Womens Health (Larchmt)* **2012**, *21*, 264–272. [CrossRef] [PubMed]
17. Amir, L.H. Managing common breastfeeding problems in the community. *BMJ* **2014**, *348*, g2954. [CrossRef] [PubMed]
18. Sultana, A.; Rahman, K.; Manjula, S. Clinical update and treatment of lactation insufficiency. *Med. J. Islamic. World Acad. Sci.* **2013**, *21*, 19–28. [CrossRef]
19. Cregan, M.D.; De Mello, T.R.; Kershaw, D.; McDougall, K.; Hartmann, P.E. Initiation of lactation in women after preterm delivery. *Acta. Obstet. Gynecol. Scand.* **2002**, *81*, 870–877. [CrossRef]
20. Brownell, E.; Howard, C.R.; Lawrence, R.A.; Dozier, A.M. Delayed onset lactogenesis ii predicts the cessation of any or exclusive breastfeeding. *J. Pediatr.* **2012**, *161*, 608–614. [CrossRef]
21. Gilmartin, C.; Amir, L.H.; Ter, M.; Grzeskowiak, L. Using domperidone to increase breast milk supply: A clinical practice survey of australian neonatal units. *J. Pharm. Pract. Res.* **2017**, *47*, 426–430. [CrossRef]
22. Grzeskowiak, L.E.; Hill, M.; Kennedy, D.S. Phone calls to an australian pregnancy and lactation counselling service regarding use of galactagogues during lactation–the Mothersafe experience. *Aust. N. Z. J. Obstet. Gynaecol.* **2018**, *58*, 251–254. [CrossRef] [PubMed]
23. Grzeskowiak, L.E.; Lim, S.W.; Thomas, A.E.; Ritchie, U.; Gordon, A.L. Audit of domperidone use as a galactogogue at an Australian tertiary teaching hospital. *J. Hum. Lact.* **2013**, *29*, 32–37. [CrossRef]
24. Smolina, K.; Morgan, S.G.; Hanley, G.E.; Oberlander, T.F.; Mintzes, B. Postpartum domperidone use in British Columbia: A retrospective cohort study. *CMAJ Open* **2016**, *4*, E13–E19. [CrossRef]
25. Mehrabadi, A.; Reynier, P.; Platt, R.W.; Filion, K.B. Domperidone for insufficient lactation in England 2002-2015: A drug utilization study with interrupted time series analysis. *Pharmacoepidemiol. Drug Saf.* **2018**, *27*, 1316–1324. [CrossRef]
26. Grzeskowiak, L.E.; Dalton, J.A.; Fielder, A.L. Factors associated with domperidone use as a galactogogue at an Australian tertiary teaching hospital. *J. Hum. Lact.* **2015**, *31*, 249–253. [CrossRef] [PubMed]
27. Wan, E.W.; Davey, K.; Page-Sharp, M.; Hartmann, P.E.; Simmer, K.; Ilett, K.F. Dose-effect study of domperidone as a galactagogue in preterm mothers with insufficient milk supply, and its transfer into milk. *Br. J. Clin. Pharmacol.* **2008**, *66*, 283–289. [CrossRef]
28. Blank, C.; Eaton, V.; Bennett, J.; James, S.L. A double blind rct of domperidone and metoclopramide as pro-lactational agents in mothers of preterm infants. Perinatal Society of Australia and New Zealand 5th Annual Conference, Canberra, Australia, 13–16 March 2001; p. 73.
29. Ingram, J.; Taylor, H.; Churchill, C.; Pike, A.; Greenwood, R. Metoclopramide or domperidone for increasing maternal breast milk output: A randomised controlled trial. *Arch. Dis. Child. Fetal. Neonatal. Ed.* **2012**, *97*, F241–F245. [CrossRef] [PubMed]
30. Campbell-Yeo, M.L.; Allen, A.C.; Joseph, K.; Ledwidge, J.M.; Caddell, K.; Allen, V.M.; Dooley, K.C. Effect of domperidone on the composition of preterm human breast milk. *Pediatrics* **2010**, *125*, e107–e114. [CrossRef]
31. Da Silva, O.P.; Knoppert, D.C.; Angelini, M.M.; Forret, P.A. Effect of domperidone on milk production in mothers of premature newborns: A randomized, double-blind, placebo-controlled trial. *Can. Med. Assoc. J.* **2001**, *164*, 17–21.
32. Fazilla, T.E.; Tjipta, G.D.; Ali, M.; Sianturi, P. Domperidone and maternal milk volume in mothers of premature newborns. *Paediatr. Indones.* **2017**, *57*, 18–22. [CrossRef]
33. Inam, I.; Hashmi, A.; Shahid, A. A comparison of efficacy of domperidone and placebo among postnatal women with inadequate breast milk production. *Pak. J. Med. Health Sci.* **2013**, *7*, 314–317.

34. Knoppert, D.C.; Page, A.; Warren, J.; Seabrook, J.A.; Carr, M.; Angelini, M.; Killick, D. The effect of two different domperidone doses on maternal milk production. *J. Hum. Lact.* **2013**, *29*, 38–44. [CrossRef]
35. Petraglia, F.; De Leo, V.; Sardelli, S.; Pieroni, M.L.; D'Antona, N.; Genazzani, A.R. Domperidone in defective and insufficient lactation. *Eur. J. Obstet. Gynaecol. Reprod. Biol.* **1985**, *19*, 281–287. [CrossRef]
36. Rai, R.; Mishra, N.; Singh, D. Effect of domperidone in 2nd week postpartum on milk output in mothers of preterm infants. *Indian J. Pediatr.* **2016**, *83*, 894–895. [CrossRef]
37. Asztalos, E.V.; Campbell-Yeo, M.; da Silva, O.P.; Ito, S.; Kiss, A.; Knoppert, D. Enhancing human milk production with domperidone in mothers of preterm infants: Results from the EMPOWER trial. *J. Hum. Lact.* **2017**, *33*, 181–187. [CrossRef] [PubMed]
38. Kauppila, A.; Anunti, P.; Kivinen, S.; Koivisto, M.; Ruokonen, A. Metoclopramide and breast feeding: Efficacy and anterior pituitary responses of the mother and the child. *Eur. J. Obstet. Gynaecol. Reprod. Biol.* **1985**, *19*, 19–22. [CrossRef]
39. Kauppila, A.; Kivinen, S.; Ylikorkala, O. A dose response relation between improved lactation and metoclopramide. *Lancet* **1981**, *317*, 1175–1177. [CrossRef]
40. Sakha, K.; Behbahan, A. Training for perfect breastfeeding or metoclopramide: Which one can promote lactation in nursing mothers? *Breastfeed. Med.* **2008**, *3*, 120–123. [CrossRef]
41. Ylikorkala, O.; Kauppila, A.; Kivinen, S.; Viinikka, L. Sulpiride improves inadequate lactation. *Br. Med. J.* **1982**, *285*, 249–251. [CrossRef]
42. Ylikorkala, O.; Kauppila, A.; Kivinen, S.; Viinikka, L. Treatment of inadequate lactation with oral sulpiride and buccal oxytocin. *Obstet. Gynecol.* **1984**, *63*, 57–60.
43. Gunn, A.J.; Gunn, T.R.; Rabone, D.L.; Breier, B.H.; Blum, W.F.; Gluckman, P.D. Growth hormone increases breast milk volumes in mothers of preterm infants. *Pediatrics* **1996**, *98*, 279–282.
44. Milsom, S.R.; Rabone, D.L.; Gunn, A.J.; Gluckman, P.D. Potential role for growth hormone in human lactation insufficiency. *Horm. Res. Paediatr.* **1998**, *50*, 147–150. [CrossRef]
45. Powe, C.E.; Allen, M.; Puopolo, K.M.; Merewood, A.; Worden, S.; Johnson, L.C.; Fleischman, A.; Welt, C.K. Recombinant human prolactin for the treatment of lactation insufficiency. *Clin. Endocrinol. (Oxf.)* **2010**, *73*, 645–653. [CrossRef]
46. Peters, F.; Schulze-Tollert, J.; Schuth, W. Thyrotrophin-releasing hormone—A lactation-promoting agent? *BJOG* **1991**, *98*, 880–885. [CrossRef]
47. Zarate, A.; Villalobos, H.; Canales, E.; Soria, J.; Arcovedo, F.; MacGregor, C. The effect of oral administration of thyrotropin-releasing hormone on lactation. *J. Clin. Endocrinol. Metab.* **1976**, *43*, 301–305. [CrossRef]
48. Nommsen-Rivers, L.; Thompson, A.; Riddle, S.; Ward, L.; Wagner, E.; King, E. Feasibility and ccceptability of metformin to augment low milk supply: A pilot randomized controlled trial. *J. Hum. Lact.* **2019**. [CrossRef]
49. Aono, T.; Shioji, T.; Aki, T.; Hirota, K.; Nomura, A.; Kurachi, K. Augmentation of puerperal lactation by oral administration of sulpiride. *J. Clin. Endocrinol. Metab.* **1979**, *48*, 478–482. [CrossRef] [PubMed]
50. De Gezelle, H.; Ooghe, W.; Thiery, M.; Dhont, M. Metoclopramide and breast milk. *Eur J. Obstet. Gynaecol. Reprod. Biol.* **1983**, *15*, 31–36. [CrossRef]
51. Fife, S.; Gill, P.; Hopkins, M.; Angello, C.; Boswell, S.; Nelson, K.M. Metoclopramide to augment lactation, does it work? A randomized trial. *J. Matern. Fetal. Med.* **2011**, *24*, 1317–1320. [CrossRef] [PubMed]
52. Hansen, W.F.; McAndrew, S.; Harris, K.; Zimmerman, M.B. Metoclopramide effect on breastfeeding the preterm infant: A randomized trial. *Obstet. Gynecol.* **2005**, *105*, 383–389. [CrossRef] [PubMed]
53. Huntingford, P.J. Intranasal use of synthetic oxytocin in management of breast-feeding. *Br. Med. J.* **1961**, *1*, 709–711. [CrossRef]
54. Ingerslev, M.; Pinholt, K. Oxytocin treatment during the establishment of lactation. *Acta. Obstet. Gynecol. Scand.* **1962**, *41*, 159–168. [CrossRef]
55. Lewis, P.; Devenish, C.; Kahn, C. Controlled trial of metoclopramide in the initiation of breast feeding. *Br. J. Clin. Pharmacol.* **1980**, *9*, 217–219. [CrossRef] [PubMed]
56. Luhman, L.A. The effect of intranasal oxytocin on lactation. *Obstet. Gynecol.* **1963**, *21*, 713–717. [PubMed]
57. Ruis, H.; Rolland, R.; Doesburg, W.; Broeders, G.; Corbey, R. Oxytocin enhances onset of lactation among mothers delivering prematurely. *Br. Med. J.* **1981**, *283*, 340–342. [CrossRef]
58. Fewtrell, M.S.; Loh, K.; Blake, A.; Ridout, D.; Hawdon, J. Randomised, double blind trial of oxytocin nasal spray in mothers expressing breast milk for preterm infants. *Arch. Dis. Child. Fetal. Neonatal. Ed.* **2006**, *91*, F169–F174. [CrossRef]

59. Tyson, J.; Perez, A.; Zanartu, J. Human lactational response to oral thyrotropin releasing hormone. *J. Clin. Endocrinol. Metab.* **1976**, *43*, 760–768. [CrossRef]
60. Grzeskowiak, L.E.; Smithers, L.G.; Amir, L.H.; Grivell, R.M. Domperidone for increasing breast milk volume in mothers expressing breast milk for their preterm infants – a systematic review and meta-analysis. *BJOG* **2018**, *125*, 1371–1378. [CrossRef]
61. Johannes, C.B.; Varas-Lorenzo, C.; McQuay, L.J.; Midkiff, K.D.; Fife, D. Risk of serious ventricular arrhythmia and sudden cardiac death in a cohort of users of domperidone: A nested case-control study. *Pharmacoepidemiol. Drug Saf.* **2010**, *19*, 881–888. [CrossRef]
62. Van Noord, C.; Dieleman, J.P.; van Herpen, G.; Verhamme, K. Domperidone and ventricular arrhythmia or sudden cardiac death: A population-based case-control study in the netherlands. *Drug Saf.* **2010**, *33*, 1003–1014. [CrossRef]
63. Sewell, C.A.; Chang, C.Y.; Chehab, M.M.; Nguyen, C.P. Domperidone for lactation: What health care providers need to know. *Obstet. Gynecol.* **2017**, *129*, 1054–1058. [CrossRef] [PubMed]
64. Bozzo, P.; Koren, G.; Ito, S. Health canada advisory on domperidone should I avoid prescribing domperidone to women to increase milk production? *Can. Fam. Physician* **2012**, *58*, 952–953. [PubMed]
65. Grzeskowiak, L. Use of domperidone to increase breast milk supply: Are women really dying to breastfeed? *J. Hum. Lact.* **2014**, *30*, 498–499. [CrossRef]
66. Doggrell, S.A.; Hancox, J.C. Cardiac safety concerns for domperidone, an antiemetic and prokinetic, and galactogogue medicine. *Expert Opin. Drug Saf.* **2014**, *13*, 131–138. [CrossRef] [PubMed]
67. Grzeskowiak, L.E. Domperidone for lactation: What health care providers really should know. *Obstet. Gynecol.* **2017**, *130*, 913. [CrossRef] [PubMed]
68. Grzeskowiak, L.E.; Amir, L.H. Pharmacological management of low milk supply with domperidone: Separating fact from fiction. *Med. J. Aust.* **2014**, *201*, 257–258. [CrossRef]
69. Biewenga, J.; Keung, C.; Solanki, B.; Natarajan, J.; Leitz, G.; Deleu, S.; Soons, P. Absence of QTc prolongation with domperidone: A randomized, double-blind, placebo-and positive-controlled thorough QT/QTc study in healthy volunteers. *Clin. Pharmacol. Drug Dev.* **2015**, *4*, 41–48. [CrossRef] [PubMed]
70. Smolina, K.; Mintzes, B.; Hanley, G.E.; Oberlander, T.F.; Morgan, S.G. The association between domperidone and ventricular arrhythmia in the postpartum period. *Pharmacoepidemiol. Drug Saf.* **2016**, *25*, 1210–1214. [CrossRef]
71. Grzeskowiak, L.E.; Smithers, L.G. Use of domperidone and risk of ventricular arrhythmia in the postpartum period: Getting to the heart of the matter. *Pharmacoepidemiol. Drug Saf.* **2017**, *26*, 863–864. [CrossRef]
72. Haase, B.; Taylor, S.N.; Mauldin, J.; Johnson, T.S.; Wagner, C.L. Domperidone for treatment of low milk supply in breast pump–dependent mothers of hospitalized premature infants a clinical protocol. *J. Hum. Lact.* **2016**, *32*, 373–381. [CrossRef]
73. Kauppila, A.; Arvela, P.; Koivisto, M.; Kivinen, S.; Ylikorkala, O.; Pelkonen, O. Metoclopramide and breast feeding: Transfer into milk and the newborn. *Eur J. Clin. Pharmacol.* **1983**, *25*, 819–823. [CrossRef]
74. Hale, T.W.; Kendall-Tackett, K.; Cong, Z. Domperidone versus metoclopramide: Self-reported side effects in a large sample of breastfeeding mothers who used these medications to increase milk production. *Clin. Lact.* **2018**, *9*, 10–17. [CrossRef]
75. Lussier, M.M.; Brownell, E.A.; Proulx, T.A.; Bielecki, D.M.; Marinelli, K.A.; Bellini, S.L.; Hagadorn, J.I. Daily breastmilk volume in mothers of very low birth weight neonates: A repeated-measures randomized trial of hand expression versus electric breast pump expression. *Breastfeed. Med.* **2015**, *10*, 312–317. [CrossRef]
76. Meier, P.P.; Engstrom, J.L. Evidence-based practices to promote exclusive feeding of human milk in very low-birthweight infants. *NeoReviews* **2007**, *8*, e467–e477. [CrossRef]
77. Borm, G.F.; Fransen, J.; Lemmens, W.A. A simple sample size formula for analysis of covariance in randomized clinical trials. *J. Clin. Epidemiol.* **2007**, *60*, 1234–1238. [CrossRef] [PubMed]
78. Powe, C.E.; Puopolo, K.M.; Newburg, D.S.; Lönnerdal, B.; Chen, C.; Allen, M.; Merewood, A.; Worden, S.; Welt, C.K. Effects of recombinant human prolactin on breast milk composition. *Pediatrics* **2011**, *127*, e359. [CrossRef]
79. Radmacher, P.G.; Adamkin, D.H. Fortification of human milk for preterm infants. *Semin. Fetal. Neonatal. Med.* **2017**, *22*, 30–35. [CrossRef]
80. Gidrewicz, D.A.; Fenton, T.R. A systematic review and meta-analysis of the nutrient content of preterm and term breast milk. *BMC Pediatr.* **2014**, *14*, 216. [CrossRef]

81. Rasmussen, K.M.; Kjolhede, C.L. Prepregnant overweight and obesity diminish the prolactin response to suckling in the first week postpartum. *Pediatrics* **2004**, *113*, e465–e471. [CrossRef]
82. Grzeskowiak, L.E.; Amir, L.H.; Smithers, L.G. Longer-term breastfeeding outcomes associated with domperidone use for lactation differs according to maternal weight. *Eur. J. Clin. Pharmacol.* **2018**, *74*, 1071–1075. [CrossRef]
83. Jialal, I.; Kaur, H.; Devaraj, S. Toll-like receptor status in obesity and metabolic syndrome: A translational perspective. *J. Clin. Endocrinol. Metab.* **2014**, *99*, 39–48. [CrossRef]
84. Keelan, J. Pharmacological inhibition of inflammatory pathways for the prevention of preterm birth. *J. Reprod. Immunol.* **2011**, *88*, 176–184. [CrossRef]
85. Ingman, W.V.; Glynn, D.J.; Hutchinson, M.R. Mouse models of mastitis–how physiological are they? *Int. Breastfeed. J.* **2015**, *10*, 12. [CrossRef]
86. Glynn, D.J.; Hutchinson, M.R.; Ingman, W.V. Toll-like receptor 4 regulates lipopolysaccharide-induced inflammation and lactation insufficiency in a mouse model of mastitis. *Biol. Reprod.* **2014**, *90*, 91. [CrossRef] [PubMed]
87. Ingman, W.V.; Glynn, D.J.; Hutchinson, M.R. Inflammatory mediators in mastitis and lactation insufficiency. *J. Mammary Gland Biol. Neoplasia* **2014**, *19*, 161–167. [CrossRef]
88. Brown, T.E.; Fernandes, P.A.; Grant, L.J.; Hutsul, J.-A.; McCoshen, J.A. Effect of parity on pituitary prolactin response to metoclopramide and domperidone: Implications for the enhancement of lactation. *J. Soc. Gynecol. Investig.* **2000**, *7*, 65–69. [CrossRef]
89. Asztalos, E.V.; Kiss, A.; da Silva, O.P.; Campbell-Yeo, M.; Ito, S.; Knoppert, D. Pregnancy gestation at delivery and breast milk production: A secondary analysis from the EMPOWER trial. *Matern. Health Neonatol. Perinatol.* **2018**, *4*, 21. [CrossRef]

8

Human Breast Milk NMR Metabolomic Profile across Specific Geographical Locations and its Association with the Milk Microbiota

Carlos Gómez-Gallego [1,*], Jose Manuel Morales [2,3,4], Daniel Monleón [2,4], Elloise du Toit [5], Himanshu Kumar [1], Kaisa M. Linderborg [6], Yumei Zhang [7], Baoru Yang [6], Erika Isolauri [8], Seppo Salminen [1] and Maria Carmen Collado [1,9,*]

1 Functional Foods Forum, Faculty of Medicine, University of Turku, 20014 Turku, Finland; kumar.himanshu@utu.fi (H.K.); sepsal@utu.fi (S.S.)
2 Laboratory of Metabolomics, Institute of Health Research-INCLIVA, 46010 Valencia, Spain; J.Manuel.Morales@uv.es (J.M.M.); daniel.monleon@uv.es (D.M.)
3 Unidad Central de Investigación en Medicina, University of Valencia, 46010 Valencia, Spain
4 Pathology Department, School of Medicine, University of Valencia, 46100 Valencia, Spain
5 Division of Medical Microbiology, Department of Pathology, University of Cape Town, 7925 Cape Town, South Africa; elloisedutoit@gmail.com
6 Food Chemistry and Food Development, Department of Biochemistry, University of Turku, 20014 Turku, Finland; kamayl@utu.fi (K.M.L.); bayang@utu.fi (B.Y.)
7 Department of Nutrition and Food Hygiene, School of Public Health, Peking University, 100191 Beijing, China; zhangyumei@bjmu.edu.cn
8 Department of Paediatrics, University of Turku and Turku University Hospital, 20520 Turku, Finland; eriiso@utu.fi
9 Department of Biotechnology, Institute of Agrochemistry and Food Technology-National Research Council (IATA-CSIC), 46980 Valencia, Spain
* Correspondence: cargom@utu.fi (C.G.-G.); mcolam@iata.csic.es (M.C.C.)

Abstract: The composition of human breast milk is highly variable, and it can be influenced by genetics, diet, lifestyle, and other environmental factors. This study aimed to investigate the impact of geographical location and mode of delivery on the nuclear magnetic resonance spectroscopy (NMR) metabolic profile of breast milk and its relationship with the milk microbiome. Human milk metabolic and microbiota profiles were determined using NMR and 16S rRNA gene sequencing, respectively, in 79 healthy women from Finland, Spain, South Africa, and China. Up to 68 metabolites, including amino acids, oligosaccharides, and fatty acid-associated metabolites, were identified in the milk NMR spectra. The metabolite profiles showed significant differences between geographical locations, with significant differences ($p < 0.05$) in the levels of galactose, lacto-*N*-fucopentaose III, lacto-*N*-fucopentaose I and 2-fucosyllactose, 3-fucosyllactose, lacto-*N*-difucohexaose II, lacto-*N*-fucopentaose III, 2-hydroxybutyrate, 3-hydroxybutyrate, proline, *N*-acetyl lysine, methyl-histidine, dimethylamine, kynurenine, urea, creatine and creatine phosphate, formate, lactate, acetate, phosphocholine, acetylcholine, LDL, VLDL, ethanolamine, riboflavin, hippurate, spermidine, spermine and uridine. Additionally, the effect of caesarean section on milk metabolome was dependent on the geographical region. Specific interrelations between human milk metabolites and microbiota were also identified. Proteobacteria, Actinobacteria, and Bacilli were most significantly associated with the milk metabolites, being either positively or negatively correlated depending on the metabolite. Our results reveal specific milk metabolomic profiles across geographical locations and also highlight the potential interactions between human milk's metabolites and microbes.

Keywords: human milk; metabolites; microbiome; mode of delivery; caesarean section; proton nuclear magnetic resonance

---

1. Introduction

Arguably, the cornerstone of healthy growth and development in children is breast feeding, since breast milk offers myriad physiological advantages when compared to other sources of nutrition. Indeed, the optimal model of infant feeding is the healthy breastfed child [1]. When compared with formula-fed infants, breastfed children exhibit a reduced risk of gastrointestinal and respiratory infections [2], allergic disease [3,4], and being overweight or obese, with the benefits actually extending beyond infancy [5,6].

Breast milk contains many biologically active compounds, such as growth factors, antimicrobial and immune-enhancing substances, oligosaccharides (HMOs), as well as a diverse and rich bacterial community [7–10].

The composition of human breast milk is determined by genetic factors, lifestyle, diet, and the age of the mother [11,12]. Furthermore, human milk's macronutrient composition varies across lactation, although it is relatively conserved between populations [13]. However, the determinants of the bioactive compounds are currently less well understood. While some components of human milk appear to be relatively stable across different locations, some, such as polyunsaturated fatty acids, vary according to the mother's diet [9,14], while others, such as polyamines [15], HMOs [16], and milk bacteria [9,17], seem to vary depending of multiple factors. The mode of birth has also been reported to be a modulating factor for human milk's composition, acting in a differential manner in different countries [9,15]. Yet, the complex interactions between the constituents of milk, the biological impact, and the consequences for the infant's health in the short- and long-term remain unclear.

In addition, the host-milk microbial interactions may be influenced by the presence and/or concentration of milk metabolites, which may in turn influence the intestinal bacterial communities as well as the immune cell populations in breastfed children due to favoring the growth of specific microbial genera [8].

The present study aimed to compare the metabolomic profile of human milk obtained from different regions and different delivery modes, as well as to ascertain the potential interaction with milk microbiota.

2. Materials and Methods

2.1. Breast Milk Sample Collection

This study's population comprised 79 healthy women volunteers representing different populations from around the world, including China (Beijing area), South Africa (Cape Town area), Finland (southwestern area), and Spain (Valencia area). The women were enrolled in the study according to previously described inclusion criteria [9]. Further, the subjects from each country (n = 20) were grouped into two sub-groups according to the mode of delivery, namely either vaginal delivery (n = 10 for each country) or caesarean section (n = 10 for China, Finland, and Spain; n = 9 for South Africa). Data regarding age of the mother and perinatal body max index (BMI) are presented in Table S1. The mothers from China had significantly lower BMI ($p < 0.001$), but there were no differences in other parameters between countries and mode of delivery. Parity was between 1 and 3, mostly 1 and 2, with no differences among countries or between mode of delivery. Exclusively breastfeeding was reported at time of the sampling.

All the participating women received written, complete, and detailed information about the study. Written informed consent was obtained from all the participants, and the ethics committees of the respective participating countries (Spain [Bioethics Committee of CSIC and the Regional

Ethics Committee for Biomedical Research, Ref: ERC-639226], Finland [Turku University Hospital, Ref: 24/1801/2013], China [Medical Research Board of Peking University, Ref: IRB00001052-16038], and South Africa [University of Cape Town, Human Research Ethics Committee, Ref: HREC 649/2016]), approved the study protocol. The study was conducted in accordance with the Declaration of Helsinki. Inclusion criteria requested exclusive breastfeeding practices at sampling time and healthy status of the mother-child pairs. Exclusion criteria included antibiotics use after birth, perinatal probiotic consumption, and presence of disease.

Prior to the sample collection, the mothers were given oral and written instructions regarding the standardized collection of samples. The mature milk samples (one month postpartum) were collected manually in the morning into a sterile tube using the same protocol in all the countries. Before the collection, the mothers' nipples and mammary areola were cleaned with soap and sterile water and then soaked in chlorohexidine in order to reduce the presence of skin bacteria. Samples were collected in the morning, from one breast, before baby feeding. The first drops of milk (approx. 500 μL) were discarded. The average collected volume was 10 mL. All the samples were kept frozen at −20 °C until delivery to the laboratory. They were then stored at −80 °C for further analysis.

The breast milk samples were thawed, carefully mixed by means of inversion, and then centrifuged at 14,000 rpm for 20 min at 4 °C. The fat was removed and the pellet was used for the total DNA extraction. Avoiding the outer layer of fat, the whey milk was transferred to a clean Falcon tube and then centrifuged again. This procedure was repeated. A clear supernatant was used for the metabolomic profile analysis.

2.2. Breast Milk Metabolite Profiling

A proton nuclear magnetic resonance (NMR) analysis of all the collected samples was performed. For each group, the milk samples (455 μL) were mixed with 45 μL of sodium-3′-trimethylsilylpropionate-2,2,3,3-d4 (TSP) solved in deuterium oxide and then placed in a 5 mm NMR tube. The final TSP concentration in each sample was 2.5 mM. All the spectra were recorded on a Bruker Avance DRX 600 spectrometer (Bruker GmbH, Rheinstetten, Germany) operating at a ^{1}H frequency of 600.13 MHz. The spectrometer was equipped with a triple resonance $^{1}H/^{13}C/^{31}P$ probe. The nominal temperature of the samples was kept at 310 K. A single-pulse pre-saturation experiment was performed for all the samples. A total of 64 transients were collected into 65 k data points for all the experiments, with a spectral width of 14 ppm. Water presaturation was performed for one second during the recycling delay for the solvent signal suppression. Prior to the Fourier transformation, the free induction decay was multiplied with a 0.3 Hz exponential line-broadening function. All the spectra were processed using MestReNova 8.1 software (Mestrelab Research S.L., Santiago de Compostela, Spain) and then transferred to MATLAB R2013a (The MathWorks Inc., Natick, MA 2013) using in-house scripts for data analysis. The metabolite spin systems and resonances were identified using data obtained from both the literature and the commercial resonances database Chenomx NMR Suite Profiler (Chenomx NMR Suite 8.1, Chenomx Inc., Edmonton, AB, Canada). The spectra were manually phase corrected and baseline adjusted, referenced to the TSP, and normalized to the total aliphatic spectral area (0.50 and 4.40 ppm) in order to eliminate any differences in the total metabolite concentration. The signals belonging to the identified metabolites were then integrated and quantified using the semi-automated ^{1}H NMR signal deconvolution routines in MestReNova 8.1 (Mestrelab Research SL, Santiago de Compostela, Spain). The final metabolite levels were calculated in arbitrary units as the area under the peak. In addition, two-dimensional NMR methods, including homonuclear correlation spectroscopy (TOCSY) and heteronuclear single quantum correlation spectroscopy (HSQC), were applied to a selected group of samples so as to confirm the assessment of the metabolites.

2.3. Breast Milk DNA Extraction and Microbial 16S rRNA Gene Sequencing

The process of microbial DNA extraction and sequencing using an Illumina MiSeq sequencer was described in a previous study by Kumar et al. [9]. The sequencing data were submitted to the

National Center for Biotechnology Information with the Sequence Read Archive accession: SRP082263 and submission ID: SUB1772296.

2.4. Statistical Analysis

A chemometrics statistical analysis was performed using in-house MATLAB scripts and the PLS_Toolbox 8.0.2 (Eigenvector Research, Inc., Wenatchee, WA, USA) statistical multivariate analysis library. The normalization of the NMR spectra was done using the total aliphatic spectral area (0.50 and 4.40 ppm) in order to eliminate any differences in the total metabolite concentration. Mean-centered and Pareto data scaling were used prior to multivariate analysis. A principal component analysis (PCA) was applied to the NMR spectra data sets. A PCA is able to identify low-dimensional embeddings of multivariate data in such a way that optimally preserves the structure of the data. The main advantage of PCA models is that the key sources of variability within the data are modeled by the so-called principal components (PCs) and, consequently, their associated scores and loadings allow for the visualization and understanding of different patterns and relations in the data. The principal components were chosen to explain at least 70% of the variance. The loading plots of the corresponding principal components were then used to detect the positions of most discriminative variables in the NMR spectra. In order to maximize the separation between the samples, a partial least squares discriminant analysis (PLS-DA) was conducted. A permutation test was performed to check the overfitting of the PLS-DA models. The multivariate chemometric models were cross-validated using ten-fold leave-one-out cross-validation. In each run, 10% of the data were left out of the training and used to test the model. The entire cross-validation process was run ten times. The spectral regions responsible for the classification of the models were identified using the variable importance in projections (VIP) coefficients obtained during the PLS-DA. The threshold used for VIP selection was $\geq$1. Spectral regions with high VIP coefficients are more important in terms of providing class separation during the analysis, while those with very small VIP coefficients provide only a small contribution to the classification.

SPSS 25.0.0.1 software (IBM Corp., Armonk, NY, USA) was employed for the statistical analysis of the milk metabolites. Differences were considered significant at $p \leq 0.05$. Due to the non-normal distribution of the data and high presence of outliers, nonparametric tests were used. Comparisons among the data between the different countries were made by applying the Kruskal-Wallis test, while comparisons between the modes of birth were made by applying the Mann-Whitney U test. The significance values in the pairwise comparison were adjusted using the Bonferroni correction for multiple tests.

Calypso online software version 8.50 was used for data normalized via cumulative sum scaling in order to generate heat maps for the Spearman's correlations between the microbial groups and milk metabolites.

3. Results

A total of 68 metabolites were identified in the human milk one month after delivery, as detailed in Table 1. The metabolites included 23 amino acids and derivatives, 18 sugars and derivatives, ten lipids and fatty acid-associated metabolites, and seven metabolites associated with energy metabolism, while the rest were linked to metabolic processes involving vitamins or nucleic acids, microbial metabolism, and food additives.

The most abundant metabolite was lactose, followed by lipids, with high amounts of the lipoproteins LDL (low-density lipoprotein) and VLDL (very low-density lipoproteins), and then, HMOs, and amino acids. The accurate relative quantitation of several metabolites by means of NMR was difficult due to the presence of multiple peaks or severe spectral overlapping, and it was thus not included in statistical analysis. Therefore, of the 68 metabolites identified, 37 were employed for statistical analysis in SPSS 25.0.0.1 software. Maternal factor and metabolites association were analyzed as shown in Table S2.

The presence of LDL and VLDL as milk metabolites can be controversial. The particles detected in milk have similar nuclear magnetic resonances (NMR), physicochemical properties and mobility than those lipoproteins detected in plasma. However, they might be also different lipid and protein conjugates with similar composition and hydrodynamic properties; lipids similar to those present in LDL and VLDL enclosed in phospholipids, free cholesterol and proteins; or free lipids similar to those enclosed in LDL and VLDL attached to large proteins. For this reason, they should be considered LDL- and VLDL-like particles.

Table 1. Human milk metabolites identified in breast milk samples and their probable origin. Chemical shifts in ppm are presented (in brackets).

Metabolite	Origin
Amino acids and derivatives	
2-Hydroxybutyrate (3.99)	endogenous
2-Hydroxyisovalerate (0.95)	endogenous
Alanine (1.47)	endogenous
Anserine (8.91)	diet
Creatinine (3.03)	endogenous
Dimethylamine (2.72)	endogenous
Glutamate (2.34)	endogenous
Glutamine (2.47)	endogenous
Carnitine (3.21)	endogenous
Histidine (7.09)	endogenous
Isoleucine (0.99)	diet
Kynurenine (6.81)	endogenous
Leucine (0.94)	diet
Methionine (2.62)	diet
Methyl-histidine (7.88)	endogenous
***N*-Acetyl lysine** (1.79)	endogenous
Phenylalanine (7.36)	endogenous
Proline (3.34)	endogenous
Taurine (3.25)	endogenous
Tryptophan (7.70)	diet
Tyrosine (3.06)	endogenous
Urea (5.77)	endogenous
Valine (0.98)	diet
Energy metabolites	
3-hydroxybutyrate (1.17)	endogenous
Citrate (2.69)	endogenous
Creatine (3.01)	endogenous
Creatine-phosphate (3.02)	endogenous
Formate (8.44)	endogenous
Lactate (1.32)	endogenous
NADH (8.46)	endogenous
Neurotransmitters, growth factors and second messengers	
4-Aminobutyrate (2.29)	endogenous
Putrescine (1.75)	microbial
Spermidine (2.61)	endogenous
Spermine (2.70)	endogenous
Fatty acids and associated metabolites	
4-Aminohippurate (2.29)	endogenous
Acetate (1.91)	endogenous
Acetylcholine (3.21)	endogenous
Butyrate (2.16)	microbial
Choline (4.06)	diet
Ethanolamine (3.13)	endogenous

Table 1. *Cont.*

Metabolite	Origin
Glycero-3-phosphocholine (3.22)	endogenous
LDL * (1.29)	endogenous
Phosphocholine (3.2)	endogenous
VLDL * (1.27)	endogenous
Sugars and derivatives	
1,6-anhydro-B-glucose (5.44)	diet
2-fucosyllactose (5.31)	endogenous
3-fucosyllactose (5.37)	endogenous
Arabinose (4.51)	microbial
Fucosyl-α-1,3-*N*-acetylglucosamine (5.14)	endogenous
Fucosyl-α-1,4-*N*-acetylglucosamine (5.01)	endogenous
Fucose (4.55)	endogenous
Galactose (4.57)	endogenous
Glucose (3.23)	endogenous
Glucose-1-phosphate (5.45)	endogenous
Lactose (3.75)	endogenous
Lactodifucotetraose (5.27)	endogenous
Lacto-*N*-difucohexaose I (5.18)	endogenous
Lacto-*N*-difucohexaose II (5.36)	endogenous
Lacto-*N*-fucopentaose I (5.31)	endogenous
Lacto-*N*-fucopentaose III (5.1)	endogenous
Myo-inositol (4.05)	endogenous
N-Acetylglucosamine (3.91)	endogenous
Vitamins and nucleosides	
Riboflavin (B2) (7.96)	diet
Uridine (5.92)	endogeonous
Others	
Ethanol (1.16)	diet
Hippurate (7.55)	microbial
Propylene glycol (1.14)	diet

Classification and probable origin inferred from "The Human Metabolome Database" [18]. Metabolites employed for statistical comparison are highlighted with bold letters. * LDL- and VLDL-like particles with similar NMR resonances, structure and mobility than plasma LDL and VLDL.

3.1. Differences in Milk Metabolites between Countries

The global metabolic profile of breast milk was found to be different between countries, as seen in Figure 1. The PLS-DA analysis showed the Spanish samples to be widely dispersed, being more similar to the Finnish and South African samples and totally separate from the Chinese samples. After the exclusion of the Spanish milk samples from the analysis, total separation with only minimal overlapping between the samples was observed. PCA plots and loadings are available as supplementary material in Figures S1 and S2.

Significant differences in the sugars and HMOs between the countries can be seen in Figure 2. When compared to the breast milk samples from Finland, the Chinese samples exhibited significantly higher levels of 3-fucosyllactose (3′FL) and lacto-*N*-fucopentaose III (LNFP III). A higher abundance of lacto-*N*-fucopentaose I (LNFP I) and 2-fucosyllactose (2′FL) was observed in Finland and Spain, respectively, while 3′FL and LNFP III were more highly abundant in South Africa and China, respectively.

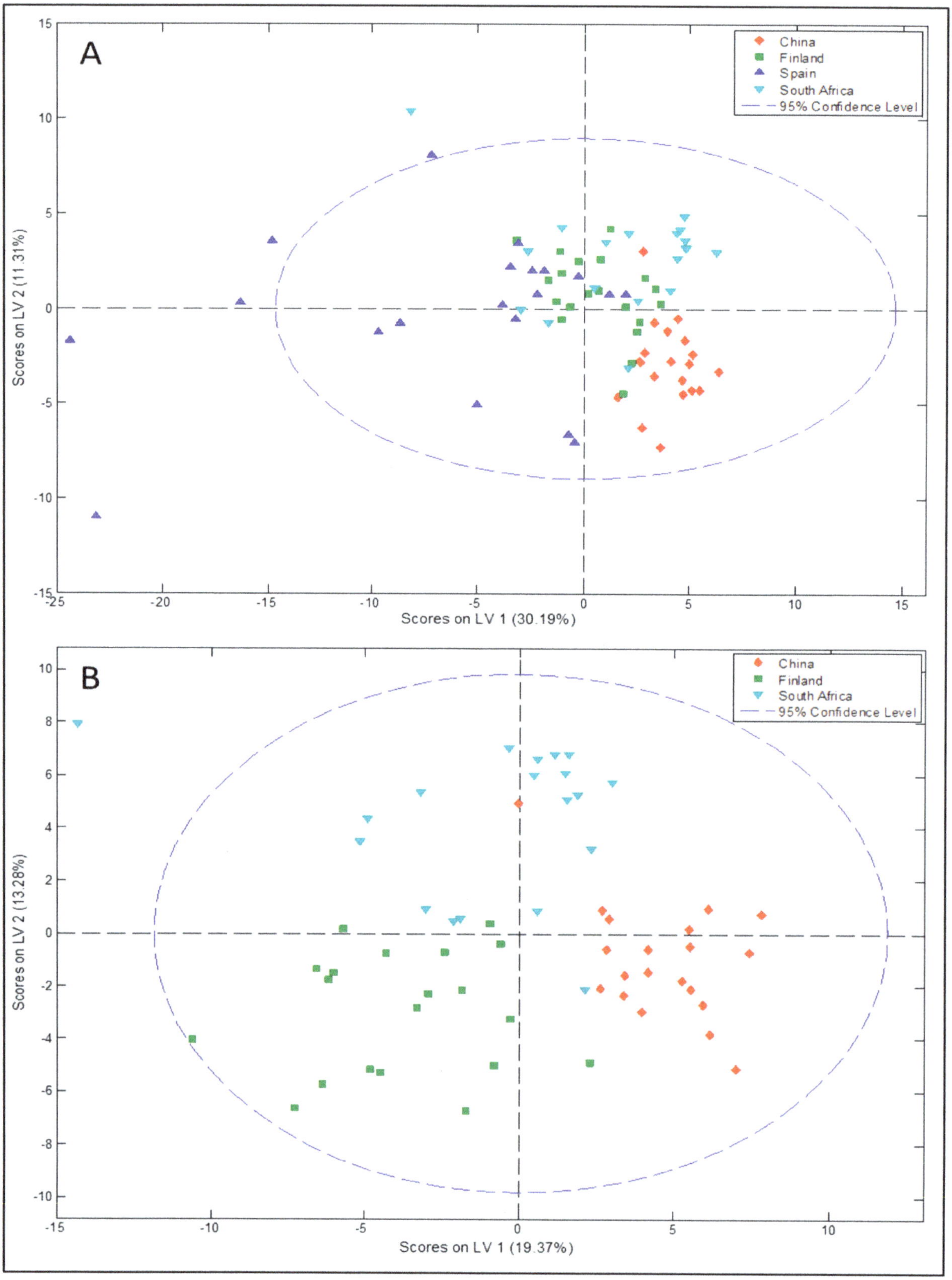

Figure 1. Partial least squares discriminant analysis (PLSDA) scores plot scaling nuclear magnetic resonance (NMR) data from all participant countries (**A**); participant countries without Spain (**B**). Countries are indicated as red diamonds (China), green squares (Finland), navy blue triangles (Spain), pale blue triangles (South Africa).

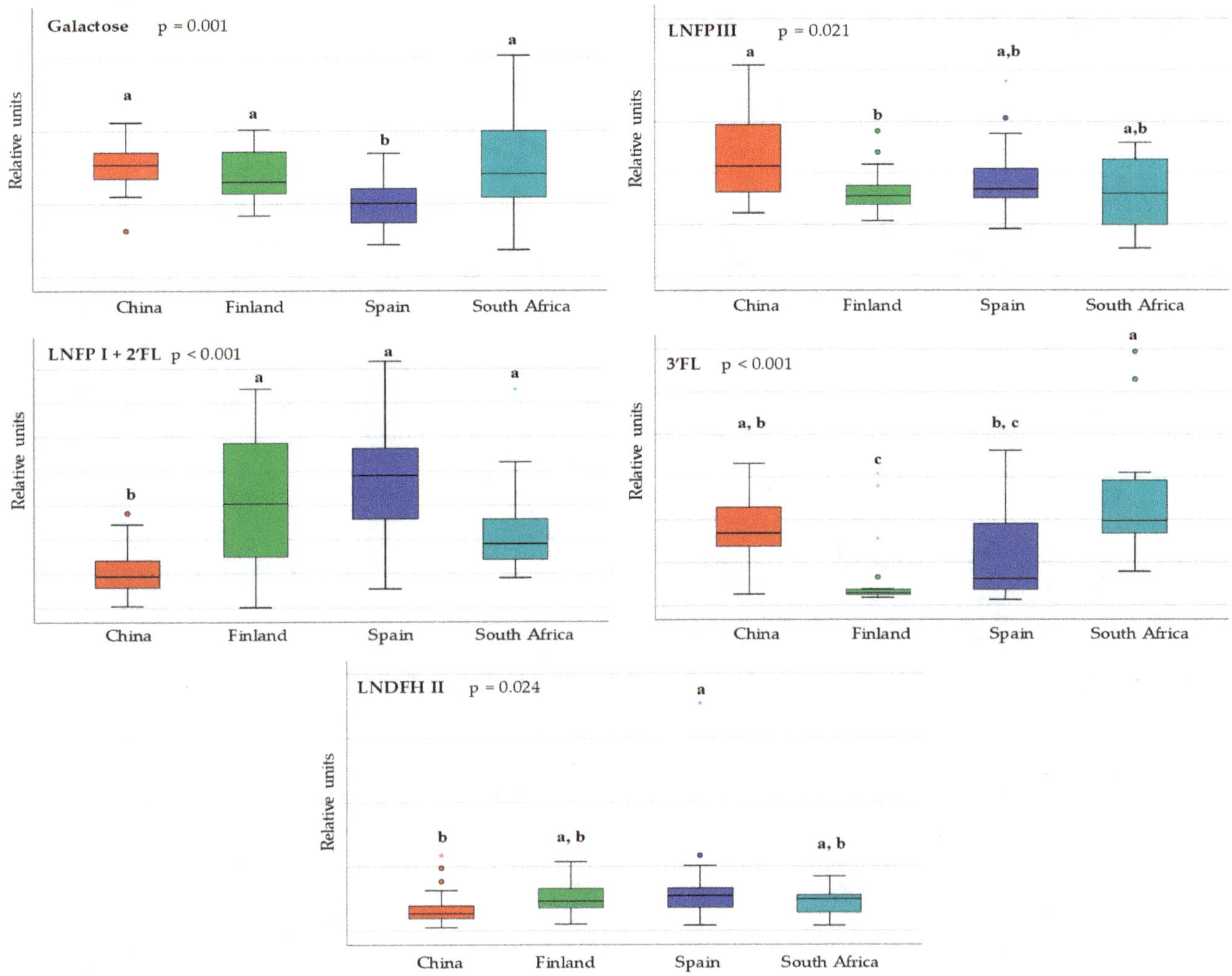

Figure 2. Box and whisker plot showing statistical significant differences in sugars and derivatives in breast milk obtained from China (red), Finland (green), Spain (blue) and South Africa (pale blue). Each bar represents the smallest observation, lower quartile (**Q1**), median, upper quartile (**Q3**) and largest observation. Differences among countries were calculated using the Kruskal-Wallis test. Unlike letters indicate statistically significant differences among countries. Circles and stars indicate outlier data. 3′FL: 3-fucosyllactose; LNFP I + 2′FL: lacto-*N*-fucopentaose I and 2-fucosyllactose; LNDFHII: lacto-*N*-difucohexaose II; LNFP III: lacto-*N*-fucopentaose III. Data are expressed in relative units.

Figure 3 shows statistically significant regional differences in the amino acids and derivatives found in the human milk samples. All of them have an endogenous origin and might therefore be the result of dietary and/or metabolic differences between geographical locations.

With regard to the content of the energy metabolites, fatty acids, and associated metabolites, the differences between countries are shown in Figures 4 and 5. The Finnish and Spanish samples were characterized by higher levels of lipoproteins (LDL and VLDL). Short-chain fatty acids (SCFA) were also detected with higher levels of acetate and formate in the Spanish samples.

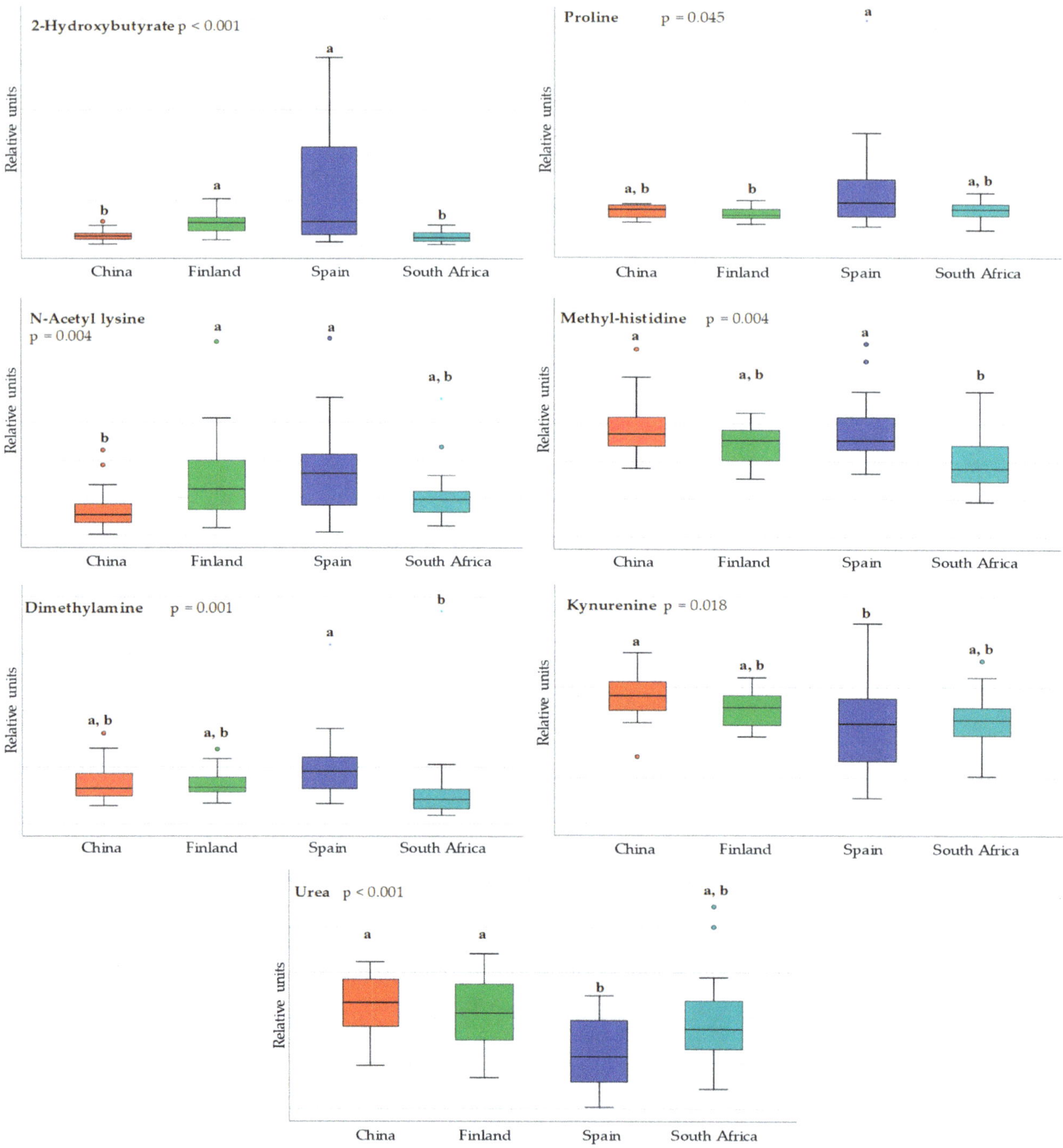

Figure 3. Box and whisker plot showing statistical significant differences in amino acids and derivatives in breast milk obtained from China (red), Finland (green), Spain (blue) and South Africa (pale blue). Data are expressed in relative units. Each bar represents the smallest observation, lower quartile (**Q1**), median, upper quartile (**Q3**) and largest observation. Differences among countries were calculated using the Kruskal-Wallis test. Unlike letters indicate statistically significant differences among countries. Circles and stars indicate outlier data.

The statistically significant differences identified in the other metabolites are presented in Figure 6. Some of them have a dietary origin, such as vitamin B2 (riboflavin), while others, such as the polyamines (spermidine and spermine), could have an endogenous, dietary, or microbial origin.

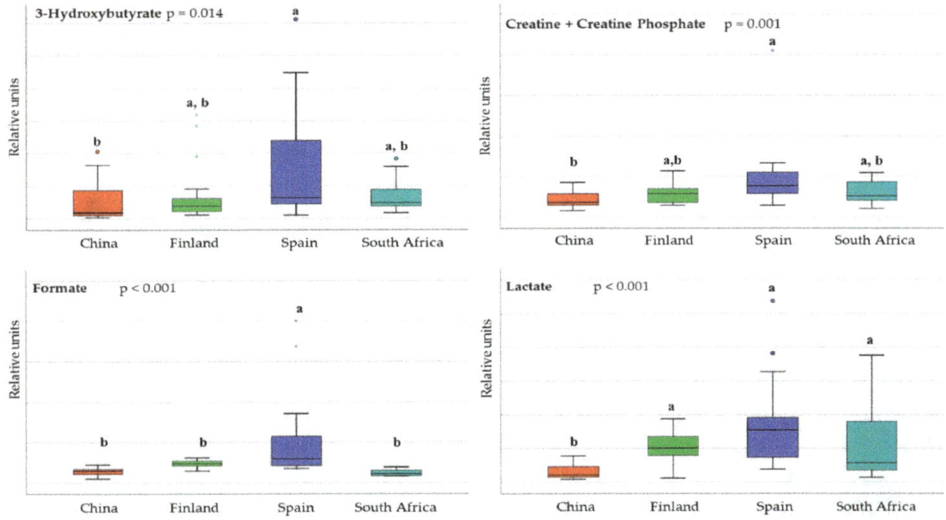

Figure 4. Box and whisker plot showing statistical significant differences in energy metabolites in breast milk in samples from China (red), Finland (green), Spain (blue) and South Africa (pale blue). Data are expressed in relative units. Each bar represents the smallest observation, lower quartile (**Q1**), median, upper quartile (**Q3**) and largest observation. Circles and stars indicate outlier data. Differences among countries were calculated using the Kruskal–Wallis test. Unlike letters indicate statistically significant differences among countries.

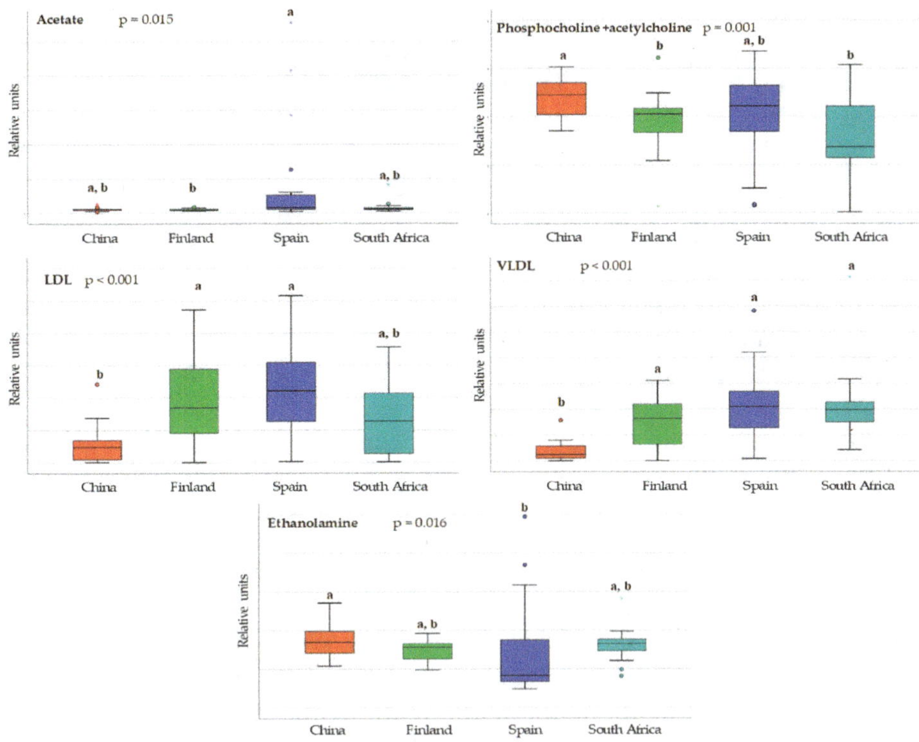

Figure 5. Box and whisker plot showing statistical significant differences in fatty acids and related metabolites in breast milk in samples from China (red), Finland (green), Spain (blue) and South Africa (pale blue). Data are expressed in relative units. Each bar represents the smallest observation, lower quartile (**Q1**), median, upper quartile (**Q3**) and largest observation. Circles and stars indicate outlier data. Differences among countries were calculated using the Kruskal–Wallis test. Unlike letters indicate statistically significant differences among countries. LDL and VLDL should be consider LDL- and VLDL-like particles with similar nuclear magnetic resonances (NMR), structure and mobility than plasma LDL and VLDL.

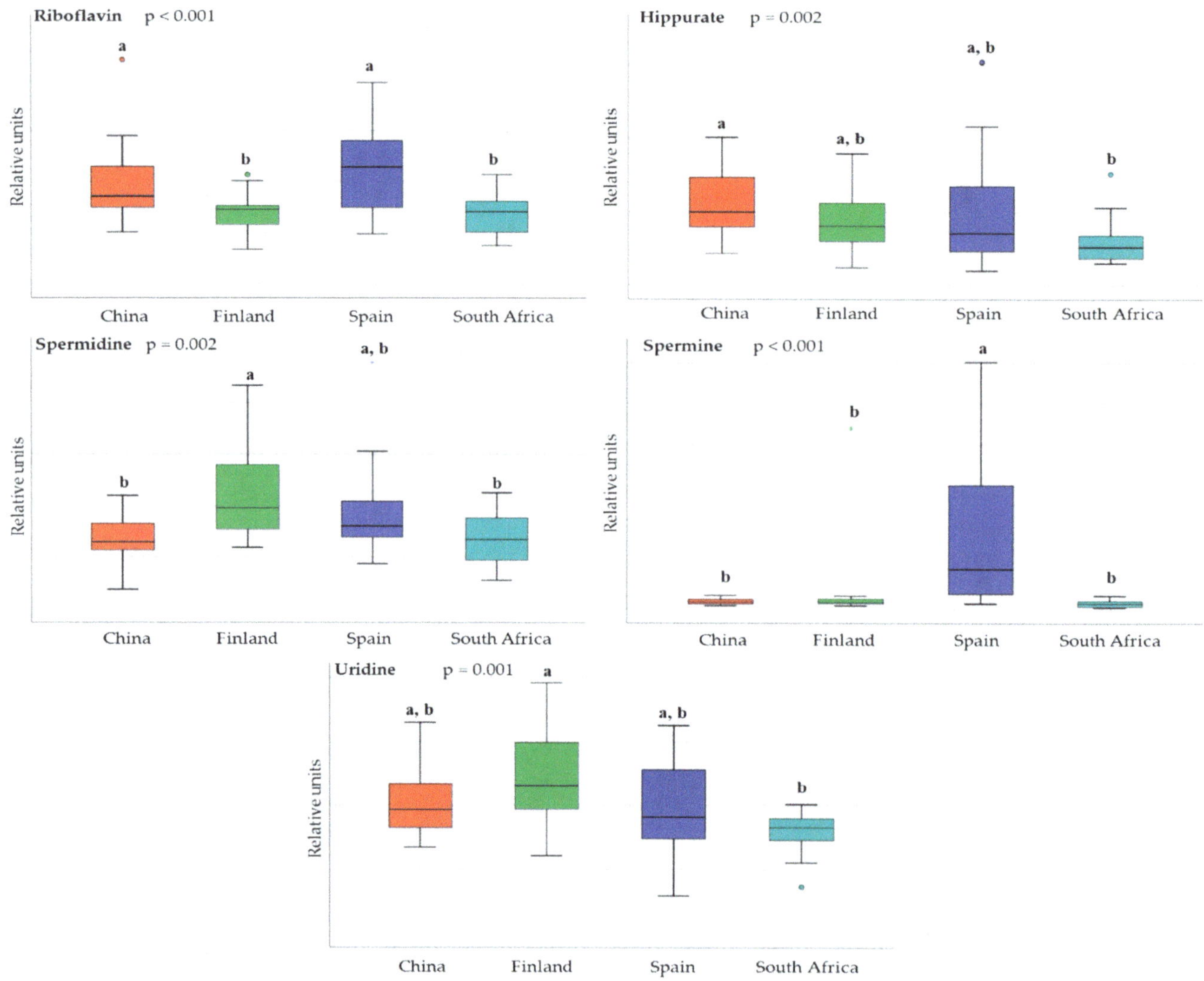

Figure 6. Box and whisker plot showing statistical significant differences in other metabolites in breast milk in samples from China (red), Finland (green), Spain (blue) and South Africa (pale bue). Data are expressed in relative units. Each bar represents the smallest observation, lower quartile (**Q1**), median, upper quartile (**Q3**) and largest observation. Circles and stars indicate outlier data. Differences among countries were calculated using the Kruskal–Wallis test. Unlike letters indicate statistically significant differences among countries.

3.2. Impact of Mode of Delivery on Human Milk Metabolites

Independent of the country, the mode of delivery has a distinct impact on the human milk metabolome, as seen in Figure 7.

When considering all the mothers included in the study, six of the 37 semi-quantified metabolites were statistically different in the milk samples obtained from the mothers who underwent vaginal delivery when compared to those who underwent caesarean section, as seen in Figure S3. The milk from the mothers who underwent vaginal delivery had higher levels of 3-hydroxybutyrate (p = 0.048) and LNFP III (p = 0.045), while the milk from the mothers who underwent caesarean section had higher relative abundances of butyrate (p = 0.043), ethanolamine (p = 0.004), proline (p = 0.018), and urea (p = 0.020). However, these differences depend on the country. In the present study, based on the mode of delivery, we found significant differences in 16 metabolites in the South African samples, 11 metabolites in the Spanish samples, four in the Finnish samples, and one in the Chinese samples, shown in Table 2, reflecting regional differences in terms of the impact of caesarean section on the milk metabolome.

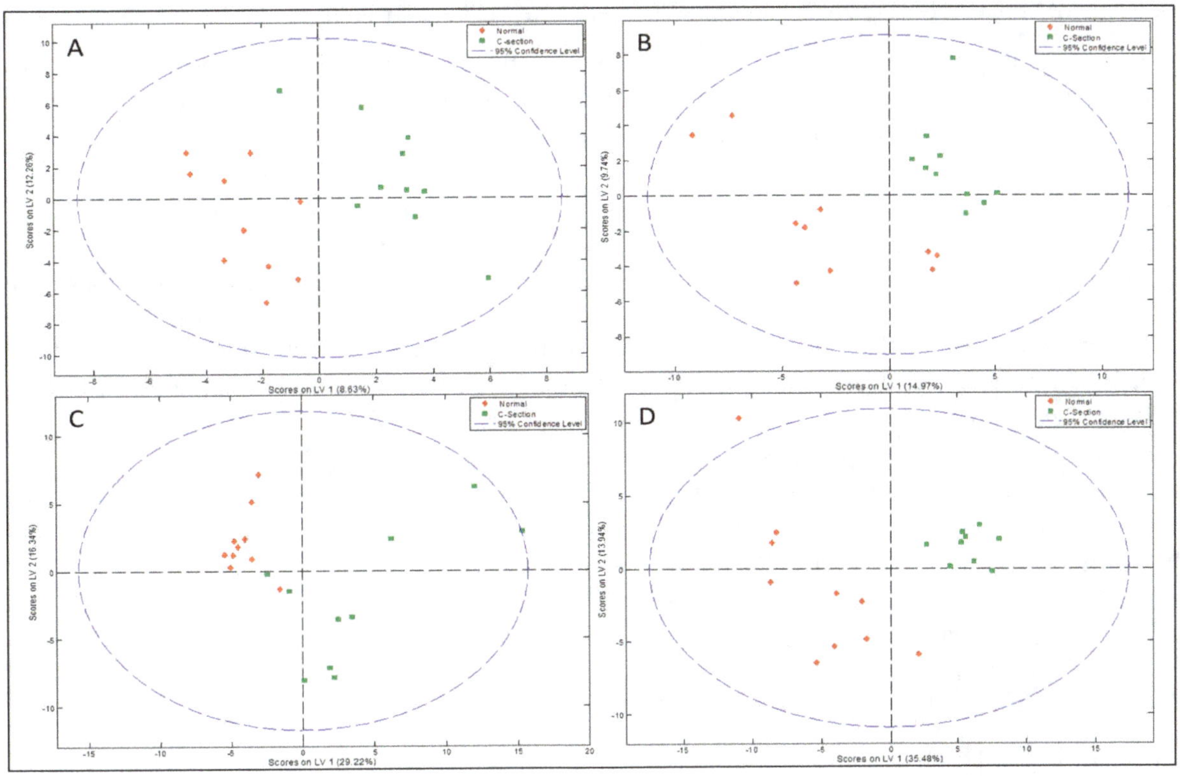

Figure 7. Partial least squares discriminant analysis scores plot scaling nuclear magnetic resonance (NMR) data from vaginal delivery samples (red) and caesarean section (green) from China (**A**), Finland (**B**), Spain (**C**), South Africa (**D**).

Table 2. Significant differences by country (*p*-value) in specific metabolites in human milk after vaginal or caesarean delivery.

Metabolite	China	Finland	Spain	South Africa
3-fucosyllactose	0.739	0.971	0.190	↑ ***0.035*** *
Alanine	0.853	0.739	0.280	↑ ***0.022*** *
Butyrate	0.579	0.579	0.436	↑ ***0.006*** *
Dimethylamine	0.971	***0.035*** *	↑ ***0.035*** *	***0.002*** *
Ethanolamine	0.631	0.579	↑ ***0.000*** *	0.661
Formate	↑ ***0.035*** *	0.684	0.796	***0.006*** *
Fucosyl-α-1,4-*N*-acetylglucosamine	0.631	***0.035*** *	0.247	***0.002*** *
Galactose	0.579	0.579	0.481	↑ ***0.002*** *
Hippurate	0.684	*0.063*	↑ ***0.009*** *	***0.022*** *
Kynurenine	0.143	*0.075*	↑ ***0.011*** *	***0.028*** *
Lactodifucotetraose	0.247	↑ ***0.035*** *	0.247	0.447
Leucine	0.631	↑ ***0.043*** *	↑ ***0.009*** *	1.000
Lacto-*N*-fucopentaose I and 2-fucosyllactose	0.353	1.000	0.971	***0.035*** *
Lacto-*N*-fucopentaose III	0.579	0.796	0.631	***0.001*** *
Methyl-histidine	0.353	0.684	↑ ***0.023*** *	***0.043*** *
Phosphocholine and acetylcholine	0.393	0.796	1.000	***0.002*** *
Proline	0.393	0.739	↑ ***0.002*** *	1.000
Propylene glycol	0.912	*0.089*	↑ ***0.023*** *	***0.004*** *
Riboflavin	0.529	0.353	↑ ***0.002*** *	0.400
Spermidine	0.579	0.353	↑ ***0.000*** *	0.604
Spermine	0.143	0.315	0.853	***0.003*** *
Urea	0.436	0.247	0.280	***0.000*** *
Uridine	0.529	0.912	***0.019*** *	0.243

* indicate *p*-values < 0.05. ↑ indicate significant higher levels in milk from caesarean section donors.

3.3. Relationship between the NMR Metabolomic Profile and Milk Microbiota

In order to explore the interrelations between the human milk metabolites and the milk microbiota profile, Spearman's rank correlations were determined and then represented in heat maps shown in Figures 8 and 9. Urea and galactose were positively correlated ($p < 0.05$) with Alpha- and Betaproteobacteria and Bacilli, although they were negatively correlated ($p < 0.05$) with Gammaproteobacteria. Yet, a group of metabolites were found to be positively correlated ($p < 0.05$) with Gammaproteobacteria, including lactate, creatine, proline, lacto-*N*-fucopentaose I, and 2-fucosyllactose VLDL, although they negatively correlated ($p < 0.05$) with Alpha- and Betaproteobacteria and Bacilli.

The Actinobacteria in the human breast milk were positively correlated ($p < 0.05$) with uridine, but negatively correlated with lacto-*N*-fucopentaose I, 2-fucosyllactose acetate, and spermidine ($p < 0.05$) as seen in Figure 8.

A few significant associations were found between the bacterial groups and HMOs, namely those related to fucosyl-α-1,4-*N*-acetylglucosamine, lactodifucotetraose, lacto-*N*-fucopentaose III, lacto-*N*-fucopentaose I, and 2-fucosyllactose, shown in Figure 9.

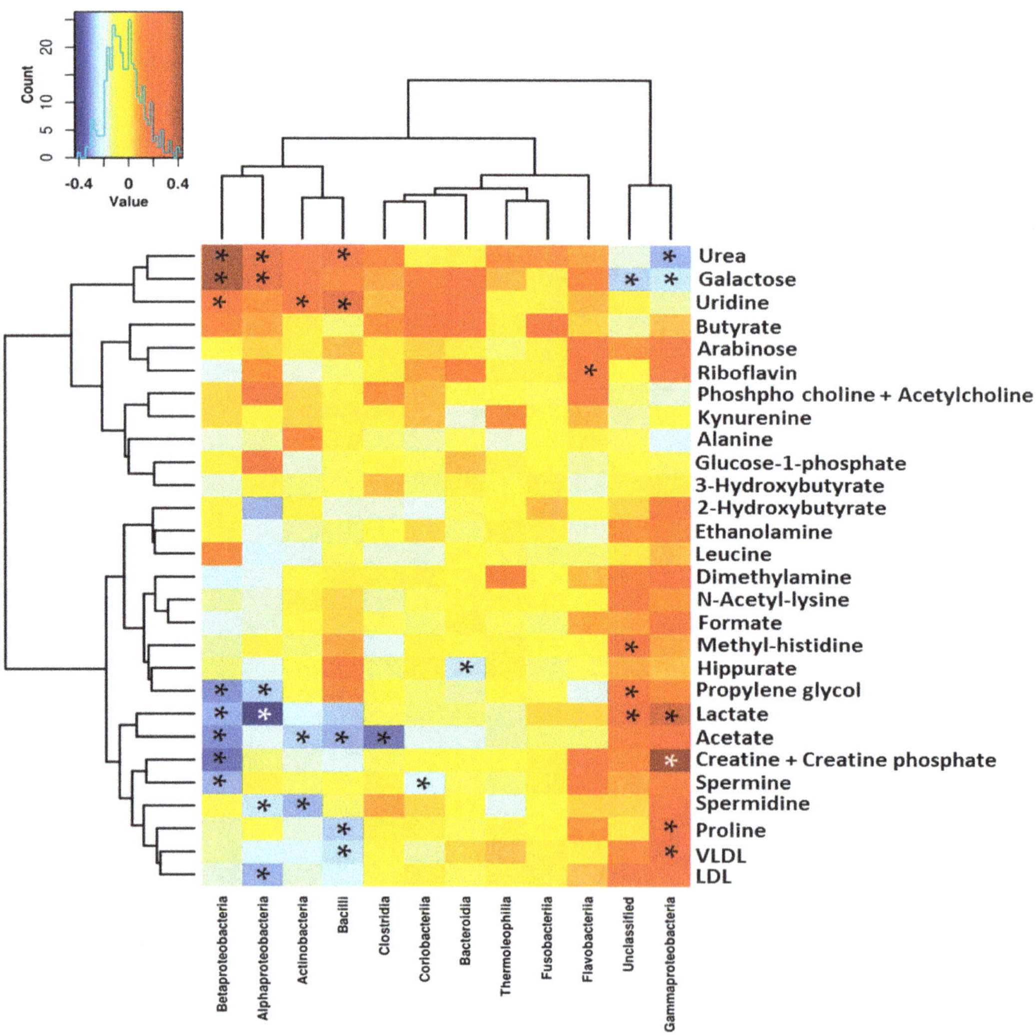

Figure 8. Heat map to show Spearman's correlation between metabolites and microbiota composition at class level. Asterisk indicates statistically significant correlation at the level of ($p < 0.05$). LDL and VLDL should be considered LDL- and VLDL-like particles with similar nuclear magnetic resonances (NMR), structure and mobility than plasma LDL and VLDL.

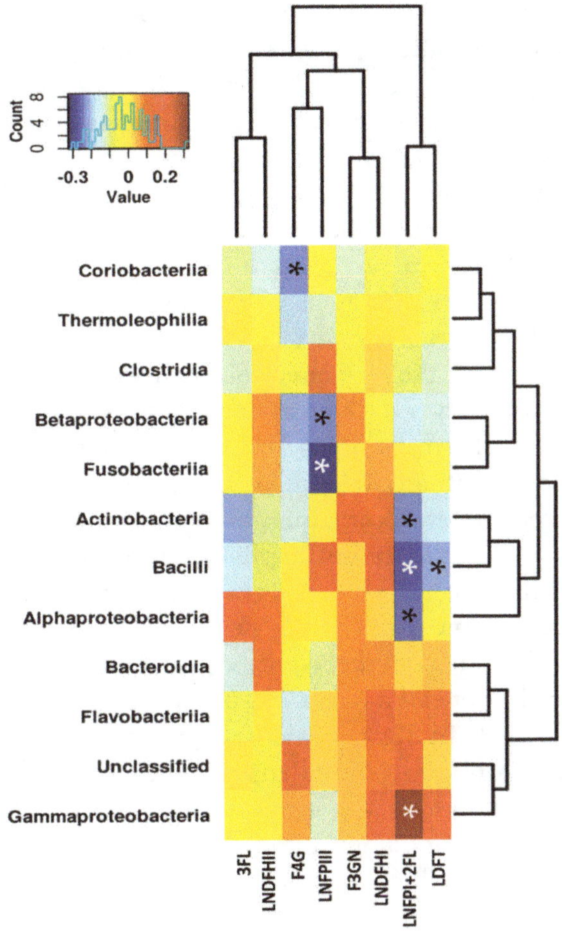

Figure 9. Heat map to show Spearman's correlation between oligosaccharides (HMOs) and microbiota composition at class level. 3FL: 3-fucosyllactose; LNDFHII: Lacto-*N*-difucohexaose; F4G: Fucosyl-α-1,4-*N*-acetylglucosamine; LNFP III: lacto-*N*-fucopentaose; F3GN: Fucosyl-α-1,3-*N*-acetylglucosamine; LNDFH I: lacto-*N*-difucohexaose I; LNFP I: lacto-*N*-fucopentaose I; 2FL: 2-fucosyllactose; LDFT: lactodifucotetraose. Asterisk indicates statistically significant correlation at the level of ($p < 0.05$).

4. Discussion

There is growing research interest in identifying and understanding the bioactive compounds found in human breast milk. The field of infant nutrition research is evolving and new methodologies are being developed to support exact knowledge concerning the composition of human milk. Moreover, a few prior studies have reported the composition of human milk using NMR-based metabolomics [1,7,19,20]. In this study, a total of 68 metabolites were identified in mature human milk. To the best of our knowledge, this is the first study to report the distinct milk metabolomics profile across different geographical locations, as well as to associate the complex interactions with human milk microbes. Spanish samples presented higher dispersion that was no associated with differences in maternal characteristics such as parity, age, or BMI between samples. Future studies to find the origin of this variability will be needed.

Different mode of delivery (vaginal vs caesarean section) influences the milk metabolite profile across locations. This study hence shows for the first time regional differences in the impact of caesarean section on human milk metabolites. The effect of caesarean section on the milk metabolome is dependent on the geographical region, with changes in different metabolites depending on the country. We suggest that the clinical intervention during caesarean and the alterations in the physiological and hormonal signals produced during normal vaginal delivery, would affected the milk metabolite profiles as already showed for milk microbiota [9]. In addition, we observed that the impact of the mode of delivery vary among geographical locations, maybe due to differences in the clinical procedures and antibiotic use [9].

Previous studies have shown inter-individual variations in human milk in terms of the macronutrients [21]. With regard to the metabolites, some of them, such as lactose, *myo*-inositol, and urea, have been reported to be conserved among mothers due to their important roles in infant growth and development, while those metabolites related to the genetic background or maternal diet are more variable, including HMOs, amino acids, choline, and vitamins [1,20]. No significant changes were found in the lactose and *myo*-inositol levels in relation to the geographical location and mode of delivery in this study, which suggests the strict regulation by the mammary gland, as has been proposed previously [1]. Yet, previous studies have found significant differences with regard to urea. For instance, Smilowitz et al. [1] analyzed 52 human milk samples collected at day 90 postpartum. They found that urea was one of the most abundant metabolites in human milk, and they further reported low variability between mothers, which suggested regulation at the level of the mammary gland, as well as an important role in developing infants as a source of nitrogen for intestinal microbiota. In the present study, the samples collected at day 30 postpartum showed differences in urea at different geographical locations in addition to relatively high variability. This may indicate differences in the regulation of the mammary gland depending on the number of days postpartum, as well as the influence of external factors, such as meat and dairy intake, or physical activity, during the early stages of lactation. The differences in the urea composition across the different geographical locations could also reflect variation in the gut microbiota composition of infants from the different locations [9,22,23]. A positive correlation between the colonic urea-nitrogen metabolism and the bifidobacteria concentration has previously been reported [24], although this association between the nitrogenated compounds and bifidobacteria might start early. We identified positive correlation between the nitrogenated compounds, such as urea, and uridine and Actinobacteria.

Similarly to urea, riboflavin has previously been reported to be a stable milk constituent in well-nourished mothers during the first month of lactation [19], although in the present study, its level varied with geographical locations. These differences might be explained by differences in maternal diet [20], and it might be extrapolated to other milk metabolites.

When compared with the other constituents, fat has previously been classified as the most variable component of breast milk due to being influenced by the time of day, inter-feeding interval, point of sampling during a feeding, stage of lactation, maternal weight, and differences between breasts [25]. In the present study, the differences in the LDL and VLDL in the milk might be partially explained by dietary impacts [26] or genetic factors, as previously reported [27]. However, their role in infant nutrition remains unclear, and the fatty acid content and their composition inside the lipoproteins might be more important for the infant than the content of lipoprotein particles. A recent study has shown the difference in the lipidomic profile across countries [9]. In this study, the lipid composition, particularly that of polyunsaturated fatty acids (PUFA), differed between the countries, with the highest level being observed in the case of omega-6 PUFA in Chinese women.

Human milk oligosaccharides, which are the third most abundant component in human milk [28,29], are a group of complex sugars that are non-digestible by infants. These HMOs contain a lactose core bound to one or more glucose, galactose, *N*-acetylglucosamine, fucose, or sialic acid residues [30]. HMOs support the competitive growth of beneficial bacterial strains within the intestine [29], inhibit the adhesion of pathogens to the infant's epithelium, and interact directly with host immune cells [30]. Each HMO fulfils different roles and activities, and each is metabolized by different bacteria [31]. In addition, specific HMOs could render epithelial cells more resistant to bacterial colonization, and they can interact with immune cells in order to reduce the expression of pro-inflammatory cytokines [32]. This means that differences in the HMOs between geographical locations may result in different roles for human milk in relation to infant health and development. It has been suggested that HMO concentrations and profiles may vary geographically [16,32].

The present study confirmed significant differences in both sugars and HMOs between countries, which was also revealed by a study by McGuire et al. [16]. Their study revealed that milk from Sweden contained more than four times more 3-fucosyllactose (3FL) and lower disialyllacto-*N*-tetraose than milk collected in rural Gambia. Similarly, our study showed significant differences in the 3FL, lacto-*N*-fucopentaose III (LNFPIII), lacto-*N*-fucopentaose I (LNFPI), and 2-fucosyllactose (2FL) levels. The HMO profile and specific oligosaccharides, such as 2FL, have also been linked to infant body composition and growth [33], the survival of children born to HIV-infected mothers [34], and allergic morbidity such as a cow milk protein allergy [33]. Furthermore, it was previously reported that specific HMOs, such as LNFPI and 3′-sialyllactose, were associated with infant morbidity and growth development, respectively, and at the same time, correlated with specific microbiota [31]. Another prior study reported an association between the total HMO concentrations and Actinobacteria (mainly *Bifidobacterium* spp.) counts [35]. More specifically, it was reported that *B. breve* was positively correlated with sialylated HMOs, while *B. longum* was positively correlated with non-fucosylated/non-sialylated HMOs. Furthermore, the same study reported positive correlations between fucosylated HMOs and the classes Verrucomicrobiae (*Akkermansia muciniphila*) and Bacilli, mainly *Staphylococcus aureus* [35]. Our results thus support the available, albeit limited, data concerning the complex interactions between microbiota and HMOs during lactation, with significant associations being found between the bacterial groups and fucosyl-α-1,4-*N*-acetylglucosamine, lactodifucotetraose, LNFPIII, LNFPI, and 2FL. According to this study, geographical variations and changes in the metabolomics profile of human milk following caesarean section may involve differences in the protective activities of HMOs.

Previous studies have indicated that the neonatal primary gut colonizers include acetate- and lactate-producing bacteria from the classes Actinobacteria (*Bifidobacterium*), Bacteroidia (*Bacteroides*) and Bacilli (*Lactobacillus*, *Streptococcus*, *Staphylococcus*, and *Enterococcus*) [36]. These bacteria have also been found to be present in human breast milk in its viable form [37,38]. In this study, higher amounts of lactate, followed by acetate and propionate, were detected in the human milk samples across locations. The origin of this lactate may be both the mammary tissue and/or milk microbiota. In the mammary gland, lactate serves as an intermediate in carbohydrates metabolism [39], while lactate and acetate are intermediate fermentation products of the microbial metabolism [40,41]. The present study found significant differences in the acetate and lactate levels between locations, which were also correlated with several bacterial groups. The impact of milk lactate on infant health is not yet known, although recent studies have suggested that lactate must be efficiently metabolized during early life in order to avoid the potential negative consequences of lactate accumulation as acidosis, neurotoxicity, and cardiac arrhythmia [42]. In addition, it is known that acetate is a product of *Bifidobacterium* metabolism, and it serves to promote the defense functions of the host cells and exert a protective effect against infection [43]. It has also been established that acetate and lactate produced by *Bifidobacterium* and *Lactobacillus* contribute to SCFA-mediated health effects, although these two microorganisms do not directly produce butyrate and/or propionate [43,44].

Interestingly, ethanol was also identified in the breast milk samples analyzed in our study. Considering that mothers do not generally drink alcoholic beverages during lactation, the presence of this compound in small amounts in human milk might be a consequence of milk microbiota metabolism. Many microorganisms, including bacteria and yeasts, produce ethanol as the major fermentation product of carbohydrates. Furthermore, recent studies have reported the presence of yeasts, such as *Saccharomyces* and *Candida*, in breast milk samples obtained from healthy women [45], and the presence of ethanol in milk might be a product of their metabolism.

It has previously been reported that specific interactions take place between milk microbes and other milk components, including macro- and micro-nutrients as well as milk cells [8,10]. In this study, we found a group of metabolites to be positively correlated with Gammaproteobacteria, including lactate, creatine, proline, lacto-*N*-fucopentaose I, and 2-fucosyllactose VLDL, as well as negatively correlated with Alpha- and Betaproteobacteria, and Bacilli.

The major limitation of this study is that we were unable to determine the effect of geographical location and caesarean section alone on the milk metabolome without the influence of other confounding variables (e.g., gestational age, diet, lifestyle, secretor status). To do so, future studies involving higher sample sizes and controlling for such variables should be performed. Despite this limitation, the present study contributes important information regarding regional variations in human milk metabolites, the impact of caesarean section, and the correlation of milk metabolites with milk microbiota. Understanding both the composition and function of the components of milk is vital to infant health. The data obtained from this study could form the basis for future studies concerning the milk metabolome and their contribution to infant health and development.

Taken together, ethnicity, diet, environment, and lifestyle could partially explain the different NMR metabolomic profiles seen in this study. It is well-known that diet influences the human metabolomics profile in the blood [46], urine [47], tissues [47], and fecal supernatants [48], and something similar may be expected in human milk. Moreover, only a few studies have investigated the relationships among the human milk microbiota and milk constituents [12,14]. Our findings confirm prior evidence showing that complex bacterial communities within milk are associated with variations in the nutritional composition and metabolites profiles [9,15].

5. Conclusions

By means of NMR, we detected 68 metabolites in human milk sampled one month postpartum. The concentrations of carbohydrates, amino acids, short-chain fatty acids, and other metabolites reflected the external environment, that is, the geographical location. In addition, the internal environment, namely the mode of delivery, also impacted the metabolite profile. Our findings support the hypothesis that human milk metabolites from healthy women vary across locations. Shifts on metabolites are associated to milk microbiota profiles suggesting a complex interlink between milk compounds. It is known that breast-feeding provides a personalized infant nutrition driving the infant gut development, immune system maturation and metabolic activities. Climate, lifestyle, environmental exposure, circadian rhythms, ethnic origin, population-specific variations and genetics would have an impact on metabolite profile explaining some of the variation observed in this study and request further research. Furthermore, our study highlights the potential interactions between human milk metabolites and microbes.

Therefore, we need to understand the pivotal relationship between environment-host-nutrition during pregnancy, lactation and early infancy due its impact for human health. This knowledge would enable the design personalized interventions to modulate milk bioactive compounds to be transferred through breastfeeding to the infants. Our data highlight the need for controlled- large-scale human studies across locations and the need to associated changes on milk bioactive compounds to infant growth, development, and health outcomes.

On this basis, we suggest the hypothesis that breast milk provides optimal immunological and metabolic guidance to the extrauterine world, although the differences reported between the locations and modes of delivery in terms of the metabolite composition might involve variations in infant development.

Supplementary Materials:
Table S1: Age and pre-pregnancy body max index (BMI) of the participants in the study. Height was measured during the first visit at hospital and weight was self-reported, Table S2: Significantly ($p < 0.05$) spearman's rank-order correlation between metabolites and maternal characteristics, Figure S1: Principal component analysis (PCA) scores plot (A) and loadings of the first principal component (B) and second principal component (C) scaling NMR data from all participant countries. Countries are indicated as red diamonds (China), green squares (Finland), navy blue triangles (Spain), pale blue triangles (South Africa), Figure S2: Principal component analysis (PCA) scores plot (A) and loadings of the first principal component (B) and second principal component (C) scaling NMR data from all participant countries without Spain. Countries are indicated as red diamonds (China), green squares (Finland), pale blue triangles (South Africa), Figure S3: Box and whisker plot showing statistical significant differences in metabolityes in breast milk samples after vaginal or caesarean delivery. LNFP III: lacto-N-fucopentaose III. Mann-Whitney U test significant level was considered at 0.05. Each bar represents the

smallest observation, lower quartile (Q1), median, upper quartile (Q3) and largest observation. Circles and stars indicate outlier data.

Author Contributions: M.C.C. and S.S. conceived the idea and designed the study. J.M.M. carried out metabolomics data analysis and C.G.-G. analyzed metabolomics data, combined with microbiota, and wrote the manuscript. All authors contributed to the interpretation of data, critically reviewed the manuscript for intellectual content and approved the final version.

Acknowledgments: We are grateful for all the participant families providing biological samples for this study.

References

1. Smilowitz, J.T.; O'Sullivan, A.; Barile, D.; German, J.B.; Lonnerdal, B.; Slupsky, C.M. The human milk metabolome reveals diverse oligosaccharide profiles. *J. Nutr.* **2013**, *143*, 1709–1718. [CrossRef] [PubMed]
2. Stuebe, A. The risks of not breastfeeding for mothers and infants. *Rev. Obstet. Gynecol.* **2009**, *2*, 222–231. [PubMed]
3. Lodge, C.J.; Tan, D.J.; Lau, M.X.; Dai, X.; Tham, R.; Lowe, A.J.; Bowatte, G.; Allen, K.J.; Dharmage, S.C. Breastfeeding and asthma and allergies: A systematic review and meta-analysis. *Acta Paediatr.* **2015**, *104*, 38–53. [CrossRef] [PubMed]
4. Luccioli, S.; Zhang, Y.; Verrill, L.; Ramos-Valle, M.; Kwegyir-Afful, E. Infant feeding practices and reported food allergies at 6 years of age. *Pediatrics* **2014**, *134* (Suppl. 1), S21–S28. [CrossRef] [PubMed]
5. Jwa, S.C.; Fujiwara, T.; Kondo, N. Latent protective effects of breastfeeding on late childhood overweight and obesity: A nationwide prospective study. *Obesity* **2014**, *22*, 1527–1537. [CrossRef] [PubMed]
6. Marseglia, L.; Manti, S.; D'Angelo, G.; Cuppari, C.; Salpietro, V.; Filippelli, M.; Trovato, A.; Gitto, E.; Salpietro, C.; Arrigo, T. Obesity and breastfeeding: The strength of association. *Women Birth* **2015**, *28*, 81–86. [CrossRef] [PubMed]
7. Longini, M.; Tataranno, M.L.; Proietti, F.; Tortoriello, M.; Belvisi, E.; Vivi, A.; Tassini, M.; Perrone, S.; Buonocore, G. A metabolomic study of preterm and term human and formula milk by proton MRS analysis: Preliminary results. *J. Matern. Fetal Neonatal Med.* **2014**, *27* (Suppl. 2), 27–33. [CrossRef] [PubMed]
8. Williams, J.E.; Price, W.J.; Shafii, B.; Yahvah, K.M.; Bode, L.; McGuire, M.A.; McGuire, M.K. Relationships among microbial communities, maternal cells, oligosaccharides, and macronutrients in human milk. *J. Hum. Lact.* **2017**, *33*, 540–551. [CrossRef] [PubMed]
9. Kumar, H.; du Toit, E.; Kulkarni, A.; Aakko, J.; Linderborg, K.M.; Yumei, Z.; Nicol, M.P.; Isolauri, E.; Yang, B.; Collado, M.C.; et al. Distinct patterns in human milk microbiota and fatty acid profiles across specific geographic locations. *Front. Microbiol.* **2016**, *7*, 1619. [CrossRef] [PubMed]
10. Boix-Amoros, A.; Collado, M.C.; Mira, A. Relationship between milk microbiota, bacterial load, macronutrients, and human cells during lactation. *Front. Microbiol.* **2016**, *7*, 492. [CrossRef] [PubMed]
11. Munblit, D.; Boyle, R.J.; Warner, J.O. Factors affecting breast milk composition and potential consequences for development of the allergic phenotype. *Clin. Exp. Allergy* **2015**, *45*, 583–601. [CrossRef] [PubMed]
12. Chung, M.Y. Factors affecting human milk composition. *Pediatr. Neonatol.* **2014**, *55*, 421–422. [CrossRef] [PubMed]
13. Ballard, O.; Morrow, A.L. Human milk composition nutrients and bioactive factors. *Pediatr. Clin. N. Am.* **2013**, *60*, 49–74. [CrossRef] [PubMed]
14. Yuhas, R.; Pramuk, K.; Lien, E.L. Human milk fatty acid composition from nine countries varies most in DHA. *Lipids* **2006**, *41*, 851–858. [CrossRef] [PubMed]
15. Gomez-Gallego, C.; Kumar, H.; Garcia-Mantrana, I.; du Toit, E.; Suomela, J.P.; Linderborg, K.M.; Zhang, Y.; Isolauri, E.; Yang, B.; Salminen, S.; et al. Breast milk polyamines and microbiota interactions: Impact of mode of delivery and geographical location. *Ann. Nutr. Metab.* **2017**, *70*, 184–190. [CrossRef] [PubMed]
16. McGuire, M.K.; Meehan, C.L.; McGuire, M.A.; Williams, J.E.; Foster, J.; Sellen, D.W.; Kamau-Mbuthia, E.W.; Kamundia, E.W.; Mbugua, S.; Moore, S.E.; et al. What's normal? Oligosaccharide concentrations and profiles in milk produced by healthy women vary geographically. *Am. J. Clin. Nutr.* **2017**, *105*, 1086–1100. [CrossRef] [PubMed]
17. Li, S.W.; Watanabe, K.; Hsu, C.C.; Chao, S.H.; Yang, Z.H.; Lin, Y.J.; Chen, C.C.; Cao, Y.M.; Huang, H.C.;

Chang, C.H.; et al. Bacterial composition and diversity in breast milk samples from mothers living in Taiwan and mainland China. *Front. Microbiol.* **2017**, *8*, 965. [CrossRef] [PubMed]

18. Wishart, D.S.; Feunang, Y.D.; Marcu, A.; Guo, A.C.; Liang, K.; Vazquez-Fresno, R.; Sajed, T.; Johnson, D.; Li, C.; Karu, N.; et al. HMDB 4.0: The human metabolome database for 2018. *Nucleic Acids Res.* **2018**, *46*, D608–D617. [CrossRef] [PubMed]
19. Sundekilde, U.K.; Downey, E.; O'Mahony, J.A.; O'Shea, C.A.; Ryan, C.A.; Kelly, A.L.; Bertram, H.C. The effect of gestational and lactational age on the human milk metabolome. *Nutrients* **2016**, *8*, 304. [CrossRef] [PubMed]
20. Spevacek, A.R.; Smilowitz, J.T.; Chin, E.L.; Underwood, M.A.; German, J.B.; Slupsky, C.M. Infant maturity at birth reveals minor differences in the maternal milk metabolome in the first month of lactation. *J. Nutr.* **2015**, *145*, 1698–1708. [CrossRef] [PubMed]
21. Mitoulas, L.R.; Kent, J.C.; Cox, D.B.; Owens, R.A.; Sherriff, J.L.; Hartmann, P.E. Variation in fat, lactose and protein in human milk over 24 h and throughout the first year of lactation. *Br. J. Nutr.* **2002**, *88*, 29–37. [CrossRef] [PubMed]
22. Kuang, Y.S.; Li, S.H.; Guo, Y.; Lu, J.H.; He, J.R.; Luo, B.J.; Jiang, F.J.; Shen, H.; Papasian, C.J.; Pang, H.; et al. Composition of gut microbiota in infants in china and global comparison. *Sci. Rep.* **2016**, *6*, 36666. [CrossRef] [PubMed]
23. Fallani, M.; Young, D.; Scott, J.; Norin, E.; Amarri, S.; Adam, R.; Aguilera, M.; Khanna, S.; Gil, A.; Edwards, C.A.; et al. Intestinal microbiota of 6-week-old infants across europe: Geographic influence beyond delivery mode, breast-feeding, and antibiotics. *J. Pediatr. Gastroenterol. Nutr.* **2010**, *51*, 77–84. [CrossRef] [PubMed]
24. De Preter, V.; Vanhoutte, T.; Huys, G.; Swings, J.; Rutgeerts, P.; Verbeke, K. Effect of lactulose and *Saccharomyces boulardii* administration on the colonic urea-nitrogen metabolism and the bifidobacteria concentration in healthy human subjects. *Aliment. Pharmacol. Ther.* **2006**, *23*, 963–974. [CrossRef] [PubMed]
25. Dror, D.K.; Allen, L.H. Overview of nutrients in human milk. *Adv. Nutr.* **2018**, *9*, 278s–294s. [CrossRef] [PubMed]
26. Jegou, M.; Gondret, F.; Lalande-Martin, J.; Tea, I.; Baeza, E.; Louveau, I. NMR-based metabolomics highlights differences in plasma metabolites in pigs exhibiting diet-induced differences in adiposity. *Eur. J. Nutr.* **2016**, *55*, 1189–1199. [CrossRef] [PubMed]
27. Garcia-Rios, A.; Perez-Martinez, P.; Mata, P.; Fuentes, F.; Lopez-Miranda, J.; Alonso, R.; Caballero, J.; Mata, N.; Perez-Jimenez, F.; Ordovas, J.M. Polymorphism at the TRIB1 gene modulates plasma lipid levels: Insight from the Spanish familial hypercholesterolemia cohort study. *Nutr. Metab. Cardiovasc. Dis.* **2011**, *21*, 957–963. [CrossRef] [PubMed]
28. Meredith-Dennis, L.; Xu, G.; Goonatilleke, E.; Lebrilla, C.B.; Underwood, M.A.; Smilowitz, J.T. Composition and variation of macronutrients, immune proteins, and human milk oligosaccharides in human milk from nonprofit and commercial milk banks. *J. Hum. Lact.* **2018**, *34*, 120–129. [CrossRef] [PubMed]
29. Chaturvedi, P.; Warren, C.D.; Altaye, M.; Morrow, A.L.; Ruiz-Palacios, G.; Pickering, L.K.; Newburg, D.S. Fucosylated human milk oligosaccharides vary between individuals and over the course of lactation. *Glycobiology* **2001**, *11*, 365–372. [CrossRef] [PubMed]
30. Kunz, C.; Rudloff, S.; Baier, W.; Klein, N.; Strobel, S. Oligosaccharides in human milk: Structural, functional, and metabolic aspects. *Annu. Rev. Nutr.* **2000**, *20*, 699–722. [CrossRef] [PubMed]
31. Davis, J.C.; Lewis, Z.T.; Krishnan, S.; Bernstein, R.M.; Moore, S.E.; Prentice, A.M.; Mills, D.A.; Lebrilla, C.B.; Zivkovic, A.M. Growth and morbidity of Gambian infants are influenced by maternal milk oligosaccharides and infant gut microbiota. *Sci. Rep.* **2017**, *7*, 40466. [CrossRef] [PubMed]
32. Thurl, S.; Munzert, M.; Boehm, G.; Matthews, C.; Stahl, B. Systematic review of the concentrations of oligosaccharides in human milk. *Nutr. Rev.* **2017**, *75*, 920–933. [CrossRef] [PubMed]
33. Sprenger, N.; Lee, L.Y.; De Castro, C.A.; Steenhout, P.; Thakkar, S.K. Longitudinal change of selected human milk oligosaccharides and association to infants' growth, an observatory, single center, longitudinal cohort study. *PLoS ONE* **2017** , *12*, e0171814. [CrossRef] [PubMed]
34. Kuhn, L.; Kim, H.Y.; Hsiao, L.; Nissan, C.; Kankasa, C.; Mwiya, M.; Thea, D.M.; Aldrovandi, G.M.; Bode, L. Oligosaccharide composition of breast milk influences survival of uninfected children born to HIV-infected

mothers in Lusaka, Zambia. *J. Nutr.* **2015**, *145*, 66–72. [CrossRef] [PubMed]

35. Aakko, J.; Kumar, H.; Rautava, S.; Wise, A.; Autran, C.; Bode, L.; Isolauri, E.; Salminen, S. Human milk oligosaccharide categories define the microbiota composition in human colostrum. *Benef. Microbes* **2017**, *8*, 563–567. [CrossRef] [PubMed]
36. De Vadder, F.; Kovatcheva-Datchary, P.; Goncalves, D.; Vinera, J.; Zitoun, C.; Duchampt, A.; Backhed, F.; Mithieux, G. Microbiota-generated metabolites promote metabolic benefits via gut-brain neural circuits. *Cell* **2014**, *156*, 84–96. [CrossRef] [PubMed]
37. Martin, R.; Langa, S.; Reviriego, C.; Jiminez, E.; Marin, M.L.; Xaus, J.; Fernandez, L.; Rodriguez, J.M. Human milk is a source of lactic acid bacteria for the infant gut. *J. Pediatr.* **2003**, *143*, 754–758. [CrossRef] [PubMed]
38. Solis, G.; de Los Reyes-Gavilan, C.G.; Fernandez, N.; Margolles, A.; Gueimonde, M. Establishment and development of lactic acid bacteria and bifidobacteria microbiota in breast-milk and the infant gut. *Anaerobe* **2010**, *16*, 307–310. [CrossRef] [PubMed]
39. Mohammad, M.A.; Maningat, P.; Sunehag, A.L.; Haymond, M.W. Precursors of hexoneogenesis within the human mammary gland. *Am. J. Physiol. Endocrinol. Metab.* **2015**, *308*, E680–E687. [CrossRef] [PubMed]
40. Belenguer, A.; Duncan, S.H.; Calder, A.G.; Holtrop, G.; Louis, P.; Lobley, G.E.; Flint, H.J. Two routes of metabolic cross-feeding between bifidobacterium adolescentis and butyrate-producing anaerobes from the human gut. *Appl. Environ. Microbiol.* **2006**, *72*, 3593–3599. [CrossRef] [PubMed]
41. Schwab, C.; Ganzle, M. Lactic acid bacteria fermentation of human milk oligosaccharide components, human milk oligosaccharides and galactooligosaccharides. *FEMS Microbiol. Lett.* **2011**, *315*, 141–148. [CrossRef] [PubMed]
42. Ewaschuk, J.B.; Naylor, J.M.; Zello, G.A. D-lactate in human and ruminant metabolism. *J. Nutr.* **2005**, *135*, 1619–1625. [CrossRef] [PubMed]
43. Fukuda, S.; Toh, H.; Taylor, T.D.; Ohno, H.; Hattori, M. Acetate-producing bifidobacteria protect the host from enteropathogenic infection via carbohydrate transporters. *Gut Microbes* **2012**, *3*, 449–454. [CrossRef] [PubMed]
44. O'Callaghan, A.; van Sinderen, D. Bifidobacteria and their role as members of the human gut microbiota. *Front. Microbiol.* **2016**, *7*, 925. [CrossRef] [PubMed]
45. Boix-Amorós, A.; Martinez-Costa, C.; Querol, A.; Collado, M.C.; Mira, A. Multiple approaches detect the presence of fungi in human breastmilk samples from healthy mothers. *Sci. Rep.* **2017**, *7*, 13016. [CrossRef] [PubMed]
46. Guertin, K.A.; Moore, S.C.; Sampson, J.N.; Huang, W.Y.; Xiao, Q.; Stolzenberg-Solomon, R.Z.; Sinha, R.; Cross, A.J. Metabolomics in nutritional epidemiology: Identifying metabolites associated with diet and quantifying their potential to uncover diet-disease relations in populations. *Am. J. Clin. Nutr.* **2014**, *100*, 208–217. [CrossRef] [PubMed]
47. Playdon, M.C.; Sampson, J.N.; Cross, A.J.; Sinha, R.; Guertin, K.A.; Moy, K.A.; Rothman, N.; Irwin, M.L.; Mayne, S.T.; Stolzenberg-Solomon, R.; et al. Comparing metabolite profiles of habitual diet in serum and urine. *Am. J. Clin. Nutr.* **2016**, *104*, 776–789. [CrossRef] [PubMed]
48. Chow, J.; Panasevich, M.R.; Alexander, D.; Vester Boler, B.M.; Rossoni Serao, M.C.; Faber, T.A.; Bauer, L.L.; Fahey, G.C. Fecal metabolomics of healthy breast-fed versus formula-fed infants before and during in vitro batch culture fermentation. *J. Proteome Res.* **2014**, *13*, 2534–2542. [CrossRef] [PubMed]

9

Lipid Profile, Lipase Bioactivity and Lipophilic Antioxidant Content in High Pressure Processed Donor Human Milk

Aleksandra Wesolowska [1,*], Joanna Brys [2,*], Olga Barbarska [1,3], Kamila Strom [3], Jolanta Szymanska-Majchrzak [4], Katarzyna Karzel [5], Emilia Pawlikowska [6], Monika A. Zielinska [7], Jadwiga Hamulka [7] and Gabriela Oledzka [3]

1 Laboratory of Human Milk and Lactation Research at Regional Human Milk Bank in Holy Family Hospital, Department of Neonatology, Faculty of Health Sciences, Medical University of Warsaw, Zwirki i Wigury Str. 63A, 02-091 Warsaw, Poland
2 Department of Chemistry, Faculty of Food Sciences, Warsaw University of Life Sciences—SGGW, Nowoursynowska St. 166, 02-787 Warsaw, Poland
3 Department of Medical Biology, Faculty of Health Sciences, Medical University of Warsaw, 14/16 Litewska St., 00-575 Warsaw, Poland
4 Department of Biochemistry, Second Faculty of Medicine, Medical University of Warsaw, Banacha 1b Str. 02-093 Warsaw, Poland
5 Faculty of Psychology, Warsaw University, Stawki 5/7, 00-183 Warsaw, Poland
6 High Pressure Physics, Polish Academy of Science, Sokolowska 29, 01-142 Warsaw, Poland
7 Department of Human Nutrition, Faculty of Human Nutrition and Consumer Sciences, Warsaw University of Life Sciences—SGGW, 159 Nowoursynowska St., 02-776 Warsaw, Poland
* Correspondence: aleksandra.wesolowska@wum.edu.pl (A.W.); joanna_brys@sggw.pl (J.B.)

Abstract: Human milk fat plays an essential role as the source of energy and cell function regulator; therefore, the preservation of unique human milk donors' lipid composition is of fundamental importance. To compare the effects of high pressure processing (HPP) and holder pasteurization on lipidome, human milk was processed at 62.5 °C for 30 min and at five variants of HPP from 450 MPa to 600 MPa, respectively. Lipase activity was estimated with QuantiChrom™ assay. Fatty acid composition was determined with the gas chromatographic technique, and free fatty acids content by titration with 0.1 M KOH. The positional distribution of fatty acid in triacylglycerols was performed. The oxidative induction time was obtained from the pressure differential scanning calorimetry. Carotenoids in human milk were measured by liquid chromatography. Bile salt stimulated lipase was completely eliminated by holder pasteurization, decreased at 600 MPa, and remained intact at 200 + 400 MPa; 450 MPa. The fatty acid composition and structure of human milk fat triacylglycerols were unchanged. The lipids of human milk after holder pasteurization had the lowest content of free fatty acids and the shortest induction time compared with samples after HPP. HPP slightly changed the β-carotene and lycopene levels, whereas the lutein level was decreased by 40.0% up to 60.2%, compared with 15.8% after the holder pasteurization.

Keywords: donor human milk; high pressure processing; carotenoids; antioxidant capacity; lipids; bile salt stimulated lipase; preterm

---

1. Introduction

Lipids in human milk are not only the main source of energy, but also of bioactive components and regulatory factors, such as vitamins and polyunsaturated fatty acids. Lipids exhibit several functions in the range of biological effects connected with neurodevelopment, immunity, digestion, metabolism regulation, cell membranes communication, and signal transduction [1]. Carotenoids, which are lipid-soluble provitamins, contribute to the anti-oxidative properties of human milk, protecting preterm infants against toxic free radicals [2]. Human milk contains a high bile salt stimulated lipase (BSSL) concentration, which enables the easy digestion of mother's milk lipids even in the absence of the enzyme in premature newborns. Human milk lipids are valuable, nourishing food with high bioavailability for newborns [3]. Therefore, expressed human milk, including donor milk, should be handled with care to minimize the loss of the unique lipid composition and lipase activity [4]. Administration of donor milk within the hospital setting often requires several preparatory stages, such as pumping, freezing, thawing, and pasteurization by heat treatment (usually holder pasteurization, HoP). The potential losses in human milk lipid content could accumulate when milk passes through all these stages from donor to recipients [5]. Earlier research indicates that heat treatment does not decrease lipid content and does not alter the fat soluble vitamins A, D, and E [6]. However, it was recently shown, using mid-infrared spectroscopy, that lipids are one of the most affected components in pooled pasteurized milk compared with raw milk donated to a milk bank [7]. It was reported earlier that the total availability of lipids in donor milk is affected by the decrease of BSSL and high adhesion to containers surface [8]. In addition, human milk processing may decrease the antioxidant properties of milk, which could have nutritional and clinical implications owing to the particular susceptibility of polyunsaturated fats to peroxidation.

One of promising preservation methods that allows the unique properties of human milk to be maintained unchanged is high pressure processing (HPP). It is a non-thermal technology that is being increasingly applied in food industries worldwide. This method consists of applying hydrostatic high pressure in short-term treatment to inactivate pathogenic microorganisms and provide nutritionally intact and sensory high-quality products [9].

The aim of our study was to evaluate high pressure processing as a promising technique for the preservation the lipid profile, antioxidant properties, and lipase enzymes activity in donor milk.

2. Materials and Methods

2.1. Ethical Approval

The Bioethics Committee of Warsaw Medical University has accepted the information about conducting this non-interventional study without reservations (admission number AKBE/59/15).

2.2. Milk Sampling

Milk samples were obtained from donors between the second and sixth week of lactation from Regional Human Milk Bank in Warsaw at Holy Family Hospital. Women were given standard instructions about the best practices for expressing breast milk. Milk samples of approximately 50 mL were collected at home or in the hospital ward using an electric or manual pump, stored in the refrigerator at the temperature of 4 °C, and delivered to the human milk bank within 24 h, while maintaining refrigerated conditions.

To carry out the study, 6 pooled samples from 3–4 donors were used. Experiments were performed in duplicate and repeated three times with similar results in the following variants:

- raw milk—control
- temperature processed milk/holder pasteurization (HoP)—comparator
- high pressure processed (HPP)—experimental

The processing influence on lipase activity and the change in human milk lipids were evaluated according to these experimental designs.

Milk samples for all analyses, except for lipase activity, were centrifuged at 4400 rpm for 15 min at 4 °C (Centrifuge 5702R, Eppendorf, Darmstadt, Germany) he lipid monolayer was carefully separated, and both supernatants and lipid monolayer were frozen for later analysis. Lipase activity assay was performed on whole milk samples.

2.3. Human Milk Processing

2.3.1. High Pressure Processing (HPP)

High pressure processing was applied to human milk samples using U 4000/65 apparatus designed and produced by Unipress Equipment at the Institute of High Pressure Physics, Polish Academy of Sciences. The maximum pressure available in the apparatus was 600 MPa and the treatment chamber had a distilled water and polypropylene glycol mixture (1:1), used as pressure-transmitting fluid. The manufacturer designed the working temperature ranges of the apparatus between −10 °C and +80 °C. In our experiments, the test condition temperature was between 19 and 21 °C. Pressure was applied in the following variants: (1) 600 MPa, 10 min; (2) 100 MPa, 10 min, interval 10 min, 600 MPa, 10 min; (3) 200 MPa, 10 min, interval 10 min, 400 MPa, 10 min; (4) 200 MPa, 10 min, interval 10 min, 600 MPa, 10 min; (5) 450 MPa, 15 min. The pressure generation time was 15–25 s and the decompression time was 1–4 s.

2.3.2. Holder Pasteurization (HoP)

Human milk samples were pasteurized according to the routine procedure performed in Regional Human Milk Bank in Warsaw at Holy Family Hospital, using Sterifeed S90 ECO Pasteurise (Medicare Colgate Ltd., Devon, UK, at 62.5 °C for 30 min.

2.4. Lipase Activity

Lipase activity was determined using the lipase assay kit (QuantiChrom Lipase Assay Kit, Bioassay Systems, Hayward, CA, USA) according to the kit instructions. Whole fat human milk samples were brought to room temperature and diluted with distilled water (1:250, *v/v*). The optical density was measured by a Biotek multiple reader at room temperature.

2.5. Lipidome Profile

2.5.1. Fat Extraction

The Folch method [10] with further improvement by Boselli [11] was applied to extract fat from the studied samples.

2.5.2. The Oxidative Induction Time

Induction time (IT) was determined by the use of PDSC (pressure differential scanning calorimetry) to evaluate the samples' oxidative stability. A differential scanning calorimeter (DSC Q20 TA Instruments, New Castle, DE, USA) coupled with a high-pressure cell was used. Fat samples of 3–4 mg were weighed into an aluminium open pan and placed in the sample chamber under oxygen atmosphere with an initial pressure of 1400 kPa. The isothermal temperature for each sample was 120 °C. Obtained diagrams were analyzed using TA Universal Analysis 2000 software (TA Instruments, New Castle, DE, USA). For each sample, the output was automatically recalculated and presented as the amount of energy per one gram. The maximum oxidation induction time was determined based on the maximum rate of heat flow.

2.5.3. Acid Values and Free Fatty Acids Content

The acid value was determined by titration of fat samples with 0.1 M ethanolic potassium hydroxide solution. Free fatty acids (FFA) concentration was calculated based on acid values and the oleic acid molar mass value. Acid values were determined according to ISO method 660:2000.

2.5.4. Fatty Acid Composition

The determination of fatty acid composition was carried out by gas chromatographic (GC) analysis of fatty acid methyl esters. Methyl esters of fatty acids were prepared through transesterification with sodium methoxide according to ISO 5509:2001. A YL6100 GC chromatograph equipped with a flame ionization detector and BPX-70 capillary column of 0.25 mm i.d. x 60 m length and 0.25 μm film thickness was used. The oven temperature was programmed as follows: 60 °C for 5 min; then it was increased by 10 °C/min to 180 °C; from 180 °C to 230 °C, it was increased by 3 °C/min; and then it was kept at 230 °C for 15 min. The temperature of the injector was 225 °C, with a split ratio of 1:50 and the detector temperature of 250 °C. Nitrogen was used as the carrier gas. The results were expressed as relative percentages of each fatty acid, calculated by external normalization of the chromatographic peak area. Fatty acids were identified by comparing the relative retention times of fatty acid methyl ester (FAME) peaks with FAME chemical standard.

2.5.5. Positional Distribution of Fatty Acid in Tag

Positional distribution of fatty acid in sn-2 and sn-1,3 positions in triacylglycerols (TAG) was based on the pancreatic lipase ability to selectively hydrolyze ester bonds in sn-1,3 positions. Briefly, 20 mg of purified pancreatic lipase (porcine pancreatic lipase, crude type II), 1 mL of Tris buffer (pH 8.0), 0.25 mL of bile salts (0.05%), and 0.1 mL of calcium chloride (2.2%) were added to 50 mL centrifuge tubes and vortexed with 0.1 g of fat sample. The mixture was incubated at 40 °C in a water bath for 5 min, after which 1 mL of 6 mol/L HCl and 1 mL of diethyl ether were added, and then the mixture was centrifuged. Diethyl ether layer was collected in test tubes and evaporated under nitrogen gas to obtain 200 uL volume. A 200 uL aliquot was loaded onto a silica gel thin layer chromatography (TLC) plate with fluorescent indicator 254 nm and developed with hexane: diethyl ether acetic acid (50:50:1, v:v:v). 2-monoacylglycerol (2-MAG) band was visualised under UV light. 2-MAG band was scraped off into a screw capped test tube, extracted twice with 1 mL of diethyl ether, and centrifuged. The ether layer was collected and entirely evaporated under nitrogen, and then the sample was dissolved in n-hexane and methylated as described above.

2.6. Carotenoids Analysis

Breastmilk carotenoids' (β-carotene, lycopene, and lutein + zeaxanthin) concentration in milk samples was assessed using high-performance liquid chromatography system (HPLC). Milk samples for the analysis were prepared on the basis of the modified method published earlier [12,13]. Analysis of the studied carotenoids was carried out at a wavelength of 471 nm for lycopene, 450 nm for β-carotene, and 445 nm for lutein + zeaxanthin using the HPLC system (Japan: 2 LC-20AD pumps, CMB-20A controller system, SIL-20AC autosampler, UV/VIS SPD-20AV detector, CTD-20AC controller, Shimadzu, Kioto, Japan) using C18 Synergi Fusion-RP 80i columns (250 × 4.60 mm, Phenomenex, CA, USA). The concentration of individual carotenoids was compared to standard curves prepared with Sigma Aldrich standards (catalogue numbers: β-carotene C4582, lutein + zeaxanthin X6250, lycopene L9879). The concentration of the studied carotenoids was expressed in nmol/L. Lutein and zeaxanthin could not be completely resolved and they were summed; therefore, all references to milk lutein concentration refer to lutein + zeaxanthin.

2.7. Statistical Analysis

Relative standard deviation for the lipase, lipidome, and lipolytic antioxidant factors results was calculated, where appropriate, for all collected data, using Microsoft Excel 2012 Software (Microsoft, Redmond, Washington, DC, USA). One-way analysis of variance (ANOVA) was performed using the Statgraphics Plus, version 5.1 (Statgraphics Technologies, Inc., The Plains, VA, USA). Differences were considered to be significant at a p-value ≤ 0.05, according to Tukey's multiple range test.

3. Results

3.1. Lipase Activity

Because of the variability of lipase activity in human milk, the results from several experiments treating different milk samples were presented as a percent of activity in different samples with respect to raw milk considered 100%. As shown in Figure 1, the enzyme activity was nearly completely eliminated by HoP (2.1% residual activity). Higher lipase activity was detected in the HPP treated samples (16.5%—600 MPa, 11%—100 + 600 MPa, 13.6%—200 + 600 MPa). Almost entire lipase activity retention was observed in pressure 200 + 400 MPa, 10 min, interval 10 min; and 450 MPa, 15 min (82.2%—200 + 400 MPa, 87.3%—450 MPa).

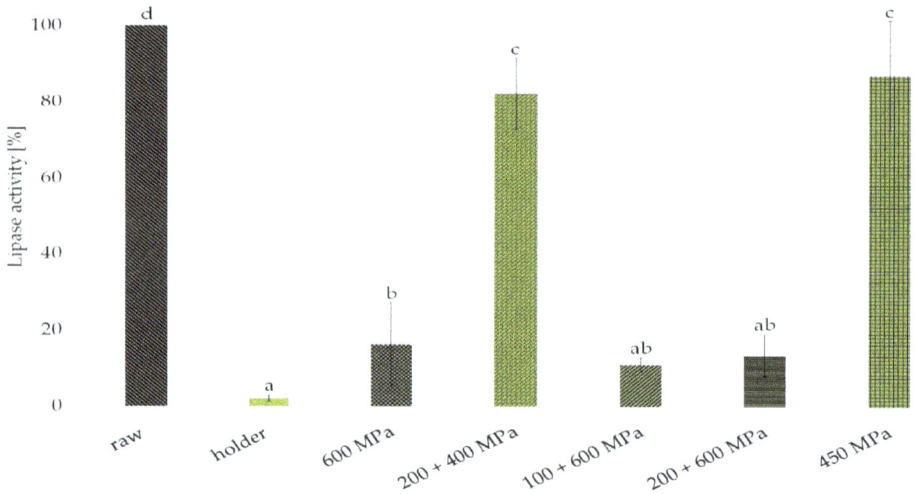

Figure 1. Lipase enzymatic activity in milk samples after holder pasteurization and variants of high pressure processing (HPP) compared with raw milk. Results are shown as a % value of raw milk with error bars representing SD. Different letters indicate that the samples are significantly different at p-value < 0.05.

3.2. FFA Content

Any type of donor milk treatment was associated with a reduction in the FFA content compared with raw milk taken as 100% (Figure 2).

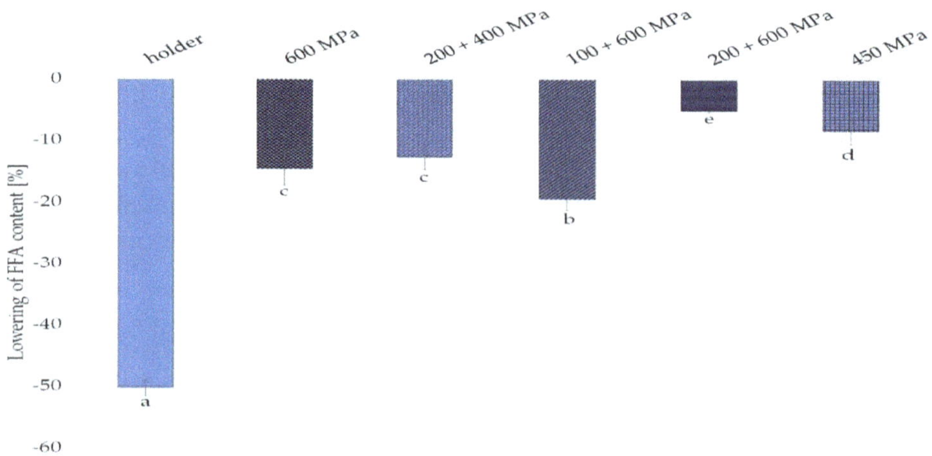

Figure 2. Decrease in free fatty acids (FFA) content compared with raw milk in fats from samples of milk after HPP and holder pasteurization. Results are shown as a % value of raw milk with error bars representing SD. Different letters indicate that the samples are significantly different at $p < 0.05$.

Holder pasteurization decreased FFA content by 50.2%. High pressure processing, depending on the variants, lowered FFA milk content by 19.5% for 100 + 600 MPa, 14.6% for 600 MPa, 12.8% for 200 + 400 MPa, 8.4% for 450 MPa, and 5.1% for 200 + 600 MPa (Figure 2).

3.3. Oxidative Stability

The PDSC measurements results of oxidative stability of sample expressed as the oxidation induction time (IT) are shown in Figure 3. Longer IT is connected with better stability. Significant differences in IT were observed especially between fat from raw and HoP milk—after heat treatment, IT was over 12 minutes shorter. The fat from samples after high pressure processing was also characterized by changed oxidative stability in comparison with the fat from raw human milk. The changes were slightly detectable in the case of 600 MPa and 200 + 600 MPa; more noticeable in 450 MPa, 15 min condition (3 minutes shorter); and about 7 min shorter induction time was observed in 200 + 400 MPa and 100 + 600 MPa (pressure 10 min, interval 10 min, pressure 10 min).

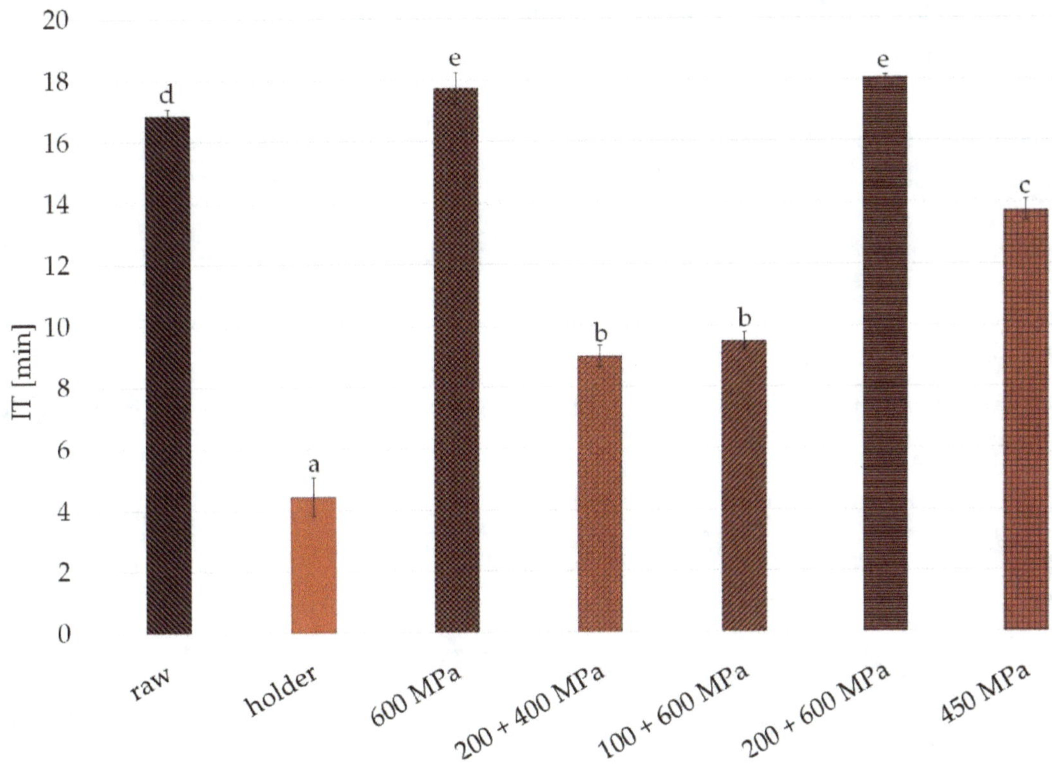

Figure 3. Oxidative stability of raw milk, in the samples after HPP and holder pasteurization. Results are shown as a % value of raw milk with error bars representing SD. Different letters indicate that the samples are significantly different at $p < 0.05$. IT, induction time.

3.4. Fatty Acid Composition

The fatty acids profile of fats from studied samples are presented in Figure 4 and Table 1. The fats from analyzed human milk contained from 10.7% to 12.2% of the polyunsaturated fatty acids (PUFA) and from 37.7% to 43.1% of the monounsaturated fatty acids (MUFA). Over 40% of all fatty acids in these fats were saturated fatty acids (SFA), of which the main representative was palmitic acid (from 23.8% to 25.1%). The main monounsaturated fatty acid present in analyzed samples of fats was oleic acid (from 34.0% to 39.4%). Polyunsaturated fatty acids found in studied samples were primarily linoleic acid (from 8.2% to 9.4%) and α-linolenic acid (1.3–1.4%). The major LCPUFA from n-6 family found in analyzed samples of fats was arachidonic acid (about 0.3–0.4%). Fats from studied human milk also contained omega-3 long chains polyunsaturated fatty acids like eicosapentaenoic acid (about 0.1%) and docosahexaenoic acid (about 0.3%). No statistically significant differences for samples after processing compared with raw milk fat were observed.

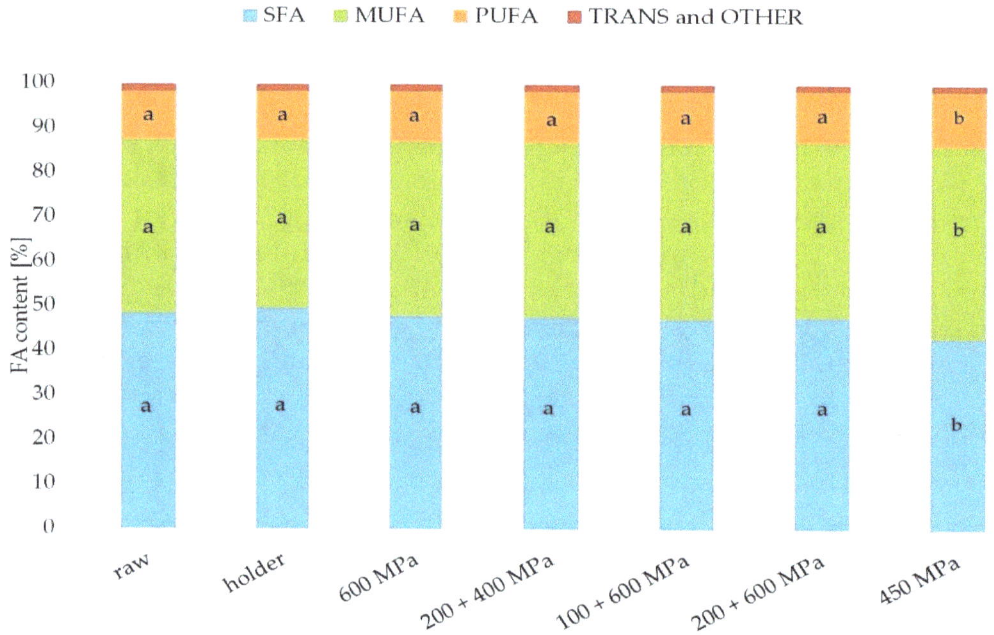

Figure 4. Content of fatty acid (SFA, saturated fatty acids; MUFA, monounsaturated fatty acids; PUFA, polyunsaturated fatty acids; TRANS, trans fatty acids) in the samples after HPP and holder pasteurization. The different lower case letters (for SFA, MUFA, and PUFA separately) indicate significantly different values ($p < 0.05$).

Table 1. Changes in fatty acid composition during high pressure processing (HPP) and holder pasteurization (mean ± SD).

Human Milk Fatty Acid Composition (%)	Raw Milk	Holder	600 MPa	200 + 400 MPa	100 + 600 MPa	200 + 600 MPa	450 MPa
Saturated fatty acids (SFA)	48.53 ± 0.94	49.77 ± 3.39	47.94 ± 0.83	47.70 ± 0.25	47.32 ± 0.08	47.72 ± 0.18	43.17 ± 0.62
C8:0	0.06 ± 0.04	0.11 ± 0.02	0.08 ± 0.04	0.04 ± 0.01	0.06 ± 0.01	0.05 ± 0.01	0.05 ± 0.00
C10:0	0.89 ± 0.09	1.07 ± 0.23	0.83 ± 0.10	0.77 ± 0.01	0.88 ± 0.02	0.85 ± 0.02	0.73 ± 0.09
C12:0	5.77 ± 0.14	6.58 ± 1.26	5.72 ± 0.36	5.28 ± 0.05	5.76 ± 0.11	5.63 ± 0.08	3.96 ± 0.51
C14:0	8.47 ± 0.40	8.89 ± 1.48	8.27 ± 0.35	8.08 ± 0.13	8.10 ± 0.07	8.15 ± 0.08	6.11 ± 0.39
C15:0	0.36 ± 0.02	0.38 ± 0.05	0.35 ± 0.02	0.35 ± 0.01	0.35 ± 0.01	0.35 ± 0.00	0.36 ± 0.01
C16:0	24.59 ± 0.49	25.13 ± 1.30	24.22 ± 0.08	24.45 ± 0.23	23.80 ± 0.01	24.14 ± 0.02	23.93 ± 0.16
C17:0	0.36 ± 0.03	0.33 ± 0.00	0.33 ± 0.01	0.34 ± 0.01	0.33 ± 0.01	0.34 ± 0.00	0.34 ± 0.01
C18:0	7.57 ± 0.03	6.94 ± 0.83	7.73 ± 0.05	7.95 ± 0.14	7.64 ± 0.09	7.81 ± 0.01	7.26 ± 0.20
C20:0	0.47 ± 0.03	0.36 ± 0.11	0.43 ± 0.01	0.46 ± 0.01	0.42 ± 0.01	0.43 ± 0.01	0.45 ± 0.01
Polyunsaturated fatty acids (PUFA)	39.07 ± 0.15	37.715 ± 2.34	39.04 ± 0.70	39.24 ± 0.42	39.46 ± 0.15	39.25 ± 0.08	43.13 ± 0.45
C20:1	0.52 ± 0.01	0.43 ± 0.13	0.52 ± 0.01	0.55 ± 0.04	0.50 ± 0.01	0.52 ± 0.01	0.72 ± 0.01
C14:1	0.25 ± 0.04	0.32 ± 0.04	0.29 ± 0.00	0.27 ± 0.01	0.28 ± 0.00	0.28 ± 0.00	0.23 ± 0.01
C15:1	0.10 ± 001	0.11 ± 0.02	0.09 ± 0.00	0.10 ± 0.01	0.09 ± 0.01	0.09 ± 0.00	0.08 ± 0.00
C16:1	2.63 ± 0.35	2.69 ± 0.25	2.44 ± 0.04	2.45 ± 0.11	2.46 ± 0.01	2.46 ± 0.01	2.49 ± 0.02
C17:1	0.20 ± 0.01	0.21 ± 0.03	0.21 ± 0.01	0.20 ± 0.01	0.23 ± 0.01	0.22 ± 0.01	0.20 ± 0.00
C18:1	35.39 ± 0.46	33.97 ± 2.50	35.49 ± 0.74	35.68 ± 0.25	35.91 ± 0.13	35.69 ± 0.09	39.41 ± 0.47
Polyunsaturated fatty acids (PUFA)	10.73 ± 1.00	11.04 ± 1.05	11.4 ± 0.12	11.53 ± 0.08	11.67 ± 0.07	11.57 ± 0.00	12.24 ± 0.30
C18:2 n-6	8.17 ± 1.15	8.75 ± 0.64	8.90 ± 0.06	8.99 ± 0.01	9.08 ± 0.04	9.05 ± 0.01	9.40 ± 0.18
C18:3 n-3	1.36 ± 0.12	1.28 ± 0.12	1.27 ± 0.01	1.30 ± 0.03	1.36 ± 0.05	1.30 ± 0.00	1.33 ± 0.06
C20:2 n-6	0.20 ± 0.01	0.18 ± 0.04	0.22 ± 0.01	0.22 ± 0.01	0.22 ± 0.01	0.22 ± 0.00	0.32 ± 0.00
C20:3 n-6	0.20 ± 0.01	0.21 ± 0.07	0.27 ± 0.03	0.25 ± 0.01	0.26 ± 0.00	0.25 ± 0.00	0.35 ± 0.01
C20:4 n-6	0.38 ± 0.01	0.34 ± 0.08	0.38 ± 0.01	0.39 ± 0.00	0.39 ± 0.00	0.38 ± 0.00	0.44 ± 0.01
C20:5 n-3	0.14 ± 0.01	0.07 ± 0.01	0.11 ± 0.04	0.11 ± 0.02	0.09 ± 0.01	0.10 ± 0.00	0.09 ± 0.03
C22:6 n-3	0.31 ± 0.01	0.22 ± 0.08	0.28 ± 001	0.27 ± 0.03	0.29 ± 0.01	0.28 ± 0.01	0.31 ± 0.00

3.5. Fatty Acid Distribution

The results regarding the percentage of fatty acids esterified at sn-2 position of TAG from fats are presented in Figure 5 and Table 2. Palmitic acid was located at sn-2 position in 64.7% TAG from raw milk fats, 66.5% fats from milk after HoP. High pressure processing causes a slight increase in the palmitic acid in sn-2 position of TAGs—to about 70% (73.6% in 600 MPa, 72.6% in 200 + 400 MPa, 70.4% 200 + 600 MPa, and 72.8% for 450 MPa). The difference was not statistically significant. Oleic acid at sn-2 was detected in 15% of TAG extracted from raw and holder pasteurized milk samples. After HPP, the percentage of oleic acid at sn-2 position of TAG diminished to 12% for 600 MPa, as well as 200 + 400 MPa and 100 + 600 MPa. In the case of 200 + 600 MPa 10 min, interval 10 min, 10 min, the percentage of the fatty acids esterified at sn-2 position of TAG was 14.1%, and almost the same for 450 MPa, 15 min. (13%).

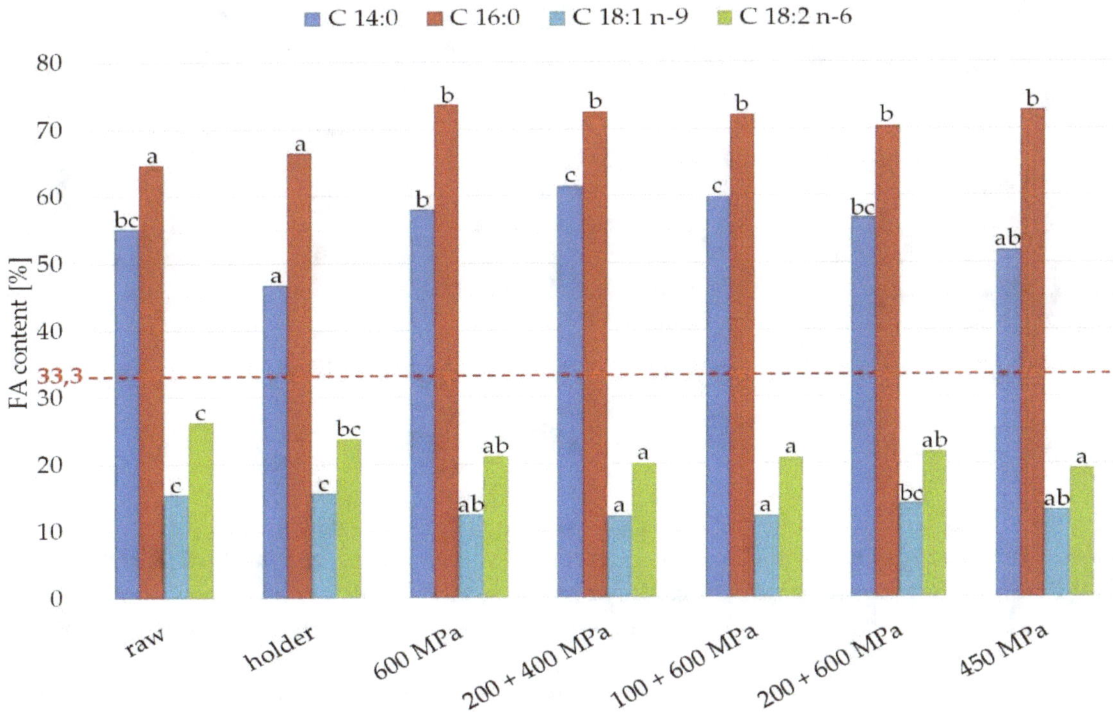

Figure 5. Fatty acid distribution in the sn-2 position of TAG from raw milk and in the samples after HPP and holder pasteurization. The different lower case letters for each fatty acid separately indicate significantly different values ($p < 0.05$). The line indicates the statistical (even) distribution of fatty acids between three TAG positions (33%).

Table 2. Changes in the fatty acid composition of sn-2 monoacylglycerols during HPP and holder pasteurization (mean ± SD; only selected fatty acids are presented).

Fatty Acid (%) in sn-2 Position of TAG	Raw Milk	Holder	600 MPa	200 + 400 MPa	100 + 600 MPa	200 + 600 MPa	450 MPa
C14:0 (myristic acid)	14.00 ± 0.71	12.50 ± 0.50	14.40 ± 0.47	14.90 ± 1.12	14.52 ± 0.62	13.90 ± 0.63	9.50 ± 0.54
C16:0 (palmitic acid)	47.70 ± 0.81	50.10 ± 1.34	53.50 ± 1.85	53.20 ± 0.59	51.50 ± 0.45	51.00 ± 1.22	52.20 ± 0.02
C18:1 (oleic acid)	16.40 ± 0.35	16.00 ± 0.18	13.40 ± 0.04	13.10 ± 1.07	13.20 ± 0.07	15.10 ± 1.65	15.40 ± 0.25
C18:2 (linoleic acid)	6.50 ± 0.28	6.20 ± 0.10	5.70 ± 0.11	5.40 ± 0.57	5.67 ± 0.28	5.90 ± 0.28	5.40 ± 0.28

3.6. Carotenoids

The studied carotenoids' concentration in raw milk was about 32.8 nmol/L for β-carotene, 85.9 nmol/L for lycopene, and 45.9 nmol/L for lutein + zeaxanthin. The content of carotenoids after processing compared with raw milk is presented in Figure 6.

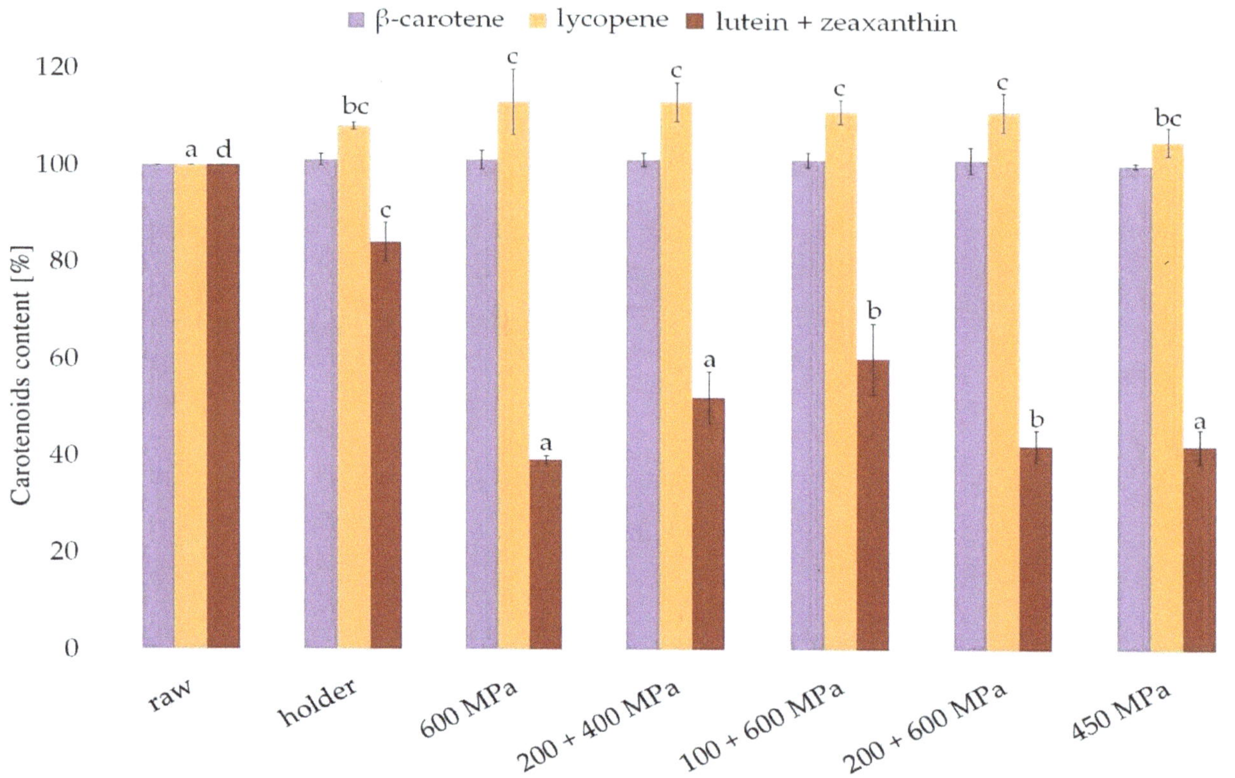

Figure 6. Content of carotenoids (β-carotene, lycopene, and lutein + zeaxanthin) in milk samples after HPP and holder pasteurization. Results are shown as a % value of raw milk with error bars representing SD. Different letters indicate that the samples are significantly different at $p < 0.05$.

β-carotene was intact after processing; therefore, the level was comparable in all milk samples. Statistically significant changes ($p \leq 0.05$) were observed in the case of lutein and zeaxanthin, as well as lycopene concentration in milk samples after processing. Pasteurization diminished the content of lutein + zeaxanthin compared with raw milk to about 84.1%, whereas HPP was so destructive as to leave 39.7% after 600 MPa, 52.9% after 200 + 400 MPa, 42.5% after 200 + 600 MPa, 60% after 100 + 600 MPa, and 42.4% after 450 MPa. In the case of lycopene, a slight content increase was observed after processing compared with raw milk—8.8% in case of pasteurization; 5.7% after 450 MPa; and 111.8% to 113.6% after other variants of high pressure processing, 200 + 400 MPa and 200 + 600 MPa, respectively.

4. Discussion

The main practical advantages of putting the baby to the breast for feeding are overall integrity of given nutrients, optimal temperature, microbiological safety, and intact bioactivity of mother's milk. Every other way of feeding involves some losses in human milk properties. Human milk is a complex body fluid with thousands of components in dynamic interplay [14–16]. For example, human milk fat breakdown by endogenous lipase is rather not noticeable when the baby is fed directly from the breast. In contrast, expressing human milk with a high lipase activity is associated with free fatty acids release from TAG, even if milk is frozen immediately. The increase of FFA levels causes pH changes that affect enzyme activity and other inherent human milk components [17–19]. In addition, unbound FFA may cause cytotoxicity in the intestinal lumen [20]. However, endogenous lipases are the prime effector of milk fats' digestion, facilitating human milk consumption in the early period of life. Therefore, it is crucial to retain enzymatic properties of human milk, especially when human milk is banked for preterms. As several previous studies proved, the activity of BSSL in donor human milk is mostly suppressed by holder pasteurization [21–23]. In contrast, high pressure processing seems to be a favorable technique for human milk preservation for this purpose [24]. Our current results concerning the residual enzymatic activity of lipase after HPP are consistent with the discovery of Demazou and co-workers, as well as the work of Pitino et al. [25,26]. All studies showed slightly diminished functional activity of this enzyme in milk after processing it in selected pressure conditions to about 80%, compared with 100% in raw milk [26]. In fact, the difference between detected enzyme activity in raw milk and milk treated in pressure of 450 MPa for 15 min and 200 + 400 MPa for 10 min with a 10 min interval was not statistically significant (Figure 1).

As human milk enzymes such as BSSL modulate the digestion to favor absorption of triglycerides hydrolysis and vitamins, human milk processing may negatively affect infants' ability to digest lipids because of the total inactivation of endogenous human milk lipases [27].

Human milk FFA content seems to be a good indicator of BSSL bioavailability in processed milk, because in the case of human milk, the FFA concentration should depend mostly on this enzyme's activity. However, available data concerning the effect of HoP on FFA concentration were inconsistent. Lepri et al. reported an 83% increase in FFA content after heat treatment [28], in contrast to several studies where no change was detected [29–32]. Only Williamson et al. report a 21% decrease in FFA concentration [33]. As shown in this study, all applied preservation techniques reduced the content of free fatty acids in fat extracted from human milk with a statistically significant difference (Figure 2). In the case of pasteurized milk, a reduction as large as 50% in the content of FFA compared with raw milk was noticed. FFA content decrease in fat from high pressure processed human milk was from 5% to 19% compared with fat from raw human milk, which is consistent with previous studies [30].

Analyzing the results, it can be observed that the differences in FFA fat content are especially significant in milk pasteurized by HoP, while after high pressure processing, the decrease in FFA content is minor. So when the enzyme was completely destroyed by heat treatment in the HoP samples, the FFA content was the lowest. This rule does not apply to high pressure samples. Among HPP variants, the largest reduction in FFA content was noticed in milk subjected to 100 + 600 MPa pressure, and lipase activity in this variant is significantly diminished. In contrast to this finding, at 200 + 600 MPa, the FFA content is almost intact while enzyme activity is severely lowered (Figure 1, Figure 2). In fact, our results of FFA and lipase activity in human milk after processing are ambiguous. The reason for this discrepancy could be a very low level of FFA in untreated human milk taken as 100%—as a result, any changes given as a percentage lead to large proportional differences [34].

Nevertheless, based on our research, we concluded that the best option seems to be 450 MPa for 15 min as the most favorable conditions for preservation of FFA concentration and lipase activity.

Oxidative stability is one of the most important factors determining the quality of foods, especially those containing high levels of unsaturated fats, including human milk. Within the fatty acid family, polyunsaturated fatty acids are highly labile molecules susceptible to oxidation, giving rise to free radicals, hydroperoxides and polymers, which might lead to loss of quality, both technological and related to their health benefits [35]. A number of methods for the assessment of oxidative stability have been developed, among which differential scanning calorimetry is one of the most frequently used. This method is very fast and convenient [36–38]. Generally, samples with longer induction times (IT) are more stable than those with a shorter induction time at the same temperature [37,39].

In our study, IT changes compared with raw milk value ranged from 5% for samples from fat after HPP in 600 MPa to 46% for HPP variant with 200–400 MPa. It appears that any kind of preservation causes changes to human milk oxidative status, but less so in selected pressure variants than in HoP (Figure 3).

Although original causes and consequences of oxidative and hydrolytic degradation processes are quite different, they seem to interact with each other and contribute to the reduction in stability of fats. Research suggests that fat FFA presence may induce oxidation as a result of a catalytic effect of carboxylic groups of FFA on the formation of free radicals. In general, the higher the level of fatty acids content, monoacylglycerols, and diacylglycerols in the fat with respect to the level of TAG, the more the oxidative stability is reduced. Pro-oxidant FFA action is thus connected with carboxylic molecular group, which accelerates the rate of hydroperoxides decomposition [35,40,41].

Analyzing the results obtained in this work, it can be concluded that the reduction in FFA content did not affect the improvement of oxidative fat stability (Figure 2, Figure 3). Pasteurized milk, despite the low content of FFA, is characterized by the shortest induction time, and thus the worst oxidative stability. Deterioration of oxidative stability in the case of pasteurized human milk could have been influenced by other factors, such as temperature, that could affect the content of antioxidants in the samples.

Human milk contains 3–5% of lipids and approximately 99% of them are TAG. The major fatty acids of TAG are palmitic acid (16:0), oleic acid (18:1), and linoleic acid (18:2 *n*-6), which constitute 25%, 30%, and 15%, respectively, of all fatty acids [42,43]. Therefore, fatty acid composition of human milk fat is unique, because the fat is characterized by a high content of saturated palmitic acid and also contains polyunsaturated fatty acids, which are not present in other milk fats [44–46].

Polyunsaturated fatty acid components of human milk are complex, including both C18 precursors, linoleic acid (18:2 *n*-6) and α-linolenic acid (18:3 *n*-3), as well as bioactive, very long chain polyunsaturated fatty acids (LCPUFA) of both *n*-6 and *n*-3 families [46,47].

Most of the studies on the effect of human milk processing, including the current study, have claimed that fatty acid composition was intact after holder pasteurization [21,30,47]. In addition, the results from our study proved no change in fatty acid profile in human milk after HPP, which is consistent with discoveries from other research studies on the effect of HPP on human milk [21,30]. It can be concluded that high pressure processing and holder pasteurization do not affect the composition of fatty acid (Figure 4, Table 1).

Moreover, the structure of human milk TAG is also unique, as 60–70% of palmitic acid is located at sn-2 position, and sn-1 and sn-3 positions are taken by 18:0, 18:1, and 18:2 fatty acids. This unique intramolecular structure is one of the key factors controlling the products formed by the gastric lipase in the stomach and by pancreatic or bile salt-stimulated lipases in the small intestinal absorption; therefore, it improves the efficiency of calcium absorption [48].

Considering the composition of fatty acid in sn-2 position of monoacylglycerols from the studied fats (Table 2), it can be seen that saturated fatty acids that occur mainly in this position are palmitic and myristic acid and unsaturated fatty acids—oleic and linoleic acids.

Analyzing the results regarding the percentage of fatty acids esterified at sn-2 position of TAG from the studied fats, it can be concluded that differences in the distribution of fatty acid in TAG were really small (Figure 5). There are no statistically significant differences between raw milk and HoP in the distribution of fatty acid in triacylglycerol molecules. These results are confirmed by many research studies [5,29–31,47,49]. According to scientists, no difference was found in the bioaccessibility of different fatty acids released from raw human milk and pasteurized human milk. If pasteurization affected the structure of triacylglycerols (TAG), the bioavailability of fatty acids found in these TAG would also change.

The percentage of palmitic acid and myristic acid at sn-2 of TAG in fats from all processed samples of human milk exceeded 33% (ranged from 64.7% to 73.6% for palmitic acid and from 46.7% to 61.4% for myristic acid), which means that these saturated fatty acids are located mainly in the internal position of TAG (Figure 5). This location increases the efficiency of calcium absorption in infants. Taking into account the percentage of unsaturated fatty acids in sn-2 position of TAG in studied fats, it can be stated that they are located mostly in external positions of TAG. The percentage of oleic acid at sn-2 of TAG in analyzed fats ranged from 12.2% to 15.7% and linoleic acids—from 19.2% to 26.3%, which confirms that they are located mainly in sn-1,3 positions of TAG (external position of TAG).

Carotenoids are principal non-enzymatic, lipophilic antioxidants that act as free radical scavengers. There is a substantial and growing body of research evidence showing an important role of carotenoids, especially lutein, in human development, related to their antioxidant and anti-inflammatory properties [50,51]. This is crucial for preterm infants, for whom carotenoid (mainly lutein) administration may decrease the risk of several prematurity disorders, including necrotizing enterocolitis, bronchopulmonary dysplasia, and retinopathy of prematurity related to elevated oxidative stress [52–54]. Carotenoids are one of the bioactive factors in human milk, and their amount is determined by maternal dietary intake; infant formulas are not fortified enough [51,55]. In our study, we found that all variants of HPP slightly changed the β-carotene and lycopene content (it is increased), whereas lutein + zeaxanthin content is decreased by 40.0% (at 600 MPa, 200 + 600 MPa, 450 MPa) up to 60.2% (at 100 + 600 MPa) compared with a 15.8% decrease in the holder pasteurized samples. It is the first time that the effect of high pressure on human milk with regard to β-carotene content has been evaluated. The only existing study comparing maternal breastmilk with donor milk has revealed the 18–53% lower amount of carotenoids after heat treatment, which is still higher than in infant formulas [55]. The increase in lycopene concentration after high pressure treatment was observed before in tomato products [56]. Human milk preservation and storage are not the only processes that affect carotenoid content. A study conducted by Tacken et al. also found that lutein is more sensitive to processing than other carotenoids [57]. In this case, tube feeding was related to the decreased concentration of lutein by 35% (even 42.6% with the phototherapy exposure), β-carotene by 26%. This relatively high decrease in lutein content may be caused by its high susceptibility to oxidation damage.

5. Conclusions

Human milk lipids are essential nutrition components for the growth and development of an infant. Commonly used holder pasteurization affects some of the nutritional and biological components of human milk and its lipid fractions [21,34]. Moreover, structural disintegration of lipid fraction of human milk by thermal pasteurization has been proven [7,27]. However, in the pilot clinical trial, the significance of those changes has not been proven with regards to important nutritional outcomes such as effectiveness of gastric emptying in the group of preterm infants [58,59]. Other studies revealed a decrease of fat absorption in preterms fed with donor milk [60]. We determined that high pressure processing, especially at 450 MPa for 15 min., minimizes changes in the lipidome and lipid related components such as lipase of donor human milk, with the exception of the destructive effect on lutein + zeaxanthin. As was previously shown, preterms' growth rate during their hospital stay depends on overall quality of lipidome [61]. Therefore, any methods of improving human milk lipids preservation, including high pressure processing of donor milk, could be beneficial in managing optimal infant weight gain and growth.

Author Contributions: A.W. and J.B. conceived and designed the experiments; O.B., K.S., J.S.-M., E.P., M.A.Z., and J.H. performed the experiments; J.B., A.W., O.B., and J.S.-M. analyzed the data; G.O. contributed reagents and materials; K.K. performed statistical analysis of this work and interpretation of data for the work; A.W., J.B., M.A.Z., and J.H. wrote the paper; O.B. prepared figure and tables for publication; G.O. revised manuscript critically for important intellectual content.

Acknowledgments: We acknowledge Elzbieta Lodykowska from the Regional Human Milk Bank in Warsaw at Holy Family Hospital for assistance with collecting milk samples and all the mothers who participated in the study.

References

1. Koletzko, B. Human milk lipids. *Ann. Nutr. Metab.* **2016**, *69*, 27–40. [CrossRef] [PubMed]
2. Tsopmo, A. Phytochemicals in Human Milk and Their Potential Antioxidative Protection. *Antioxidants* **2018**, *7*, 32. [CrossRef] [PubMed]
3. Koletzko, B.; Rodríguez-Palmero, M.; Demmelmair, H.; Fidler, N.; Jensen, R.; Sauerwald, T.; Mis, N.F. Physiological aspects of human milk lipids. *Early Hum. Dev.* **2001**, *65*, S3–S18. [CrossRef]
4. Nessel, I.; Khashu, M.; Dyall, S.C. The effects of storage conditions on long-chain polyunsaturated fatty acids, lipid mediators, and antioxidants in donor human milk—A review. *Prostaglandins Leukot. Essent. Fatty Acids* **2019**, *149*, 8–17. [CrossRef] [PubMed]
5. Fidler, N.; Sauerwald, T.U.; Demmelmair, H.; Koletzko, B. Fat Content and Fatty Acid Composition of Fresh, Pasteurized, or Sterilized Human Milk. *Adv. Exp. Med. Biol.* **2001**, *501*, 485–495. [PubMed]
6. Van Zoeren-Grobben, D.; Schrijver, J.; Berg, H.V.D.; Berger, H.M. Human milk vitamin content after pasteurisation, storage, or tube feeding. *Arch. Dis. Child.* **1987**, *62*, 161–165. [CrossRef]
7. Cavazos-Garduño, A.; Serrano-Niño, J.; Solís-Pacheco, J.; Gutierrez-Padilla, J.; González-Reynoso, O.; García, H.; Aguilar-Uscanga, B. Effect of pasteurization, freeze-drying and spray drying on the fat globule and lipid profile of human milk. *J. Food Nutr. Res.* **2016**, *4*, 296–302.
8. Hamosh, M.; Henderson, T.R.; Ellis, L.A.; Mao, J.-I.; Hamosh, P. Digestive Enzymes in Human Milk: Stability at Suboptimal Storage Temperatures. *J. Pediatr. Gastroenterol. Nutr.* **1997**, *24*, 38–43. [CrossRef]
9. Peila, C.; Emmerik, N.E.; Giribaldi, M.; Stahl, B.; Ruitenberg, J.E.; van Elburg, R.M.; Moro, G.E.; Bertino, E.; Coscia, A.; Cavallarin, L. Human Milk Processing: A Systematic Review of Innovative Techniques to Ensure the Safety and Quality of Donor Milk. *J. Pediatr. Gastroenterol. Nutr.* **2017**, *64*, 353–361. [CrossRef]
10. Iverson, S.J.; Lang, S.L.C.; Cooper, M.H. Comparison of the bligh and dyer and folch methods for total lipid determination in a broad range of marine tissue. *Lipids* **2001**, *36*, 1283–1287. [CrossRef]
11. Boselli, E.; Velazco, V.; Caboni, M.F.; Lercker, G. Pressurized liquid extraction of lipids for the determination of oxysterols in egg-containing food. *J. Chromatogr. A* **2001**, *917*, 239–244. [CrossRef]
12. Macias, C.; Schweigert, F.J. Changes in the Concentration of Carotenoids, Vitamin A, Alpha-Tocopherol and Total Lipids in Human Milk throughout Early Lactation. *Ann. Nutr. Metab.* **2001**, *45*, 82–85. [CrossRef] [PubMed]
13. Zielinska, M.A.; Hamulka, J.; Wesolowska, A. Carotenoid Content in Breastmilk in the 3rd and 6th Month of Lactation and Its Associations with Maternal Dietary Intake and Anthropometric Characteristics. *Nutrients* **2019**, *11*, 193. [CrossRef] [PubMed]
14. Ballard, O.; Morrow, A.L. Human Milk Composition: Nutrients and Bioactive Factors. *Pediatr. Clin. N. Am.* **2013**, *60*, 49–74. [CrossRef] [PubMed]
15. Andreas, N.J.; Kampmann, B.; Le-Doare, K.M. Human breast milk: A review on its composition and bioactivity. *Early Hum. Dev.* **2015**, *91*, 629–635. [CrossRef] [PubMed]
16. Bardanzellu, F.; Fanos, V.; Strigini, F.A.L.; Artini, P.G.; Peroni, D.G. Human Breast Milk: Exploring the Linking Ring Among Emerging Components. *Front. Pediatr.* **2018**, *6*, 215. [CrossRef] [PubMed]
17. Vázquez-Román, S.; Escuder-Vieco, D.; Martín-Pelegrina, M.; Muñoz-Amat, B.; Fernández-Álvarez, L.; Brañas-García, P.; Lora-Pablos, D.; Beceiro-Mosquera, J.; Pallás-Alonso, C. Effect of refrigerated storage on the pH and bacterial content of pasteurized human donor milk. *J. Dairy Sci.* **2018**, *101*, 10714–10719. [CrossRef] [PubMed]
18. Ogundele, M.O. Effects of storage on the physicochemical and antibacterial properties of human milk. *Br. J. Biomed. Sci.* **2002**, *59*, 205–211. [CrossRef]
19. Ahrabi, A.F.; Handa, D.; Codipilly, C.N.; Shah, S.; Williams, J.E.; McGuire, M.A.; Potak, D.; Aharon, G.G.; Schanler, R.J. Effects of Extended Freezer Storage on the Integrity of Human Milk. *J. Pediatr.* **2016**, *177*, 140–143. [CrossRef]
20. Penn, A.H.; Altshuler, A.E.; Small, J.W.; Taylor, S.F.; Dobkins, K.R.; Schmid-Schönbein, G.W. Effect of Digestion and Storage of Human Milk on Free Fatty Acid Concentration and Cytotoxicity. *J. Pediatr. Gastroenterol. Nutr.* **2014**, *59*, 365–373. [CrossRef]
21. Pitino, M.A.; Alashmali, S.M.; Hopperton, K.E.; Unger, S.; Pouliot, Y.; Doyen, A.; O'Connor, D.L.; Bazinet, R.P. Oxylipin concentration, but not fatty acid composition, is altered in human donor milk pasteurised using both thermal and non-thermal techniques. *Br. J. Nutr.* **2019**, *122*, 47–55. [CrossRef] [PubMed]

22. Peila, C.; Moro, G.E.; Bertino, E.; Cavallarin, L.; Giribaldi, M.; Giuliani, F.; Cresi, F.; Coscia, A. The Effect of Holder Pasteurization on Nutrients and Biologically-Active Components in Donor Human Milk: A Review. *Nutrients* **2016**, *8*, 477. [CrossRef]
23. Ewaschuk, J.B.; Unger, S. Human milk pasteurization: Benefits and risks. *Curr. Opin. Clin. Nutr. Metab. Care* **2015**, *18*, 269–275.
24. Wesolowska, A.; Sinkiewicz-Darol, E.; Barbarska, O.; Bernatowicz-Lojko, U.; Borszewska-Kornacka, M.K.; Van Goudoever, J.B. Innovative Techniques of Processing Human Milk to Preserve Key Components. *Nutrients* **2019**, *11*, 1169. [CrossRef] [PubMed]
25. Pitino, M.A.; Unger, S.; Doyen, A.; Pouliot, Y.; Aufreiter, S.; Stone, D.; Kiss, A.; O'Connor, D.L. High Hydrostatic Pressure Processing Better Preserves the Nutrient and Bioactive Compound Composition of Human Donor Milk. *J. Nutr.* **2019**, *149*, 497–504. [CrossRef]
26. Demazeau, G.; Plumecocq, A.; Lehours, P.; Martin, P.; Couëdelo, L.; Billeaud, C. A New High Hydrostatic Pressure Process to Assure the Microbial Safety of Human Milk While Preserving the Biological Activity of Its Main Components. *Front. Public Health* **2018**, *6*, 306. [CrossRef]
27. De Oliveira, S.C.; Bourlieu, C.; Ménard, O.; Bellanger, A.; Henry, G.; Rousseau, F.; Dirson, E.; Carrière, F.; Dupont, D.; Deglaire, A. Impact of pasteurization of human milk on preterm newborn in vitro digestion: Gastrointestinal disintegration, lipolysis and proteolysis. *Food Chem.* **2016**, *211*, 171–179. [CrossRef] [PubMed]
28. Lepri, L.; Del Bubba, M.; Maggini, R.; Donzelli, G.P.; Galvan, P. Effect of pasteurization and storage on some components of pooled human milk. *J. Chromatogr. B Biomed. Sci. Appl.* **1997**, *704*, 1–10. [CrossRef]
29. Henderson, T.R.; Fay, T.N.; Hamosh, M. Effect of pasteurization on long chain polyunsaturated fatty acid levels and enzyme activities of human milk. *J. Pediatr.* **1998**, *132*, 876–878. [CrossRef]
30. Moltó-Puigmartí, C.; Permanyer, M.; Castellote, A.I.; López-Sabater, M.C.; Castellote-Bargalló, A.I. Effects of pasteurisation and high-pressure processing on vitamin C, tocopherols and fatty acids in mature human milk. *Food Chem.* **2011**, *124*, 697–702. [CrossRef]
31. Romeu-Nadal, M.; Castellote, A.; Gayà, A.; López-Sabater, M.C. Effect of pasteurisation on ascorbic acid, dehydroascorbic acid, tocopherols and fatty acids in pooled mature human milk. *Food Chem.* **2008**, *107*, 434–438. [CrossRef]
32. Borgo, L.A.; Araújo, W.M.C.; Conceição, M.H.; Resck, I.S.; Mendonça, M.A. Are fat acids of human milk impacted by pasteurization and freezing? *Nutr. Hosp.* **2015**, *31*, 1386–1393.
33. Williamson, S.; Finucane, E.; Ellis, H.; Gamsu, H.R. Effect of heat treatment of human milk on absorption of nitrogen, fat, sodium, calcium, and phosphorus by preterm infants. *Arch. Dis. Child.* **1978**, *53*, 555–563. [CrossRef]
34. Gao, C.; Miller, J.; Middleton, P.F.; Huang, Y.-C.; McPhee, A.J.; Gibson, R.A. Changes to breast milk fatty acid composition during storage, handling and processing: A systematic review. *Prostaglandins Leukot. Essent. Fat. Acids* **2019**, *146*, 1–10. [CrossRef] [PubMed]
35. Martin, D.; Reglero, G.; Señoráns, F.J. Oxidative stability of structured lipids. *Eur. Food Res. Technol.* **2010**, *231*, 635–653. [CrossRef]
36. Kowalski, B.; Gruczyńska, E.; Maciaszek, K. Kinetics of rapeseed oil oxidation by pressure differential scanning calorimetry measurements. *Eur. J. Lipid Sci. Technol.* **2000**, *102*, 337–341. [CrossRef]
37. Tan, C.P.; Man, Y.C. Recent developments in differential scanning calorimetry for assessing oxidative deterioration of vegetable oils. *Trends Food Sci. Technol.* **2002**, *13*, 312–318. [CrossRef]
38. Bryś, J.; Wirkowska, M.; Gorska, A.; Ostrowska-Ligeza, E.; Bryś, A. Application of the calorimetric and spectroscopic methods in analytical evaluation of the human milk fat substitutes. *J. Therm. Anal. Calorim.* **2014**, *118*, 841–848. [CrossRef]
39. Kowalski, B.; Tarnowska, K.; Gruczynska, E.; Bekas, W. Chemical and Enzymatic Interesterification of Beef Tallow and Rapeseed Oil Blend with Low Content of Tallow. *J. Oleo Sci.* **2004**, *53*, 479–488. [CrossRef]
40. Miyashita, K.; Takagi, T. Study on the oxidative rate and prooxidant activity of free fatty acids. *J. Am. Oil Chem. Soc.* **1986**, *63*, 1380–1384. [CrossRef]
41. Hamam, F.; Shahidi, F. Enzymatic acidolysis of an arachidonic acid single-cell oil with capric acid. *J. Am. Oil Chem. Soc.* **2004**, *81*, 887–892. [CrossRef]
42. Mu, H. Production and nutritional aspects of human milk fat substitutes. *Lipid Technol.* **2010**, *22*, 126–129. [CrossRef]

43. Visentainer, J.V.; Santos, O.O.; Maldaner, L.; Zappielo, C.; Neia, V.; Visentainer, L.; Pelissari, L.; Pizzo, J.; Rydlewski, A.; Silveira, R.; et al. Lipids and Fatty Acids in Human Milk: Benefits and Analysis. In *Biochemistry and Health Benefits of Fatty Acids*; IntechOpen: London, UK, 2018.
44. Bryś, J.; Flores, L.F.V.; Górska, A.; Wirkowska-Wojdyła, M.; Ostrowska-Ligęza, E.; Bryś, A. Use of GC and PDSC methods to characterize human milk fat substitutes obtained from lard and milk thistle oil mixtures. *J. Therm. Anal. Calorim.* **2017**, *130*, 319–327. [CrossRef]
45. Lien, E.L. The role of fatty acid composition and positional distribution in fat absorption in infants. *J. Pediatr.* **1994**, *125*, S62–S68. [CrossRef]
46. Salamon, S.; Csapó, J. Composition of the mother's milk II. Fat contents, fatty acid composition. A review. *Acta Univ. Sapientiae Aliment.* **2009**, *2*, 196–234.
47. Delgado, F.J.; Cava, R.; Delgado, J.; Ramírez, R. Tocopherols, fatty acids and cytokines content of holder pasteurised and high-pressure processed human milk. *Dairy Sci. Technol.* **2014**, *94*, 145–156. [CrossRef]
48. Nielsen, N.S.; Yang, T.; Xu, X.; Jacobsen, C. Production and oxidative stability of a human milk fat substitute produced from lard by enzyme technology in a pilot packed-bed reactor. *Food Chem.* **2006**, *94*, 53–60. [CrossRef]
49. Baack, M.L.; Norris, A.W.; Yao, J.; Colaizy, T. Long Chain Polyunsaturated Fatty Acid Levels in U.S. Donor Human Milk: Meeting the Needs of Premature Infants? *J. Perinatol.* **2012**, *32*, 598–603. [CrossRef]
50. Giampietri, M.; Lorenzoni, F.; Moscuzza, F.; Boldrini, A.; Ghirri, P. Lutein and Neurodevelopment in Preterm Infants. *Front. Mol. Neurosci.* **2016**, *10*, 4034. [CrossRef]
51. Zielińska, M.A.; Wesołowska, A.; Pawlus, B.; Hamułka, J. Health Effects of Carotenoids during Pregnancy and Lactation. *Nutrients* **2017**, *9*, 838. [CrossRef]
52. Manzoni, P.; Guardione, R.; Bonetti, P.; Priolo, C.; Maestri, A.; Mansoldo, C.; Mostert, M.; Anselmetti, G.; Sardei, D.; Bellettato, M. Lutein and zeaxanthin supplementation in preterm very low-birth-weight neonates in neonatal intensive care units: A multicenter randomized controlled trial. *Am. J. Perinatol.* **2013**, *30*, 25–32. [CrossRef]
53. Rubin, L.P.; Chan, G.M.; Barrett-Reis, B.M.; Fulton, A.B.; Hansen, R.; Ashmeade, T.; Oliver, J.; Mackey, A.; Dimmit, R.; Hartmann, E. Effect of carotenoid supplementation on plasma carotenoids, inflammation and visual development in preterm infants. *J. Perinatol.* **2012**, *32*, 418–424. [CrossRef]
54. Costa, S.; Giannantonio, C.; Romagnoli, C.; Vento, G.; Gervasoni, J.; Persichilli, S.; Zuppi, C.; Cota, F. Effects of lutein supplementation on biological antioxidant status in preterm infants: A randomized clinical trial. *J. Matern. Neonatal Med.* **2013**, *26*, 1311–1315. [CrossRef]
55. Hanson, C.; Lyden, E.; Furtado, J.; Van Ormer, M.; Anderson-Berry, A. A Comparison of Nutritional Antioxidant Content in Breast Milk, Donor Milk, and Infant Formulas. *Nutrients* **2016**, *8*, 681. [CrossRef]
56. Oey, I.; Van Der Plancken, I.; Van Loey, A.; Hendrickx, M. Does high pressure processing influence nutritional aspects of plant based food systems? *Trends Food Sci. Technol.* **2008**, *19*, 300–308. [CrossRef]
57. Tacken, K.J.M.; Vogelsang, A.; Dikkeschei, B.D.; Van Lingen, R.A.; Slootstra, J.; Van Zoeren-Grobben, D. Loss of triglycerides and carotenoids in human milk after processing. *Arch. Dis. Child. Fetal Neonatal Ed.* **2009**, *94*, 447–450. [CrossRef]
58. Bellanger, A.; Ménard, O.; Pladys, P.; Dirson, E.; Kroell, F.; De Oliveira, S.C.; Le Gouar, Y.; Dupont, D.; Deglaire, A.; Bourlieu, C. Impact of human milk pasteurization on gastric digestion in preterm infants: A randomized controlled trial. *Am. J. Clin. Nutr.* **2017**, *105*, 379–390.
59. Perrella, S.L.; Hepworth, A.R.; Gridneva, Z.; Simmer, K.N.; Hartmann, P.E.; Geddes, D.T. Gastric emptying and curding of pasteurized donor human milk and mother's own milk in preterm infants. *J. Pediatr. Gastroenterol. Nutr.* **2015**, *61*, 125–129.
60. Andersson, Y.; Sävman, K.; Bläckberg, L.; Hernell, O. Pasteurization of mother's own milk reduces fat absorption and growth in preterm infants. *Acta Paediatr.* **2007**, *96*, 1445–1449. [CrossRef]
61. Alexandre-Gouabau, M.-C.; Moyon, T.; Cariou, V.; Antignac, J.-P.; Qannari, E.M.; Croyal, M.; Soumah, M.; Guitton, Y.; David-Sochard, A.; Billard, H.; et al. Breast Milk Lipidome Is Associated with Early Growth Trajectory in Preterm Infants. *Nutrients* **2018**, *10*, 164. [CrossRef]

10

Validation of the Breastfeeding Score—A Simple Screening Tool to Predict Breastfeeding Duration

Hanne Kronborg * and Michael Væth

Department of Public Health, Faculty of Health, Aarhus University, 8000 Aarhus, Denmark; vaeth@ph.au.dk
* Correspondence: hk@ph.au.dk

Abstract: Easy to use screening tools to identify mothers in risk of early breastfeeding cessation are needed. The purpose was to validate a revised version of the breastfeeding score, consisting of four questions addressing completed education, earlier breastfeeding duration, self-efficacy, and sense of security not knowing the exact amount of milk the baby ingests. We used two cohorts from 2004 (n = 633) and 2017 (n = 579) to explore the predictive validity of the breastfeeding score to identify mothers at risk of breastfeeding cessation within the first 17 weeks postpartum. The analyses included sensitivity and specificity, clinically relevant cut-points, and calibrations plots. A cut-point ≥5 points identified 61% of first-time and 42% of multiparous mothers in the validation cohort 2017 to be at risk of early breastfeeding cessation with a sensitivity and specificity of 80% and 60% for first-time, and 69% and 82% for multiparous, respectively. The corresponding numbers in the 2004 cohort were almost identical. The area under the receiver operating characteristic (ROC) curves were 0.77 and 0.78 and the calibration plots showed good agreement for the two cohorts. The breastfeeding score indicated good ability to discriminate between mothers at risk of early exclusive breastfeeding cessation. The simple form of the tool makes it easy to use in daily practice.

Keywords: breastfeeding; infant; parity; maternal behavior; educational status; self-efficacy; risk factors; prognosis; sensitivity and specificity; practice

---

1. Introduction

Breastfeeding has been shown to be beneficial for the health of both the mother and infant, not only in the postnatal period, but also later in life [1]. However, breastfeeding rates are still below the recommended in western societies [2]. One third of new mothers experience that establishment of breastfeeding is complicated by early breastfeeding problems [3,4]. From ongoing Cochrane reviews, we know that professional support in the early postpartum period helps mothers to successfully establish breastfeeding [5]. The challenge is to identify the mothers at risk of early breastfeeding cessation and thus in need of early support. Usable screening tools have to be simple to use in practice and reliable to discriminate between mothers.

Successful breastfeeding depends on multiple factors [6–8], and a tool to predict breastfeeding duration should therefore include different kinds of indicators. The challenge is still to establish a link from the risk profile of predictors for early cessation of breastfeeding to a practical tool (index) providing valid information for professionals to initiate preventive efforts. Consensus has not yet been reached on which indicators or indexes are the most reliable. Numerous postpartum screening tools developed during the last decades include behavioral and observational factors connected to breastfeeding [9]; others include more self-reported psychosocial factors [10]. So far, the tools have primarily been evaluated for construct and content validity and psychometric properties, and, to a lesser extent, for their predictive validity [10–13]. Moreover, a number of tools are comprehensive and contain a large number of variables, making them less useful in practice [10–13]. The Breastfeeding

Self-Efficacy Scale-Short Form (BSES-SF), including 14 items measuring perceived self-efficacy towards breastfeeding, has been the tool that has shown the best ability to predict breastfeeding success [12,14]. Still, the question remains whether it is possible to produce a reliable self-reported tool with fewer questions to predict early breastfeeding cessation.

In 2007, we introduced a breastfeeding score, developed on the basis of data from a cohort of breastfeeding mothers from 1999 and validated using cohort data from 2004 [15]. This breastfeeding score was based on four simple questions and showed a strong prediction of the breastfeeding cessation in the first four months postpartum. Thus, the tool complied with demands of both simplicity and reliability. The aim of the present study was to validate a revised version of the breastfeeding score using new and expanded data.

2. Materials and Methods

The validation process followed the method suggested by Altman et al. [16–18]. The breastfeeding score was first tested in a temporal validation on a second dataset collected independently of the first dataset which was used in the development process. In the present study, we also validated the revised version of the breastfeeding score on a third dataset of mothers from different geographical areas where we had no exclusion criteria.

2.1. Three Cohorts Included in the Derivation and Validation Process

The breastfeeding score was obtained from the derivation cohort collected in 1999 [19], which included 471 Danish-speaking mothers who had given birth to a single child with a gestational age ≥37 weeks. The temporal validation was performed on a cohort of 723 mothers from 2004 [20], which constituted the comparison group from a randomized trial with the same inclusion criteria and data obtained from the same area as the derivation cohort. Detailed description of the cohorts can be found elsewhere [19,20].

The external validation cohort from 2017 (n = 612) consisted of the comparison group in a community-based randomized trial [21,22]. The aim of the trial was to test the effect of the Newborn Behavioral Observation method with the comparison group treated as usual. The health visitor recruited mothers from the beginning of January 2017 until the end of January 2018 at the first home visit one to two weeks after birth. There were no exclusion criteria, except exclusion of mothers who were unable to manage own legal affairs. The validation cohort from 2017 thus included first-time mothers, premature births, twin births, postpartum depressed mothers, and mothers with a different ethnic background than Danish. The study was performed in four Danish municipalities, representing several geographical regions of Denmark [22]. The comparison groups were chosen as validation cohorts to avoid impact from the interventions studied in the randomized trials.

2.2. Data Collection

Data in all three cohorts were collected from self-reported questionnaires. Questions included in the breastfeeding score were identical in wording and were collected approximately two weeks postpartum. The duration of exclusive breastfeeding was defined as only ingesting mother's milk according to indicators for assessing breastfeeding practices from the WHO [23]. Data on breastfeeding duration were collected by the local health visitors in the derivation cohort and self-reported in the validation cohorts. The follow-up periods were 17 and 26 weeks for the 1999 and 2004 cohorts, and nine months for the 2017 cohort. Data were obtained by mail in the first two cohorts, and by a web-based system in the 2017 cohort.

2.3. Ethical Approval

Permission to conduct the cohort studies in 1999 and 2004 was obtained from the Science Ethic Committee for the Counties of Ringkoebing, Ribe and Soenderjylland (ref. 2047-99) and (ref. 2480-03), and the Danish Data Protection Agency (j.nr. 2013-41-1866, 1344) and (j.nr. 2003-41-3306), respectively. According to the cohort study 2017 the Central Denmark Region Committee on Health Research Ethics found no need for ethical approval (ref.no.172/2016) as there was no biomedicine involved in the project. Written consent was obtained from all participating mothers. Approval was obtained from the Danish Data Protection Agency (ref.no. 62908/2016).

2.4. Risk Factors Included in the Breastfeeding Score

Originally, the breastfeeding score included the following four risk factors: duration of schooling, previous breastfeeding experience, self-efficacy concerning breastfeeding, and mother's confidence not knowing the exact amount of milk the baby ingests when breastfeeding [15,19]. These factors represent information within sociodemographic, pre and perinatal as well as psychosocial domains.

In the current validation, we chose to change the sociodemographic variable from years of schooling to level of education. Originally, we used the distinction between having completed primary or secondary school (high school) [19]. Today, more than 70% finish secondary school in Denmark, and the level of further education is thus more informative. Furthermore, we changed the variable name from confidence to sense of security (not knowing the exact amount of milk the baby ingests when breastfeeding). The variable name was changed primarily to achieve a more descriptive translation of the content of the question and secondly to make a clearer distinction from the self-efficacy variable. The wording of the question (in Danish) was not changed. Thus, the current validation included the following four risk factors: Completed education measured at levels: none, short, skilled, theoretical bachelor, master. Earlier breastfeeding duration measured in weeks: none for primipara, 0–5, 6–17, >17 for multipara. Self-efficacy measured on a five-point Likert scale from very certain to very uncertain. Sense of security not knowing the exact amount of milk the baby ingests measured on a five-point Likert scale from very secure to very unsecure. Questions and their categorization appear from Table 1.

2.5. Statistical Methods

Initially, descriptive analyses of the risk factors in the three cohorts were performed, and Chi^2 tests were used to compare the derivation and validation cohorts, as seen in Table 1. Next, we used Cox regression analysis to assess the influence of the four risk factors on exclusive breastfeeding cessation in the first 17 weeks postpartum in the derivation cohort. For comparison, data from the two validation cohorts were analysed in the same way. The hazard ratios (HR) estimated the ratio of the cessation rate of exclusive breastfeeding for a given category of the risk factor relative to the cessation rate for the reference category. Integer scores roughly proportional to the log (HR) estimates in the derivation cohort were subsequently obtained for each category of the four risk factors. Finally, for each mother, the breastfeeding score was computed as the sum of the scores for the categories to which she belonged, providing a possible risk score of 0–12 points, as seen in Table 2. The scoring thus obtained was subsequently validated on the two independently collected dataset to evaluate the robustness of the prediction of the breastfeeding score as suggested by Altman et al. [16,17].

Table 1. Characteristics of mothers in the derivation and validation cohorts with complete information on the four questions included in the breastfeeding score.

Characteristics	Derivation Cohort 1999	Validation Cohort 2004	p Value *	Validation Cohort 2017	p Value *
	n = 391	n = 633		n = 579	
	n (%)	n (%)		n (%)	
Sociodemographic Factors					
Maternal age: How old are you?					
17–23	36 (9)	43 (7)		34 (6)	
24–31	245 (63)	391 (62)	0.32	323 (56)	0.002
>32	109 (28)	196 (31)		222 (38)	
Vocational Education: Which vocational education have you completed?					
None–short-skilled	256 (65)	373 (59)	0.04	195 (34)	<0.001
Theoretical bachelor–master	135 (35)	260 (41)		384 (66)	
Smoking: Do you smoke now after giving birth?					
Yes	78 (20)	113 (18)	0.40	33 (6)	<0.001
No	313 (80)	520 (82)		546 (94)	
Perinatal factors					
Parity: How many children have you given birth to?					
Primipara	157 (40)	257 (41)	0.91	276 (48)	0.02
Multipara	233 (60)	376 (59)		303 (53)	
Previous breastfeeding experience: How many weeks did you breastfeed your previous child without giving it anything else?					
None, primipara	157 (40)	257 (41)		276 (48)	
0–5 weeks	31 (8)	40 (6)	0.09	70 (12)	<0.001
6–17 weeks	104 (27)	137 (22)		83 (14)	
>17 weeks	99 (25)	199 (31)		150 (26)	
Psychosocial factors					
Self-efficacy with respect to breastfeeding: How certain are you that you can complete four months of exclusive breastfeeding					
Medium to very uncertain (1–3)	131 (33)	153 (24)	<0.001	189 (33)	0.78
Certain to very certain (4–5)	260 (67)	480 (76)		390 (67)	
Sense of security not knowing the exact amount of milk the baby ingests: I feel fine about not knowing exactly how much milk my child gets when being breastfed					
Is not true (1–2)	181 (46)	240 (38)	0.01	246 (42)	0.24
Is fairly–exactly true (3–5)	210 (54)	393 (62)		333 (58)	

Note: p value * from a comparison with derivation cohort.

Table 2. Risk factors associated with breastfeeding cessation in the first 17 weeks after delivery.

Risk Factors	Prognostic Index						
	Derivation Cohort 1999			Validation Cohort 2004		Validation Cohort 2017	
	Log HR	95% CI	Scores	Log HR	95% CI	Log HR	95% CI
Completed Vocational Education							
None–short–skilled	0.32	−0.04–0.69	1	0.51	0.24–0.79	0.24	0.00–0.48
Theoretical bachelor–master	ref.	ref.	0	ref.	ref.	ref.	ref.
Previous breastfeeding experience:							
None, primipara	0.89	0.25–1.53	3	1.02	0.62–1.42	0.49	0.11–0.87
0–5 weeks	1.79	1.05–2.52	6	1.49	0.96–2.03	0.85	0.39–1.31
6–17 weeks	1.14	0.49–1.79	4	0.77	0.33–1.21	0.78	0.34–1.22
>17 weeks	ref.	ref.	0	ref.	ref.	ref.	ref.
Self-efficacy with respect to breastfeeding							
Uncertain	0.82	0.48–1.17	3	0.98	0.70–1.25	1.11	0.85–1.38
Certain	ref.	ref.	0	ref.	ref.	ref.	ref.
Sense of security not knowing the exact amount of milk the baby ingests							
Insecure	0.72	0.35–1.08	2	0.51	0.24–0.77	0.71	0.46–97
Secure	ref.	ref.	0	ref.	ref.	ref.	ref.

Cox regression analysis of data from 391 mothers with complete information in the derivation cohort, and assigned scores included in the breastfeeding score for each category of the four risk factors. For comparison, the corresponding Cox regression analyses of data from 633 and 579 mothers in the validation cohorts.

The two validation cohorts were used to investigate the breastfeeding score's ability to predict maternal risk of early breastfeeding cessation defined as cessation of exclusive breastfeeding before the end of week 17. Subsequently, we used receiver operating characteristic (ROC) curves to explore the diagnostic validity of the breastfeeding score and to identify a suitable cut-point, as seen in Figure 1. Moreover, the validity of the breastfeeding score was evaluated by calibration plots, as seen in Figure 2, and analyses, describing numbers and proportions of mothers who stopped breastfeeding within 17 weeks according to their breastfeeding score, as seen in Table 3.

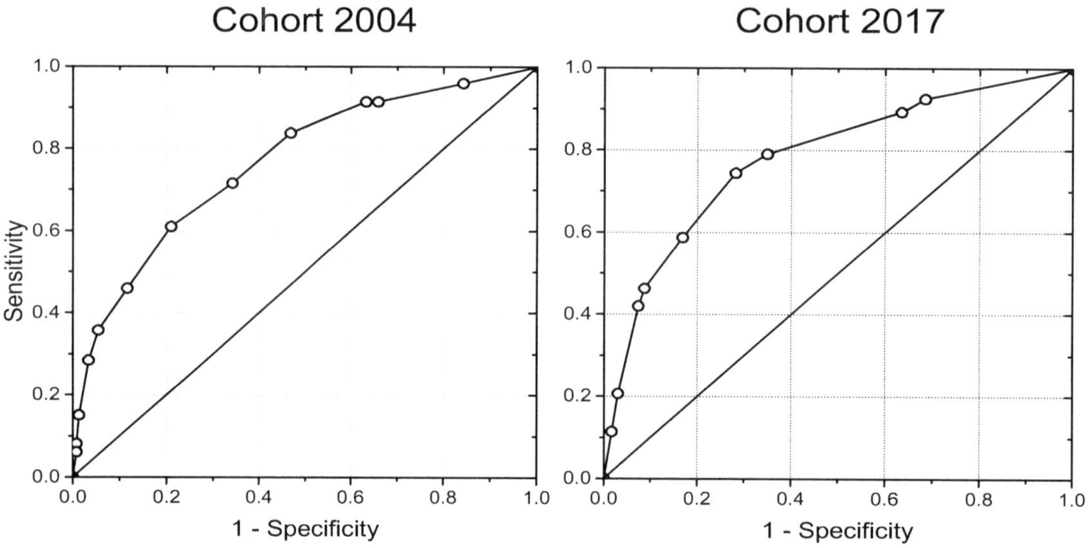

Figure 1. Receiver operating characteristic (ROC) curves for the breastfeeding scores in the validation 2004 (n = 633) and 2017 (n = 579) cohorts.

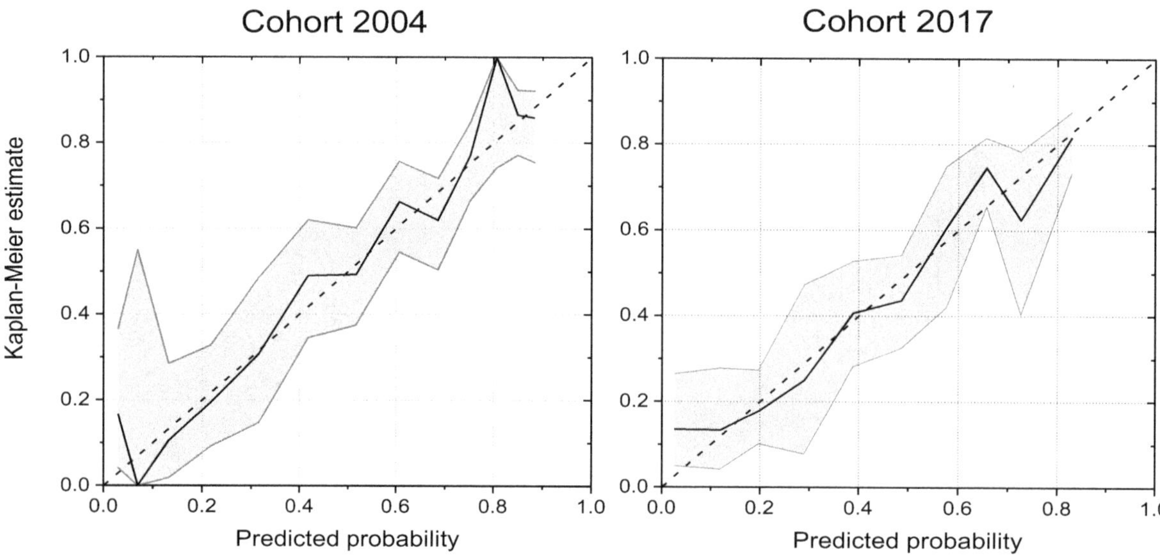

Figure 2. Calibrations plots with 95% confidence intervals for the breastfeeding scores in the validation cohorts 2004 (n = 633) and 2017 (n = 579).

Table 3. Primiparous and multiparous mothers in the validation cohorts divided into risk groups according to their breastfeeding scores. Numbers and proportions of mothers who stopped breastfeeding within 17 weeks in each risk group.

Breastfeeding Score	Validation Cohort 2004			Validation Cohort 2017		
	n (%)	No. Stopped	% (95% CI)	n (%)	No. Stopped	% (95% CI)
Primipara						
0–4 points	103 (40)	32	31 (22–41)	109 (39)	29	27 (19–36)
5–19 points	154 (60)	92	60 (0.52–0.68)	167 (61)	113	68 (60–75)
Multipara						
0–4 points	222 (59)	38	17 (12–23)	177 (58)	43	24 (18–31)
5–19 points	154 (41)	84	55 (46–63)	126 (42)	96	76 (68–83)

3. Results

In the derivation and validation cohorts, we had 391 (83%), 633 (88%), and 579 (95%) mothers, respectively, with complete information on the included risk factors in the breastfeeding score. Among mothers in these cohorts, 194 (41%), 246 (39%), and 281 (49%) had stopped exclusive breastfeeding within 17 weeks after birth. A comparison of the distribution of the risk factors in the three cohorts showed that the educational level changed over time with an increasing proportion of mothers with a long-term education. Moreover, the age of the mothers at birth increased and fewer were smoking. Earlier breastfeeding duration among multipara only showed minor differences, whereas mothers in the validation cohort 2017 had reported similar levels of self-efficacy and sense of security towards breastfeeding as mothers in the derivation cohort 1999; mothers in the validation cohort 2004 reported slightly higher levels, as seen in Table 1.

Table 2 presents results of the Cox regression analysis in the three cohorts with log hazard ratios quantifying risk of breastfeeding cessation for each category relative to the reference category of the four risk factors. Scores assigned to each category of the four risk factors from the derivation cohort are also shown.

The ROC curves, seen in Figure 1, illustrate the association between sensitivity and specificity for different cut-points of the breastfeeding score, when mothers in the validation cohorts had been allocated points depending on their replies concerning the risk factors early after birth. The areas under the ROC curves were 0.77 (CI: 0.73–0.81) and 0.78 (CI: 0.74–0.82), respectively, for the validation cohorts from 2004 and 2017. A detailed calculation for the sensitivity and specificity with associated cut-points showed that a cut-point ≥5 gave the highest sensitivity and specificity. A cut-point ≥5 points predicted that 61% of first-time mothers and 42% of multiparous mothers in the validation cohort 2017 had a high risk of early breastfeeding cessation before 17 weeks with a sensitivity and specificity of 80% and 60% for first-time and 69% and 82% for multiparous mothers, respectively. The corresponding numbers for a cut-point ≥5 in the validation cohort 2004 were almost identical, pointing out that 60% of first-time and 41% of multiparous mothers were at risk; sensitivity and specificity were 74% and 53% for first-time mothers and 69% and 72% for multiparous mothers, respectively.

In both validation cohorts, the calibration plot with confidence intervals, as seen in Figure 2, showed a good agreement between the observed and predicted probability of breastfeeding cessation before the end of week 17 postpartum. From Table 3, it appears that 80% of first-time mothers and 69% of multiparous mothers with a risk score of 5–19 points stopped exclusive breastfeeding before 17 weeks in the validation cohort 2017. The corresponding numbers for mothers with a risk score of 5–19 points in the validation cohort 2004 were 68% and 70%, respectively.

4. Discussion

Validation of the revised version of the breastfeeding score in a general population of Danish mothers confirmed its ability to identify new mothers at risk of early breastfeeding cessation.

The breastfeeding score combines four risk factors to a simple score. The score showed a high ability to discriminate between mothers with different risks and had a good predictive performance.

The updating of the breastfeeding score with a replacement of the sociodemographic risk factor from completed primary or secondary school to completed level of further education included recalibration of the relative weight of the four risk factors included in the breastfeeding score, as suggested by Moons et al. [18]. The use of retrospective data when testing the performance of the breastfeeding score made it possible not only to compare observed events of early breastfeeding cessation with the prediction from the breastfeeding score, but also to assess the ability of the breastfeeding score to discriminate and calibrate between risk groups and thereby assess the clinical usefulness of the score [18]. Self-reported data on the risk factors used to validate the breastfeeding score were collected early after birth independently of collection of data on the outcome of exclusive breastfeeding. Although mothers generally recall their breastfeeding duration quite accurately [24], the collection of data on breastfeeding duration by health professionals must be considered more reliable, which was the case in the derivation cohort. The transferability of the breastfeeding score was supported by the validation of the cohort from 2017, consisting of an unselected study population of new mothers living in different geographical areas of Denmark, with a diverse population of mothers reflecting the Danish background population according to age and level of education [25].

The four included risk factors in the breastfeeding score represented different domains of the multifactorial structure of breastfeeding. Level of completed education contributed with information on maternal sociodemographic background, well-known to influence breastfeeding duration [6]. Previous breastfeeding experience contributed with information on the pre and perinatal period, including first time motherhood and the success of breastfeeding for the multiparous mother expressed by the duration of exclusive breastfeeding of the previous child. Mothers tend to breastfeed for just as long as or a little longer than they did with a previous child [26]. Self-efficacy and sense of security concerning breastfeeding contributed with information on the psychosocial aspects of breastfeeding, which have been shown to be essential predictors of breastfeeding duration [7,19,27]. The general self-efficacy towards breastfeeding expressed the mothers' confidence in overcoming any difficulties and achieving success [28]. Thereby, the predictor expressed maternal ability and strengths to overcome early problems and continue breastfeeding. Sense of security towards breastfeeding gathered information about the insecurity many mothers experience when they start breastfeeding. Concerns may be related to having enough milk [29] and getting used to a responsive feeding style with an infant-led approach [30,31]. Breastfeeding implies to learn how to read the infant's cues on hunger and satiety to have a sense of security because the amount of milk the infant ingests is not visible. The inclusion of predictors from different domains of the multifactorial construct of breastfeeding may explain why the breastfeeding score maintains its predictive ability over time in different populations of new mothers.

The breastfeeding score indicated a high predictive value. The Self-efficacy Scale-Short Form (BSES-SF) has been found to predict the exclusive breastfeeding to 16 weeks in smaller study samples [12,14]. A direct comparison of the predictive values of the two screening tools are not possible, as we have not been able to find a comprehensive validation of the BSES-SF. The cut-point of five revealed a good ability to discriminate between subgroups by pointing to 60% of first-time mothers and 40% of multiparous mothers to be at risk of early breastfeeding cessation. The outcome of exclusive breastfeeding was determined based on mothers who stopped breastfeeding within 17 weeks, because this is the minimum recommended duration of exclusive breastfeeding according to the European Committees on Nutrition ESPGHAN and EFSA [32,33]. The relatively high proportion of mothers at risk of early breastfeeding cessation reflected the high proportion of mothers who generally stop exclusive breastfeeding before four months [1]. Cochrane reviews have repeatedly shown positive effects of supporting mothers in the breastfeeding act [5]. The breastfeeding score may ensure that the intervention is addressed to the insecure mothers who wish to breastfeed by pointing to mothers at risk of early cessation and in need for early support. From a public health perspective, it is especially important to identify the insecure first-time mothers and support them in establishing breastfeeding, considering the association between breastfeeding duration of the first and later infants [27].

From a practical point of view, the breastfeeding score is easy to use with a simple scoring system, which does not require technical assistance. The breastfeeding score aims to identify women with increased need for additional support when establishing breastfeeding. A short questionnaire can be used to obtain the breastfeeding score as it is based on self-reported questions. An example of a questionnaire is enclosed in Table 4. Because the breastfeeding score is self-reported, any health professional with an interest in identifying mothers in need of additional support when establishing breastfeeding can use the score. The time after discharge to home is the optimal time to screen the mother, since at that time she has experiences with breastfeeding and is therefore able to answer the questions more reliably in relation to her experiences.

Table 4. Practical application of the breastfeeding score. The written postpartum questionnaire for mothers.

The purpose of the questions is to give you the breastfeeding guidance that meet your needs ***Just enter a number or cross in the box that best suits your situation***		
Basic information Which education have you completed?	❑ ❑	none / short / skilled bachelor / master
Your experiences with breastfeeding This is my first child If you have given birth earlier, how many weeks did you breastfeed your previous child without giving it anything else than your milk?	❑ ✎	yes weeks
Your expectations to breastfeeding How certain are you that you can complete four months of exclusive breastfeeding?	❑ ❑ ❑ ❑ ❑	very uncertain very certain
How does the following apply to you? I feel fine about not knowing exactly how much milk my baby gets when being breastfed?	❑ ❑ ❑ ❑ ❑	is not true exactly true

The breastfeeding score is an addition to the health professional's own assessment. The health professional often knows the educational level of the mother in advance, but less about the mothers' experiences with and expectations to breastfeeding. When used in a Danish setting, health visitors describe the questions included in the screening tool as suitable to initiate and open a dialogue about how mothers experience breastfeeding and create basis for further guidance on areas of importance. Moreover, the simple scoring system connected to the answers of the questions makes it easy to calculate the mother's score. A practical application with a key for reading the score is enclosed in Table 5. A cut-point of five will identify the first-time mother who expresses a low level of self-efficacy or sense of security towards breastfeeding, and, likewise, the multiparous mother with previous short breastfeeding experience. To prove these benefits, the breastfeeding score needs further process evaluation among health professionals using the breastfeeding score in their daily practice in different settings.

Table 5. Practical application of the breastfeeding score. Key for reading the score.

When the mother has completed the questionnaire, her answers are converted into a total score. The individual questions are awarded points according to the system below.		
Completed vocational education	none / short / skilled	1
	bachelor / master	0
Previous breastfeeding experience	None, first-time mother	3
	0–5 weeks	6
	6–17 weeks	4
	>17 weeks	0
Self-efficacy with respect to breastfeeding	Medium to very uncertain, 1–3	3
	Certain to very certain, 4–5	0
Sense of security not knowing the exact amount of milk the baby ingests	Is not true, 1–2	2
	Is fairly–exactly true, 3–5	0
The points are added up to a total score Overall score: 0–5 = mothers are offered standard care Overall score: 6–19 = mothers are offered additional support during establishment of breastfeeding		

The validation of the breastfeeding score was carried out in Denmark, a country with a well-educated population and a long tradition for initiating breastfeeding after birth and for breastfeeding for a relatively long period of time [34]. There is no reason to believe the questions included in the breastfeeding score will be understood or perceived differently in other western societies with a culture similar to the Danish; however, additional studies are needed to confirm the prognostic value of using the breastfeeding score in other settings.

5. Conclusions

The breastfeeding score, consisting of four risk factors representing the sociodemographic, perinatal, and psychosocial domains of breastfeeding, showed a high predictive value and a good ability to discriminate between mothers at risk of exclusive breastfeeding cessation before 17 weeks postpartum. Both the temporal and external validation of the breastfeeding score supported the predictive value of the four questions asked shortly after birth. The construction with a simple score connected to the answers of the four questions makes the breastfeeding score easy to use in daily practice.

Author Contributions: H.K. conceived the study idea and wrote the original draft of the article. Both authors were involved in data analysis, writing, reviewing and editing of the article. Both authors have read and approved the final version

Acknowledgments: The authors thank the families and health visitors who participated in the studies and thereby made the present study possible. The authors also wish to thank Ingeborg H. Kristensen, PhD, Department of Public Health at Aarhus University, for valuable and indispensable work in conjunction with the 2017 cohort study.

References

1. Bahl, R.; Barros, A.J.; França, G.V.; Horton, S.; Krasevec, J.; Murch, S.; Sankar, M.J.; Walker, N.; Rollins, N.C. Lancet Breastfeeding Series Group. Breastfeeding in the 21st century: Epidemiology, mechanisms, and lifelong effect. *Lancet* **2016**, *387*, 475–490.
2. Rollins, N.C.; Bhandari, N.; Hajeebhoy, N.; Horton, S.; Lutter, C.K.; Martines, J.C.; Piwoz, E.G.; Richter, L.M.; Victora, C.G. Lancet Breastfeeding Series Group. Why invest, and what will it take to improve breastfeeding practices? *Lancet* **2016**, *387*, 491–504. [CrossRef]

3. Kronborg, H.; Vaeth, M. How effective breastfeeding technique and pacifier use related to breastfeeding problems and breastfeeding duration? *Birth* **2009**, *36*, 34–42. [CrossRef] [PubMed]
4. Wagner, E.A.; Chantry, C.J.; Dewey, K.G.; Nommsen-Rivers, L.A. Breastfeeding concerns at 3 and 7 days postpartum and feeding status at 2 months. *Pediatrics* **2013**, *132*, e865–e875. [CrossRef]
5. McFadden, A.; Gavine, A.; Renfrew, M.J.; Wade, A.; Buchanan, P.; Taylor, J.L.; Veitch, E.; Rennie, A.M.; Crowther, S.A.; Neiman, S.; et al. Support for healthy breastfeeding mothers with healthy term babies. *Cochrane Database Syst. Rev.* **2017**, *28*, CD001141. [CrossRef]
6. Cohen, S.S.; Alexander, D.D.; Krebs, N.F.; Young, B.E.; Cabana, M.D.; Erdmann, P.; Hays, N.P.; Bezold, C.P.; Levin-Sparenberg, E.; Turini, M.; et al. Factors Associated with Breastfeeding Initiation and Continuation: A Meta-Analysis. *J. Pediatr.* **2018**, *203*, 190–196. [CrossRef]
7. De Jager, E.; Broadbent, J.; Fuller-Tyszkiewicz, M.; Skouteris, H. The role of psychosocial factors in exclusive breastfeeding to six months postpartum. *Midwifery* **2014**, *30*, 657–666. [CrossRef]
8. Colombo, L.; Crippa, B.L.; Consonni, D.; Bettinelli, M.E.; Agosti, V.; Mangino, G.; Bezze, E.N.; Mauri, P.A.; Zanotta, L.; Roggero, P.; et al. Breastfeeding Determinants in Healthy Term Newborns. *Nutrients* **2018**, *10*, 48. [CrossRef]
9. Sartorio, B.T.; Coca, K.P.; Marcacine, K.O.; Abuchaim, É.S.V.; Abrão, A.C.F.V. Breastfeeding assessment instruments and their use in clinical practice. *Rev. Gaucha Enferm.* **2017**, *38*, e64675.
10. Casal, C.S.; Lei, A.; Young, S.L.; Tuthill, E.L. A Critical Review of Instruments measuring Breastfeeding Attitudes, Knowledge, and Social Support. *J. Hum. Lact.* **2017**, *33*, 21–47. [CrossRef]
11. Moran, V.H.; Dinwoodie, K.; Bramwell, R.; Dykes, F. A critical analysis of the content of the tools that measure breast-feeding interaction. *Midwifery* **2000**, *16*, 260–268. [CrossRef] [PubMed]
12. Tuthill, E.L.; McGrath, J.M.; Graber, M.; Cusson, R.M.; Young, S.L. Breastfeeding Self-efficacy: A Critical Review of Available Instruments. *J. Hum. Lact.* **2016**, *32*, 35–45. [CrossRef] [PubMed]
13. Ho, Y.J.; McGrath, J.M. A review of the psychometric properties of breastfeeding assessment tools. *J. Obstet. Gynecol. Neonatal Nurs.* **2010**, *39*, 386–400. [CrossRef] [PubMed]
14. Wutke, K.; Dennis, C.L. The reliability and validity of the Polish version of the Breastfeeding Self-Efficacy Scale-ShortForm: Translation and psychometric assessment. *Int. J. Nurs. Stud.* **2007**, *44*, 1439–1446. [CrossRef] [PubMed]
15. Kronborg, H.; Vaeth, M.; Olsen, J.; Iversen, L.; Harder, I. Early breastfeeding cessation: Validation of a prognostic breastfeeding score. *Acta Paediatr.* **2007**, *96*, 688–692. [CrossRef]
16. Altman, D.G.; Royston, P. What do we mean by validating a prognostic model? *Stat. Med.* **2000**, *19*, 453–473. [CrossRef]
17. Altman, D.G.; Vergouwe, Y.; Royston, P.; Moons, K.G. Prognosis and prognostic research: Validating a prognostic model. *BMJ* **2009**, *28*, b605. [CrossRef]
18. Moons, K.G.M.; Altman, D.G.; Vergouwe, Y.; Royston, P. Prognosis and prognostic research: Application and impact of prediction models in clinical practice. *BMJ* **2009**, *338*, b606. [CrossRef]
19. Kronborg, H.; Vaeth, M. The influence of psychosocial factors on the duration of breastfeeding. *Scand. J. Public Health* **2004**, *32*, 210–216. [CrossRef]
20. Kronborg, H.; Vaeth, M.; Olsen, J.; Iversen, L.; Harder, I. Effect of early postnatal breastfeeding support: A cluster-randomized community based trial. *Acta Paediatr.* **2007**, *96*, 1064–1070. [CrossRef]
21. Kristensen, I.H.; Vinter, M.; Nickell, I.K.; Kronborg, H. Health visitors' competences before and after implementing the newborn behavioral observations (NBO) system in a community setting: A cluster randomised study. *Public Health Nurs.* **2019**. [CrossRef] [PubMed]
22. Kristensen, I.H.; Kronborg, H. What are the effects of supporting early parenting by enhancing parents' understanding of the infant? Study protocol for a cluster-randomized community-based trial of the Newborn Behavioral Observation (NBO) method. *BMC Public Health* **2018**, *18*, 832. [CrossRef] [PubMed]
23. World Health Organisation (WHO). *Indicators for Assessing Breastfeeding Practices*; Division of Child Health and Development: Geneva, Switzerland, 1991; WHO/CDD/SER/91.14, Corr. 1; Available online: https://www.who.int/maternal_child_adolescent/documents/cdd_ser_91_14/en/ (accessed on 2 October 2019).
24. Natland, S.T.; Andersen, L.F.; Nilsen, T.I.; Forsmo, S.; Jacobsen, G.W. Maternal recall of breastfeeding duration

twenty years after delivery. *BMC Med. Res. Methodol.* **2012**, *12*, 1471–2288. [CrossRef] [PubMed]
25. Statistics Denmark. Live Birth by Municipality, Age of Mothers, and Sex of Child. Available online: https://www.statistikbanken.dk/FODIE (accessed on 29 October 2019).
26. Bai, D.L.; Fong, D.Y.; Tarrant, M. Previous breastfeeding experience and duration of any and exclusive breastfeeding among multiparous mothers. *Birth* **2015**, *42*, 70–77. [CrossRef] [PubMed]
27. Kronborg, H.; Foverskov, E.; Væth, M.; Maimburg, R.D. The role of intention and self-efficacy on the association between breastfeeding of first and second child, a Danish cohort study. *BMC Pregnancy Childbirth* **2018**, *18*, 454. [CrossRef] [PubMed]
28. Bandura, A. Theoretical Perspectives and The Nature and Structure of Self-Efficacy. In *Self-Efficacy the Exercise of Control*; Freeman, W.H. and Company: New York, NY, USA, 1997; pp. 5–42.
29. Li, R.; Fein, S.B.; Chen, J.; Grummer-Strawn, L.M. Why mothers stop breastfeeding: mothers' self-reported reasons for stopping during the first year. *Pediatrics* **2008**, *122*, S69–S76. [CrossRef]
30. Brown, A.; Arnott, B. Breastfeeding duration and early parenting behaviour: The importance of an infant-led, responsive style. *PLoS ONE* **2014**, *9*, e83893. [CrossRef]
31. Little, E.E.; Legare, C.H.; Carver, L.J. Mother infant Physical Contact Predicts Responsive Feeding among U.S. Breastfeeding Mothers. *Nutrients* **2018**, *10*, 1251. [CrossRef]
32. Agostoni CDecsi TFewtrell, M. Complementary feeding: A commentary by the ESPGHAN Committee on Nutrition. *J. Pediatr. Gastroenterol. Nutrients* **2008**, *46*, 99–110. [CrossRef]
33. European Food Safety Authority, EFSA. *Scientific Opinion on the Appropriate Age for Introduction of Complementary Feeding of Infants*; EFSA Panel on Dietetic Products, NDA Nutrition and Allergies: Parma, Italy, 2019; Available online: http://www.efsa.europa.eu/en/efsajournal/doc/1423.pdf (accessed on 2 October 2019).
34. Kronborg, H.; Foverskov, E.; Væth, M. Breastfeeding and introduction of complementary food in Danish infants. *Scand. J. Public Health* **2015**, *43*, 138–145. [CrossRef]

11

Sex-Specific Human Milk Composition: The Role of Infant Sex in Determining Early Life Nutrition

Laura Galante [1], Amber M. Milan [1], Clare M. Reynolds [1], David Cameron-Smith [1,2,3], Mark H. Vickers [1] and Shikha Pundir [1,*]

1 Liggins Institute, the University of Auckland, Auckland 1142, New Zealand; l.galante@auckland.ac.nz (L.G.); a.milan@auckland.ac.nz (A.M.M.); c.reynolds@auckland.ac.nz (C.M.R.); d.cameron-smith@auckland.ac.nz (D.C.-S.); m.vickers@auckland.ac.nz (M.H.V.)

2 Riddet Institute, Massey University, Palmerston North 4442, New Zealand

3 Food & Bio-Based Products Group, AgResearch, Palmerston North 4442, New Zealand

* Correspondence: s.pundir@auckland.ac.nz

Abstract: Male and female infants respond differentially to environmental stimuli, with different growth and neurodevelopmental trajectories. Male infants are more likely to be disadvantaged when subjected to adversity and show a higher risk of perinatal complications. However, the underlying causes of this sex-bias are not well defined and optimising the early life nutritional care may be necessary to minimise the "male disadvantage" that may be experienced early in life. Experimental models have demonstrated that animal milk composition differs according to offspring sex, suggesting that the tailoring of early life nutrition may be one mechanism to maximise health protection and development to infants of both sexes. However, evidence for a sex-specificity in human milk composition is limited and conflicting, with studies documenting higher milk energy content for either male or female infants. These data show sex differences, however, there has been limited compositional analysis of the current data nor strategies proposed for how sex-specific compositional differences in early life nutrition may be used to improve infant health. The present narrative review highlights that an improved understanding of sex-specific human milk composition is essential for promoting optimal infant growth and development.

Keywords: human milk; sex-specificity; infant growth; early life nutrition; postnatal outcomes; breastfeeding

---

1. Introduction

Human milk (HM) is the gold standard for infant nutrition, providing the necessary building blocks required for postnatal growth and development [1,2]. The biochemical composition of HM is highly dynamic and varies between mothers and within the same mother throughout the different stages of lactation [3–6] and within a feed, such that foremilk and hindmilk have differing biochemical compositions [7]. HM composition changes most notably during the transition from colostrum to mature milk, with the intermediate of transitional milk, as lactation proceeds [8]. However, the dynamic regulation of HM composition is also impacted by maternal, environmental, and infant factors. Changes in maternal diet significantly influence HM macronutrient composition, particularly within the lipid fraction. This is evident in mothers consuming a western-style diet, where high dietary consumption of omega-6 is directly reflected in the HM lipid profile [9]. Further, maternal BMI has also documented impacts on HM lipid profile with different fatty acid profile between obese and lean mothers [10,11]. Along with macronutrient composition, non-nutritive milk bioactives are also impacted by maternal factors such as stress [12] and BMI [13]. HM bioactives, such as growth [14] and satiety factors [15,16], and different classes of hormones, such as steroids [17], play important roles in human physiology, including the regulation of energy intake [18,19] and somatic growth [20,21]. Interestingly, most of these bioactive compounds have been reported to follow sex-specific secretion pathways in adults, children [22,23], and in cord blood [24,25], yet, little is known about their sex-specific distribution in HM.

Despite international recognition of the importance of breastfeeding, not all infants can be exclusively breastfed. Some mothers indeed encounter challenges in establishing and/or maintaining lactation over the first six months of life [26–29], which results in early weaning or formula-feeding for their infants. Nutritional and hormonal exposures during the first 1000 days of life are known to be important for both short- and long-term health outcomes [30]. In this context, the observation that male and female infants have a sexually-dimorphic response to their early nutritional environment [31] suggests that there are sex-specific requirements during this early phase of life for optimal growth and development. Yet, there are currently no practice guidelines establishing different nutritional strategies or requirements for male and female infants [32]. For this reason, a better understanding of whether male and female infants receive different nutritional and hormonal intakes through maternal HM would provide important information around the potential need to tailor nutritional strategies for clinical and community settings in a sex-specific manner.

The present work constitutes a narrative review of the existing evidence regarding sex-specificity in HM composition in relation to sex-specific health outcomes such as the higher perinatal risk of mortality and morbidity observed in male neonates.

2. The "Male Disadvantage": A Consequence of Sex-Specific Requirements?

Differences in perinatal outcomes between males and females have been recognised since the 1970's as the "male disadvantage" [33]. The concept arose from the observation that male infants in the United States had a higher risk of neonatal mortality compared to females, and that this was not related to specific disease processes. Newborn males are known to be more vulnerable than females to postnatal complications including respiratory distress syndrome [34], neonatal anaemia and mineral deficiencies, particularly in high-risk populations such as low birthweight (LBW) infants [35]. Stevenson et al., later examined the "male disadvantage" to understand whether technological advances in neonatal care, such as improved ventilation, enhanced surfactant therapies and administration of antenatal steroids, would improve outcomes in male infants. However, despite an overall decrease in mortality following the implementation of these strategies, a sex-bias was still observed in male infants [36].

At present, sex-specific differences in perinatal health outcomes, including neurological, metabolic and respiratory complications, with males having higher risk for poorer health [37,38], remain of concern as a cause of higher mortality and morbidity in male newborns. While the main cause for this bias is unknown, the observation that female and male offspring react differently to early life nutritional stimuli [39,40] may be a crucial factor in our understanding of the mechanisms underlying these differences in postnatal outcomes. Research carried out on ovine model has shown that offspring of different sexes respond differently to a standard supplemental nutrition [41]. When newborn lambs were randomised to receive maternal milk and either milk fortifiers or water for two weeks they showed differential outcomes compared to same-sex controls, with supplemented males displaying increased insulin in response to the intravenous glucose tolerance test (IVGTT) received at four months. Conversely, insulin was lower after the IVGTT in supplemented females compared to female controls. Divergent responses to infant feeding have also been documented in humans. Lucas et al., demonstrated that in humans, male preterm neonates were more responsive than females to preterm formula with higher protein, energy content and micronutrients to meet higher preterm requirements. These infants displayed higher Bayley's test scores, indicative of improved neurodevelopment, at 18 months of age, in comparison to male infants receiving a standard term formula [31]. Given the evidence of sex-specific infant outcomes based on differences in early life nutritional support, an improved understanding of the innate compositional differences in HM produced for these infants is essential to establishing requirements and guidelines for supplemental support.

3. Sex-Specific Composition of Maternal Milk

Evidence from animal models (Table 1) suggests that infant sex is a predictive determinant of maternal milk composition. Primate [41–43] and bovine [44] models have demonstrated that mothers produce different milk for male and female singleton offspring. For example, macaque (*Macaca mulatta*) mothers of male offspring produced a lower volume of milk but with a higher energy content, whereas mothers of female offspring had greater volume of milk which was less energy-dense, resulting in similar total energy content of the milk produced for both sexes [42]. Yet, milk produced for female macaque offspring had higher calcium content [41]. In a bovine model, mothers have been shown to produce considerably more milk and of higher energy content for their female offspring [44]. Evidence of sex-specific milk production has also been reported for other ruminants, as well as marsupials. Wild eastern kangaroos (*Macropus giganteus*) [45] and Tammar wallabies (*Macropus eugenii*) [46] were found to produce milk with higher protein for male offspring but same energy content and volume for offspring of different sex. Similarly, Iberian red deer (*Cervus elaphus hispanicus*) mothers were observed to produce greater yields of milk with higher energy content for male calves, reflected by higher protein, fat and lactose content [47]. While these studies provide evidence that the sex of offspring has an impact on the nutritional composition of maternal milk across very different *taxa*, the range of milk-borne compounds analysed in each study is limited and no information is available around hormonal concentration in milk produced for male and female offspring. Furthermore, the mechanisms driving sex-specific milk synthesis are currently unclear and need to be investigated in order to enable a better understanding of the phenomenon.

Table 1. Overview of animal studies on sex-specificity in maternal milk.

	Species	Sample Size	Offspring Age at Collection	Sex-Specific Difference	Study
Primates	Rhesus Macaque (*Macaca mulatta*)	106	3–4 months	↑ energy and ↑ fat for males	Hinde, 2007 [43]
		114 (62 F, 52 M)		↓ volume ↑ energy density for males	Hinde, 2009 [42]
		104 (61 F, 43 M)		↑ calcium for females	Hinde et al., 2013 [41]
Ruminants	Holstein breed of cow (*Bos Taurus*)	113,750 (data from lactation records)	not reported	↑ volume for females	Hinde et al., 2014 [44]
	Red deer (*Cervus elaphus hispanicus*)	91 (44 M, 47 F)	2, 6, 10 and 14 weeks	↑ volume, ↑ protein, ↑ fat and ↑ lactose for males	Landete-Catillejos et al., 2005 [47]
Marsupials	Kangaroo (*Macropus giganteus*)	91	6–10 months	↑ protein for males	Quesnel et al., 2017 [45]
	Wallaby (*Macropus eugenii*)	2 milking sessions: 15 in July (6 M, 9 F), 11 in October (4 M, 7 F)	4–8 months	↑ protein for males	Robert and Braun, 2012 [46]

F, female offspring; M, male offspring; ↑, higher compared to the opposite sex; ↓, lower compared to the opposite sex.

Despite data derived from experimental models, there remains a paucity of data around the potential for sex-specificity in HM composition in regards to nutrients and bioactive compounds. The potential for a sex-specificity has however been suggested by clinical research on twins [48]. In this setting, opposite-sex twins, that receive HM which cannot simultaneously be tailored for both sexes, have been hypothesised to have different outcomes in comparison with same-sex twins in regards to postnatal growth [48]. Kanazawa and Segal observed indeed that breastfed opposite-sex twins were on average 1 inch shorter and 12 pounds lighter than same-sex twins during adolescence and early adulthood. This may suggest that the sex-specificity of HM might have a role in the early growth of the infant and exerts effects that persist throughout the life course of the individual.

Nonetheless to date only six human studies have reported on the relationship between HM composition and infant sex [49–54]. These studies primarily focused on macronutrient profile and energy content of HM and reported conflicting relationships in regard to infant sex. In particular, one study on Filipino mothers found no association between HM composition and infant sex [52]. Another study reported that American mothers of male infants produce HM with a greater energy content [49]; whereas, other research groups found that HM was higher in energy for female infants in Korean and Kenyan mothers [50,51]. Interestingly, the study on Kenyan mothers reported a conditional association between female sex and higher fat content in HM, that was displayed only by mothers with low socioeconomic status [50], supporting the Trivers-Willard hypothesis of unequal parental investment between female and male offspring depending on maternal condition [55]. Mirroring experimental models, HM for female infants in Iraqi mothers was found to have a higher calcium content; yet phosphorus content and total volume were reduced relative to the HM produced for male infants [53]. However, these studies reported several limitations and were conducted in different contexts and with very different sampling and analytical methods, as summarized in Table 2, which likely explain the disparity in findings. Nevertheless, despite being limited by collection methods, Fujita's study [50] highlights the fact that HM composition is affected not only by multiple factors but also by the interactions between factors. A similar conditional association of the infant sex with HM composition has been reported by Fields et al., while looking at the influence of maternal BMI on HM composition [54]. Here, similarly to what was observed in Kenyan mothers, where fat content in HM was conditionally altered for female infants by the socioeconomic status of the family, Fields et al., found that insulin and leptin concentrations in maternal HM were the highest for mothers of females only when maternal BMI was very high [54].

Importantly, there is emerging research demonstrating a sex-specific differential effect of animal milk bioactives on offspring outcomes. As an example, elevated cortisol in the milk of lactating macaques has been found to correlate with a more nervousness and less confident temperament, impacting male offspring to a greater extent than female [56]. However, existing evidence supporting the idea of a sex-specific response to the nutrition received during early life (Table 3) is limited. The available findings often relate to subjects at risk, such as those born preterm or small for gestational age [31,57] and only assess the effect of the nutrition received immediately after birth [40]. Furthermore, in most of these studies the compositional analysis of maternal milk is not included, preventing the possibility of any association between specific milk-borne compounds and sex-specific response. This suggests the need for further research to fully understand the impact of nutritional and hormonal intakes during this sensitive period on sex-specific infant growth and development.

Table 2. Summary of human research on sex-specific human milk (HM) composition.

Study	Country	Sample Size	Collection Methods	Infant Age at Collection	Findings	Limitations
Yahya et al., 2009 [53]	Iraq	109 (52 M, 57 F)	Foremilk collected	Not specified	↑ calcium for females, ↑ volume and phosphorus for males	Composition not representative of hindmilk
Powe et al., 2010 [49]	United States of America	25	Breast was emptied by pump expression (mother's pump or study pump).	2–5 months	↑ energy content (derived by carbohydrates, protein and lipid content) for males	Small sample size, inconsistent sampling time and use of instruments for milk collection, inconsistency of stage of lactation at sampling
Hahn et al., 2016 [51]	South Korea	478 (244 M, 234 F)	Sample collected during day time	0–3 months	↑ carbohydrate and energy content for females	Inconsistent sampling time, Absence of information on maternal diet and anthropometry, inconsistency of stage of lactation at sampling
Fujita et al., 2012 [50]	Kenya	83 (47 M, 36 F)	Foremilk collected in the morning by manual expression	Not specified	↑ fat for females only in mothers with a low socioeconomic status	Composition not representative of hindmilk
Quinn, 2013 [52]	Philippines	103 (52 M, 51 F)	Sample collected in the morning by manual expression after mother nursed the infants for approximately 3 minutes	0–18 months	No significant differences were found between male and female infants in HM composition	Composition not representative of foremilk, inconsistency in stage of lactation at sampling
Fields et al., 2017 [54]	Australia	37(16 M, 21 F)	Breast emptied by pump expression	1 and 6 months	↑ insulin and leptin for females born to obese mothers	Small sample size

F, female infant; M, male infant; ↑, higher compared to the opposite sex.

Table 3. Overview of animal and human studies on sex-specific response to early life nutrition.

		Sample Size	Nutrition	Sex-Specific Response	Limitations	Study
Animal	Sheep (*Ovis aries*)	42	Ewe's milk + milk fortifiers vs. Ewe's milk + water	↑ Insulin response in supplemented males, ↓ insulin response in supplemented females	Absence of direct estimates of milk composition and feeding behaviours	Jaquiery et al., 2016 [40]
	Rhesus Macaque (*Macaca mulatta*)	108	Maternal milk with ↑ cortisol	Males were more nervous and less confident	Absence of other hormonal measurements and lack of sensitive methodology to measure cortisol in milk	Hinde et al., 2015 [56]
Human		752	HM vs. FM	Breastfed same-sex twins were on average 1 inch taller and 12 pounds heavier than opposite-sex twins	Absence of HM compositional analyses and subjects' body composition	Kanazawa and Segal, 2017 [48]
		424	Preterm FM vs. term FM	Preterm males fed preterm formula had ↑ Bayley's test scores at 18 months	Absence of full term control group	Lucas et al., 1990 [31]
		76	Standard vs. high-nutrient diet	Male adolescents fed with high-nutrient diet after preterm birth had larger caudate nucleus volume and verbal IQ	Small sample size, absence of a full term control group	Isaacs et al., 2008 [57]

↑, higher compared to control and opposite sex; ↓, lower compared to control and opposite sex; IQ, intelligence quotient; FM, formula milk.

4. Conclusions

Evidence to date suggests that infants of different sex may have different nutritional and hormonal requirements. This underpins a need for sex-specific nutritional strategies for male and female infants, in order to optimise their growth and development. Experimental and limited clinical observations that maternal HM composition changes dependent on male or female sex, support this hypothesis. However, these reported sex-specific differences in HM composition require validation and clarification in additional human cohorts. These studies should aim to describe sex-specific differences in HM composition across the course of lactation and correlate differences with sex-specificity of infant outcomes, including sex-specific growth trajectories and sex-specific morbidity risk.

Author Contributions: L.G. wrote the manuscript. A.M.M., C.M.R., D.C.-S., M.H.V., and S.P. critically evaluated and edited the manuscript.

References

1. Dieterich, C.M.; Felice, J.P.; O'Sullivan, E.; Rasmussen, K.M. Breastfeeding and health outcomes for the mother-infant dyad. *Pediatr. Clin. N. Am.* **2013**, *60*, 31–48. [CrossRef] [PubMed]
2. Martin, C.R.; Ling, P.R.; Blackburn, G.L. Review of infant feeding: Key features of breast milk and infant formula. *Nutrients* **2016**, *8*, 279. [CrossRef] [PubMed]
3. Zou, X.Q.; Guo, Z.; Huang, J.H.; Jin, Q.Z.; Cheong, L.Z.; Wang, X.G.; Xu, X.B. Human milk fat globules from different stages of lactation: A lipid composition analysis and microstructure characterization. *J. Agric. Food Chem.* **2012**, *60*, 7158–7167. [CrossRef] [PubMed]
4. Dewey, K.G.; Finley, D.A.; Lönnerdal, B. Breast milk volume and composition during late lactation (7–20 months). *J. Pediatr. Gastroenterol. Nutr.* **1984**, *3*, 713–720. [CrossRef] [PubMed]
5. Jiang, J.; Wu, K.; Yu, Z.; Ren, Y.; Zhao, Y.; Jiang, Y.; Xu, X.; Li, W.; Jin, Y.; Yuan, J.; et al. Changes in fatty acid composition of human milk over lactation stages and relationship with dietary intake in Chinese women. *Food Funct.* **2016**, *7*, 3154–3162. [CrossRef] [PubMed]
6. Saarela, T.; Kokkonen, J.; Koivisto, M. Macronutrient and energy contents of human milk fractions during the first six months of lactation. *Acta Paediatr.* **2005**, *94*, 1176–1181. [CrossRef] [PubMed]
7. Mizuno, K.; Nishida, Y.; Taki, M.; Murase, M.; Mukai, Y.; Itabashi, K.; Debari, K.; Liyama, A. Is increased fat content of hindmilk due to the size or the number of milk fat globules? *Int. Breastfeed J.* **2009**, *4*, 7. [CrossRef] [PubMed]
8. Ballard, O.; Morrow, A.L. Human milk composition: Nutrients and bioactive factors. *Pediatr. Clin. N. Am.* **2013**, *60*, 49–74. [CrossRef] [PubMed]
9. Martin, M.A.; Lassek, W.D.; Gaulin, S.J.C.; Evans, R.W.; Woo, J.G.; Geraghty, S.R.; Davidson, B.S.; Morrow, A.L.; Kaplan, H.S.; Gurven, M.D. Fatty acid composition in the mature milk of Bolivian forager-horticulturalists: Controlled comparisons with a US sample. *Matern. Child Nutr.* **2012**, *8*, 404–418. [CrossRef] [PubMed]
10. Mäkelä, J.; Linderborg, K.; Niinikoski, H.; Yang, B.; Lagström, H. Breast milk fatty acid composition differs between overweight and normal weight women: the STEPS Study. *Eur. J. Nutr.* **2013**, *52*, 727–735. [CrossRef] [PubMed]
11. Panagos, P.G.; Vishwanathan, R.; Penfield-Cyr, A.; Matthan, N.R.; Shivappa, N.; Wirth, M.D.; Hebert, J.R.; Sen, S. Breastmilk from obese mothers has pro-inflammatory properties and decreased neuroprotective factors. *J. Perinatol. J. Calif. Perinat. Assoc.* **2016**, *36*, 284–290. [CrossRef] [PubMed]
12. Thibeau, S.; D'Apolito, K.; Minnick, A.F.; Dietrich, M.S.; Kane, B.; Cooley, S.; Groer, M. Relationships of maternal stress with milk immune components in African American mothers of healthy term infants. *Breastfeed Med.* **2016**, *11*, 6–14. [CrossRef] [PubMed]
13. Houseknecht, K.L.; McGuire, M.K.; Portocarrero, C.P.; McGuire, M.A.; Beerman, K. Leptin is present in human milk and is related to maternal plasma leptin concentration and adiposity. *Biochem. Biophys. Res. Commun.* **1997**, *240*, 742–747. [CrossRef] [PubMed]

14. Blum, J.W.; Baumrucker, C.R. Insulin-like growth factors (IGFs), IGF binding proteins, and other endocrine factors in milk: Role in the newborn. *Adv. Exp. Med. Biol.* **2008**, *606*, 397–422. [CrossRef] [PubMed]
15. Çatlı, G.; Olgaç Dündar, N.; Dündar, B.N. Adipokines in breast milk: An update. *J. Clin. Res. Pediatr. Endocrinol.* **2014**, *6*, 192–201. [CrossRef] [PubMed]
16. Savino, F.; Sorrenti, M.; Benetti, S.; Lupica, M.M.; Liguori, S.A.; Oggero, R. Resistin and leptin in breast milk and infants in early life. *Early Hum. Dev.* **2012**, *88*, 779–782. [CrossRef] [PubMed]
17. Pundir, S.; Wall, C.R.; Mitchell, C.J.; Thorstensen, E.B.; Lai, C.T.; Geddes, D.T.; Cameron-Smith, D. Variation of Human Milk Glucocorticoids over 24 hour Period. *J. Mammary Gland Biol. Neoplasia* **2017**, *22*, 85–92. [CrossRef] [PubMed]
18. Klok, M.D.; Jakobsdottir, S.; Drent, M.L. The role of leptin and ghrelin in the regulation of food intake and body weight in humans: A review. *Obes. Rev. J. Int. Assoc. Study Obes.* **2007**, *8*, 21–34. [CrossRef] [PubMed]
19. Dallman, M.F.; Warne, J.P.; Foster, M.T.; Pecoraro, N.C. Glucocorticoids and insulin both modulate caloric intake through actions on the brain. *J. Physiol.* **2007**, *583*, 431–436. [CrossRef] [PubMed]
20. Laron, Z. Insulin-like growth factor 1 (IGF-1): A growth hormone. *Mol. Pathol.* **2001**, *54*, 311–316. [CrossRef] [PubMed]
21. Murray, P.G.; Clayton, P.E. Endocrine control of growth. *Am. J. Med. Genet. C Semin. Med. Genet.* **2013**, *163C*, 76–85. [CrossRef] [PubMed]
22. Geary, M.P.P.; Pringle, P.J.; Rodeck, C.H.; Kingdom, J.C.P.; Hindmarsh, P.C. Sexual dimorphism in the growth hormone and insulin-like growth factor axis at birth. *J. Clin. Endocrinol. Metab.* **2003**, *88*, 3708–3714. [CrossRef] [PubMed]
23. Rosenbaum, M.; Leibel, R.L. Role of gonadal steroids in the sexual dimorphisms in body composition and circulating concentrations of leptin. *J. Clin. Endocrinol. Metab.* **1999**, *84*, 1784–1789. [CrossRef] [PubMed]
24. Vatten, L.J.; Nilsen, S.T.; Ødegård, R.A.; Romundstad, P.R.; Austgulen, R. Insulin-like growth factor I and leptin in umbilical cord plasma and infant birth size at term. *Pediatrics* **2002**, *109*, 1131–1135. [CrossRef] [PubMed]
25. Pardo, I.M.; Geloneze, B.; Tambascia, M.A.; Pereira, J.L.; Barros Filho, A.A. Leptin as a marker of sexual dimorphism in newborn infants. *J. Pediatr.* **2004**, *80*, 305–308. [CrossRef]
26. Chapman, D.J.; Pérez-escamilla, R. Identification of risk factors for delayed onset of lactation. *J. Am. Diet Assoc.* **1999**, *99*, 450–454. [CrossRef]
27. Hruschka, D.J.; Sellen, D.W.; Stein, A.D.; Martorell, R. Delayed onset of lactation and risk of ending full breast-feeding early in rural guatemala. *J. Nutr.* **2003**, *133*, 2592–2599. [CrossRef] [PubMed]
28. Grajeda, R.; Pérez-Escamilla, R. Stress during labor and delivery is associated with delayed onset of lactation among urban Guatemalan women. *J. Nutr.* **2002**, *132*, 3055–3060. [CrossRef] [PubMed]
29. Hauck, Y.L.; Fenwick, J.; Dhaliwal, S.S.; Butt, J.A. Western Australian survey of breastfeeding initiation, prevalence and early cessation patterns. *Matern. Child Health J.* **2011**, *15*, 260–268. [CrossRef] [PubMed]
30. Ford, N.D.; Behrman, J.R.; Hoddinott, J.F.; Maluccio, J.A.; Martorell, R.; Ramirez-Zea, M.; Stein, A.D. Exposure to improved nutrition from conception to age 2 years and adult cardiometabolic disease risk: A modelling study. *Lancet Glob. Health* **2018**, *6*, 875–884. [CrossRef]
31. Lucas, A.; Morley, R.; Cole, T.J.; Lucas, P.J.; Gore, S.M.; Crowle, P.; Pearse, R.; Boon, A.J.; Powell, R. Early diet in preterm babies and developmental status at 18 months. *Lancet* **1990**, *335*, 1477–1481. [CrossRef]
32. Harding, J.E.; Cormack, B.E.; Alexander, T.; Alsweiler, J.M.; Bloomfield, F.H. Advances in nutrition of the newborn infant. *Lancet Lond. Engl.* **2017**, *389*, 1660–1668. [CrossRef]
33. Naeye, R.L.; Burt, L.S.; Wright, D.L.; Blanc, W.A.; Tatter, D. Neonatal mortality, the male disadvantage. *Pediatrics* **1971**, *48*, 902–906. [PubMed]
34. Brothwood, M.; Wolke, D.; Gamsu, H.; Benson, J.; Cooper, D. Prognosis of the very low birthweight baby in relation to gender. *Arch. Dis. Child* **1986**, *61*, 559–564. [CrossRef] [PubMed]
35. Libster, R.; Hortoneda, J.B.; Laham, F.R.; Casellas, J.M.; Israele, V.; Polack, N.R.; Delgado, M.F.; Klein, M.I.; Polack, F.P. Breastfeeding prevents severe disease in full term female infants with acute respiratory infection. *Pediatr. Infect. Dis. J.* **2009**, *28*, 131. [CrossRef] [PubMed]

36. Stevenson, D.K.; Verter, J.; Fanaroff, A.A.; Oh, W.; Ehrenkranz, R.A.; Shankaran, S.; Donovan, E.F.; Wright, L.L.; Lemons, J.A.; Tyson, J.E.; et al. Sex differences in outcomes of very low birthweight infants: The newborn male disadvantage. *Arch. Dis. Child Fetal. Neonatal. Ed.* **2000**, *83*, 182–185. [CrossRef]
37. Peacock, J.L.; Marston, L.; Marlow, N.; Calvert, S.A.; Greenough, A. Neonatal and infant outcome in boys and girls born very prematurely. *Pediatr. Res.* **2012**, *71*, 305–310. [CrossRef] [PubMed]
38. García-Patterson, A.; Aulinas, A.; Sojo, L.; Ginovart, G.; Adelantado, J.M.; de Leiva, A.; Corcoy, R. Poorer perinatal outcome in male newborns of women with pregestational diabetes mellitus. *Diabet. Med. J. Br. Diabet. Assoc.* **2011**, *28*, 436–439. [CrossRef] [PubMed]
39. Cheng, T.S.; Loy, S.L.; Cheung, Y.B.; Chan, J.K.Y.; Pang, W.W.; Godfrey, K.M.; Gluckman, P.D.; Kwek, K.; Saw, S.M.; Chong, Y.-S.; et al. Sexually dimorphic response to feeding mode in the growth of infants. *Am. J. Clin. Nutr.* **2016**, *103*, 398–405. [CrossRef] [PubMed]
40. Jaquiery, A.L.; Park, S.S.; Phua, H.H.; Berry, M.J.; Meijler, D.; Harding, J.E.; Oliver, M.H.; Bloomfield, F.H. Brief neonatal nutritional supplementation has sex-specific effects on glucose tolerance and insulin regulating genes in juvenile lambs. *Pediatr. Res.* **2016**, *80*, 861–869. [CrossRef] [PubMed]
41. Hinde, K.; Foster, A.B.; Landis, L.M.; Rendina, D.; Oftedal, O.T.; Power, M.L. Daughter dearest: Sex-biased calcium in mother's milk among rhesus macaques. *Am. J. Phys. Anthropol.* **2013**, *151*, 144–150. [CrossRef] [PubMed]
42. Hinde, K. Richer milk for sons but more milk for daughters: Sex-biased investment during lactation varies with maternal life history in rhesus macaques. *Am. J. Hum. Biol.* **2009**, 512–519. [CrossRef] [PubMed]
43. Hinde, K. First-time macaque mothers bias milk composition in favor of sons. *Curr. Biol.* **2007**, *17*, 958–959. [CrossRef] [PubMed]
44. Hinde, K.; Carpenter, A.J.; Clay, J.S.; Bradford, B.J. Holsteins favor Heifers, not bulls: Biased milk production programmed during pregnancy as a function of fetal sex. *PLoS ONE* **2014**, *9*, e86169. [CrossRef] [PubMed]
45. Quesnel, L.; MacKay, A.; Forsyth, D.M.; Nicholas, K.R.; Festa-Bianchet, M. Size, season and offspring sex affect milk composition and juvenile survival in wild kangaroos. *J. Zool.* **2017**, *302*, 252–262. [CrossRef]
46. Robert, K.A.; Braun, S. Milk Composition during lactation suggests a mechanism for male biased allocation of maternal resources in the tammar wallaby (*Macropus eugenii*). *PLoS ONE* **2012**, *7*, e51099. [CrossRef] [PubMed]
47. Landete-Castillejos, T.; García, A.; López-Serrano, F.R.; Gallego, L. Maternal quality and differences in milk production and composition for male and female Iberian red deer calves (*Cervus elaphus hispanicus*). *Behav. Ecol. Sociobiol.* **2005**, *57*, 267–274. [CrossRef]
48. Kanazawa, S.; Segal, N.L. Same-sex twins are taller and heavier than opposite-sex twins (but only if breastfed): Possible evidence for sex bias in human breast milk. *J. Exp. Child Psychol.* **2017**, *156*, 186–191. [CrossRef] [PubMed]
49. Powe, C.E.; Knott, C.D.; Conklin-Brittain, N. Infant sex predicts breast milk energy content. *Am. J. Hum. Biol. Off. J. Hum. Biol. Assoc.* **2010**, *22*, 50–54. [CrossRef] [PubMed]
50. Fujita, M.; Roth, E.; Lo, Y.-J.; Hurst, C.; Vollner, J.; Kendell, A. In poor families, mothers' milk is richer for daughters than sons: A test of Trivers–Willard hypothesis in agropastoral settlements in Northern Kenya. *Am. J. Phys. Anthropol.* **2012**, *149*, 52–59. [CrossRef] [PubMed]
51. Hahn, W.-H.; Song, J.-H.; Song, S.; Kang, N. mi. Do gender and birth height of infant affect calorie of human milk? An association study between human milk macronutrient and various birth factors. *J. Matern. Fetal Neonatal. Med.* **2017**, *30*, 1608–1612. [CrossRef] [PubMed]
52. Quinn, E.A. No evidence for sex biases in milk macronutrients, energy, or breastfeeding frequency in a sample of filipino mothers. *Am. J. Phys. Anthropol.* **2013**, *152*, 209–216. [CrossRef] [PubMed]
53. Yahya, A.; Altufaily, C.A.B.P. The effect of infant gender on the quality of breast milk. *Kufa Med. J.* **2009**, *1*, 12.
54. Fields, D.A.; George, B.; Williams, M.; Whitaker, K.; Allison, D.B.; Teague, A.; Demerath, E.W. Associations between human breast milk hormones and adipocytokines and infant growth and body composition in the first 6 months of life. *Pediatr. Obes.* **2017**, 1. [CrossRef] [PubMed]
55. Trivers, R.L.; Willard, D.E. Natural selection of parental ability to vary the sex ratio of offspring. *Science* **1973**, *179*, 90–92. [CrossRef] [PubMed]

56. Hinde, K.; Skibiel, A.L.; Foster, A.B.; Del Rosso, L.; Mendoza, S.P.; Capitanio, J.P. Cortisol in mother's milk across lactation reflects maternal life history and predicts infant temperament. *Behav. Ecol.* **2015**, *26*, 269–281. [CrossRef] [PubMed]
57. Isaacs, E.B.; Gadian, D.G.; Sabatini, S.; Chong, W.K.; Quinn, B.T.; Fischl, B.R.; Lucas, A. The effect of early human diet on caudate volumes and IQ. *Pediatr. Res.* **2008**, *63*, 308–314. [CrossRef] [PubMed]

12

Do a Few Weeks Matter? Late Preterm Infants and Breastfeeding Issues

Beatrice Letizia Crippa [1,2,*], Lorenzo Colombo [1,2], Daniela Morniroli [1,2], Dario Consonni [3], Maria Enrica Bettinelli [4], Irene Spreafico [5], Giulia Vercesi [1,2], Patrizio Sannino [5], Paola Agnese Mauri [2,6], Lidia Zanotta [1,2], Annalisa Canziani [2,6], Paola Roggero [1,2], Laura Plevani [1], Donatella Bertoli [5], Stefania Zorzan [5], Maria Lorella Giannì [1,2] and Fabio Mosca [1,2]

1. Neonatal Intensive Care Unit, Fondazione IRCCS Cà Granda Ospedale Maggiore Policlinico, via Commenda 12, 20122 Milan, Italy; lorenzo.colombo@mangiagalli.it (L.C.); daniela.morniroli@gmail.com (D.M.); giulia.vercesi@policlinico.mi.it (G.V.); lidia.zanotta@policlinico.mi.it (L.Z.); paola.roggero@unimi.it (P.R.); laura.plevani@mangiagalli.it (L.P.); maria.gianni@unimi.it (M.L.G.); fabio.mosca@mangiagalli.it (F.M.)
2. Department of Clinical Sciences and Community Health, University of Milan, Via San Barnaba 8, 20122 Milan, Italy; paola.mauri@unimi.it (P.A.M.); annalisacanziani.ac@gmail.com (A.C.)
3. Epidemiology Unit, Fondazione IRCCS Ca' Granda Ospedale Maggiore Policlinico, Via San Barnaba 8, 20122 Milan, Italy; dario.consonni@unimi.it
4. Mother and Child Unit, Università degli Studi di Milano, ATS Città Metropolitana di Milano, 20122 Milan, Italy; MBettinelli@ats-milano.it
5. Direzione Professioni Sanitarie, Fondazione IRCCS Cà Granda Ospedale Maggiore Policlinico, via Commenda 12, 20122 Milan, Italy; irenespreafico@gmail.com (I.S.); patrizio.sannino@policlinico.mi.it (P.S.); donatella.bertoli@policlinico.mi.it (D.B.); stefania.zorzan@policlinico.mi.it (S.Z.)
6. Dipartimento Donna-Bambino-Neonato, Fondazione IRCCS Cà Granda Ospedale Maggiore Policlinico, via Commenda 12, 20122 Milan, Italy

* Correspondence: beatriceletizia.crippa@gmail.com

Abstract: The late preterm infant population is increasing globally. Many studies show that late preterm infants are at risk of experiencing challenges common to premature babies, with breastfeeding issues being one of the most common. In this study, we investigated factors and variables that could interfere with breastfeeding initiation and duration in this population. We conducted a prospective observational study, in which we administered questionnaires on breastfeeding variables and habits to mothers of late preterm infants who were delivered in the well-baby nursery of our hospital and followed up for three months after delivery. We enrolled 149 mothers and 189 neonates, including 40 pairs of twins. Our findings showed that late preterm infants had a low rate of breastfeeding initiation and early breastfeeding discontinuation at 15, 40 and 90 days of life. The mothers with higher educational levels and previous positive breastfeeding experience had a longer breastfeeding duration. The negative factors for breastfeeding were the following: Advanced maternal age, Italian ethnicity, the feeling of reduced milk supply and having twins. This study underlines the importance of considering these variables in the promotion and protection of breastfeeding in this vulnerable population, thus offering mothers tailored support.

Keywords: breastfeeding; late preterm; protective factors; promotion of breastfeeding; breastfeeding support

---

1. Introduction

Late preterms are defined as infants born from 34 0/7 to 36 6/7 weeks of gestational age (GA) and comprise approximately 75% of all preterm births [1]. Late preterm births are increasing overall due to the increased use of reproductive technologies and, therefore, the occurrence of multiple pregnancies, in combination with advances in obstetric surveillance and interventions, which could lead to the choice of preterm delivery for babies at risk of perinatal complications (intrauterine growth restriction, placental insufficiency or monochorionic multiple pregnancies) [2,3]. Compared with infants born at term, late preterm infants are at increased risk of neonatal morbidity (i.e., hypoglycemia, hypothermia, jaundice, delayed oral feeding, readmission to the hospital, transient tachypnoea, neuro-developmental delays and mortality) [2]. This population has immature organs and systems, including the brain; a compromised immunomodulatory response; and an increased susceptibility to inflammatory injury and oxidative stress [4,5]. For this reason, breast milk with its bioactive components and its combination of nutritional, anti-infective, anti-inflammatory, anti-oxidative, epigenetic, and gut-colonizing substances is particularly important for these infants [4–7].

Despite these benefits, late preterm infants have a decreased likelihood of breastfeeding initiation and shortened breastfeeding duration compared to term newborns [2,4,8]. To date, few studies have investigated the modifiable factors affecting breastfeeding and discussed the best approaches to promoting and supporting breastfeeding in this vulnerable population [2,4,8]. Kair et al. determined barriers and facilitators of breastfeeding continuation among a large cohort of late preterm infants and compared preterm infants admitted to the well-baby nursery to those admitted to the neonatal intensive care unit (NICU), concluding that NICU admission was not associated with early breastfeeding cessation [6]. Moreover, the experience of breastfeeding late preterm infants was investigated in a cohort of 44 mothers who were interviewed by phone up to 12 months after delivery [9]. Reduced milk supply, difficulties in latching, feelings of failure, and inadequate lactation support from health care providers after discharge have been identified as the most challenging difficulties encountered by the mothers [9].

The purpose of our research is to investigate the variables that could affect breastfeeding duration in a population of late preterm infants admitted to a well-baby nursery and followed up for three months after birth.

2. Materials and Methods

A prospective, observational, single-center study was carried out in the well-baby nursery of Fondazione IRCCS Ca' Granda Ospedale Maggiore Policlinico in Milan, Italy. The Ethics Committee of the "Fondazione Istituto di Ricovero e Cura a Carattere Scientifico Cà Granda Ospedale Maggiore Policlinico" endorsed the present study, and parents provided written informed consent.

We enrolled all consenting mothers with an adequate comprehension of the Italian language who had given birth to late preterm infants admitted to the well-baby nursery from October to December 2017. According to our internal protocol, late preterm infants with a GA from 34 0/7 to 36 6/7 weeks (estimated based on the last menstrual period) and birth weight $\geq$ 1800 g were admitted to the well-baby nursery, provided that their clinical conditions were stable. This means no need of intravenous infusions, noninvasive respiratory support, or any type of invasive assistance, whereas monitoring of vital parameters and/or the need of incubator were possible in the nursery in the first 24 h of life. We did not enroll a control group of term neonates. The exclusion criteria were the following: Hospitalization in the NICU, congenital anomalies, genetic syndromes, respiratory diseases, neurologic problems, metabolic disorders, or gastrointestinal problems. Before discharge, a structured questionnaire for each infant, including twins, was administered to mothers by one of five health care professionals. The questionnaire used was created by the public health organization of the city of Milan (ATS Città di Milano) for monitoring and comparing breastfeeding habits during the Baby-Friendly Hospital Initiative (BFHI) accreditation [10] of the city's hospitals. It included closed-ended questions and took fifteen minutes to administer.

The questionnaire assessed sociodemographic characteristics (maternal age, education, ethnicity), basic characteristics of newborns (GA, birth weight), previous experiences (participation in a prenatal class and previous experience with breastfeeding), type of delivery, peripartum experiences (skin-to-skin contact for at least two hours after birth and rooming-in, defined as the baby being kept in the mother's room for at least 23 h a day), factors affecting lactation (latching difficulties; use of a pacifier; the feeling of reduced milk supply, defined as a subjective maternal perception of having not enough milk to satisfy the baby; breastfeeding on demand or scheduled breastfeeding), and mode of feeding.

Our breastfeeding policy was based on the principles of the BFHI [10]. For this reason, the process of breastfeeding on demand was always explained to mothers and actively promoted by all health care professionals. In contrast, scheduled feeding, defined as feeding the baby at set intervals, was always the mother's choice. The mode of breastfeeding was reported according to the World Health Organization (WHO) definitions [11]: "Exclusive breastfeeding" indicates no food or drink other than breast milk; and "predominant breastfeeding" indicates that the infant's predominant source of nourishment was breast milk but that the infant also received other liquids (i.e., water and water-based drinks). "Mixed feeding" refers to the use of both breast milk and formula.

We used obstetric charts and infants' computerized medical charts (Neocare, i & t Informatica e Tecnologia Srl, Italy) to collect the basic characteristics of the newborns (i.e., birth weight and GA), mode of breastfeeding, and accurate reports of the skin-to-skin contact time and rooming-in time. All the other data were obtained from the questionnaires.

The mothers completed the first follow-up questionnaire during the visit after discharge, within the first seven days of their infants' lives. Then, structured phone interviews were conducted at 15, 40, and 90 days after birth. The data on the variables subject to changes over time (i.e., latching difficulties, use of a pacifier, mode of feeding) were also collected during each follow-up period. These interviews lasted approximately fifteen minutes. The health care providers in charge of collecting the data during the hospitalization were the same providers responsible for the administration of the questionnaires and phone interviews. With regard to twins, mothers completed the first follow-up questionnaire and the subsequent phone interviews separately for each infant.

To take into account intra-individual correlations over time and the probability of exclusive breastfeeding according to selected variables (including those related to sociodemographic features, clinical characteristics, delivery, peripartum, and past or current lactation determinants), odds ratios (ORs) and 95% confidence intervals (CIs) were calculated with univariate and multiple generalized estimation equation (GEE) logistic regression models. The statistical analyses were performed using Stata 15 (StataCorp LLC, College Station, TX, USA, 2017).

3. Results

The total eligible population included 149 mothers and 189 neonates, including 40 pairs of twins. Seventeen percent of these neonates (32 neonates) were born at 34 weeks of GA, 33.3% (63 neonates) were born at 35 weeks of GA, and 49.7% (94 neonates) were born at 36 weeks of GA. Neonatal birth weight ranged from 2050 g to 2990 g. Only 119 mothers completed the study, with a final dropout rate of 20%. The basic characteristics of the mothers are shown in Table 1.

The minimum maternal age was 20 years, and the maximum age was 49 years. Italians represented 82.5% of the study population: Among them, 56.8% had a degree and 51.2% attended a prenatal class. However, in the population of foreign mothers, there was a lower educational level (30.8% had a degree and 34.6% attended a prenatal class). In contrast to the Italian mothers, foreign mothers were more likely to breastfeed on demand (27% vs. 18%) and to have had positive breastfeeding experiences (57.7% vs. 45.5%). Most of the population did not experience skin-to-skin contact (95.5%) or rooming-in (88.6%).

Table 2 shows the proportion of different types of feeding over the first three months of life.

At discharge, only 16.8% of mothers exclusively breastfed their babies, and the rate increased to a maximum of 40.3% at 15 days of life. Mixed feeding peaked at discharge (78.8%) and decreased over time, while the rate of formula feeding progressively increased. Among the lactation factors also reported in Table 2, incorrect latching of the baby on the breast (even if only reported by the mother) was more common during the first days after birth, while the perception of reduced milk supply occurred later.

Table 1. Population features.

	Foreign Mothers (n = 26)		Italian Mothers (n = 123)		Total (n = 149)	
	n	%	n	%	n	%
Sociodemographic features						
Maternal age						
20–29 years	8	30.8	8	6.5	16	10.7
30–34 years	10	38.5	37	30.1	47	31.5
35–39 years	5	19.2	41	33.3	46	30.9
40–49 years	3	11.5	37	30.1	40	26.8
Education						
High school diploma	18	69.2	53	43.1	71	47.7
Degree	8	30.8	70	56.9	78	52.3
Previous experiences						
Prenatal classes						
Yes	9	34.6	63	51.2	72	48.3
No	17	65.4	60	48.8	77	51.7
Previous breastfeeding experience						
Positive	7	27	22	18	29	19.4
None	19	73	88	71.5	107	71.8
Negative	0	0	13	10.5	13	8.8
Delivery and peripartum experiences						
Mode of delivery						
Eutocic	8	30.8	35	28.4	43	28.9
Vacuum/forceps	0	0	6	4.9	6	4.0
Emergency cesarean section	8	30.8	36	29.3	44	29.5
Elective cesarean section	10	38.4	46	37.4	56	37.6
Twins	8	20	32	80	40	100
Skin-to-skin contact						
Yes	2	7.7	5	4.1	7	4.7
No	24	92.3	118	95.9	142	95.3
Rooming-in						
Yes	5	19.2	12	9.8	17	11.4
No	21	80.1	111	90.2	132	88.6
Lactation factors						
Type of breastfeeding						
Scheduled	11	42.3	67	54.5	78	52.3
On demand	15	57.7	56	45.5	71	47.7

Table 2. Follow-up findings.

Variable	Before Discharge * (n = 149)	First Visit after Discharge (n = 138)	15 Days of Life (n = 134)	40 Days of Life (n = 127)	90 Days of Life (n = 119)
	n (%)	n (%)	n (%)	n (%)	n (%)
Lactation factors					
Latching difficulty	44 (29.5)	29 (21)	28 (20.9)	13 (10.2)	8 (6.7)
Pacifier	42 (28.1)	45 (32.6)	51 (38)	69 (54.3)	72 (60.5)
Feeling of reduced milk supply	5 (3.3)	6 (4.4)	10 (7.4)	12 (9.4)	5 (4.2)
Type of feeding					
Exclusive breastfeeding	25 (16.8)	53 (38.4)	54 (40.3)	43 (33.8)	37 (31.1)
Predominant breastfeeding	0 (0.0)	0 (0.0)	0 (0.0)	2 (1.7)	6 (5.0)
Mixed feeding	113 (75.8)	71 (51.5)	64 (47.8)	46 (36.2)	25 (21.0)
Formula feeding	11 (7.4)	14 (10.1)	16 (11.9)	36 (28.3)	51 (42.9)
Lost to follow up	0	11(7.3)	15 (10)	22 (14.8)	30 (20)

* "Before discharge" refers to the 24 h period before discharge.

For each investigated variable, no difference was found in the answers provided by the mothers with regard to twins.

According to univariate and multivariate regression (Table 3), the factors found to be protective for exclusive breastfeeding were a previous positive experience of breastfeeding and maternal education. Maternal age over 35 years, Italian ethnicity, the feeling of reduced milk supply, and twin pregnancies were risk factors for the early cessation of breastfeeding.

Table 3. Factors affecting breastfeeding: results of univariate and multivariate logistic regressions.

	OR Crude (95% CI)	OR Adjusted * (95% CI)
Sociodemographic features		
Maternal age		
Maternal age < 30 years	1.0 (reference)	1.0 (reference)
Maternal age 30–34 years	1.5 (0.6–3.9)	0.8 (0.2–2.9)
Maternal age 35–39 years	0.5 (0.2–1.4)	0.3 (0.1–0.9)
Maternal age > 40 years	0.3 (0.1–0.8)	0.2 (0.0–0.7)
Education		
High school diploma	1.0 (reference)	1.0 (reference)
Degree	1.2 (0.6–2.1)	2.2 (1.0–5.0)
Ethnicity		
Foreign mothers	1.0 (reference)	1.0 (reference)
Italian ethnicity	0.4 (0.2–0.7)	0.2 (0.0–0.7)
Previous experiences		
Prenatal classes		
No prenatal classes	1.0 (reference)	1.0 (reference)
Prenatal classes	1.5 (0.8–2.9)	1.5 (0.7–3.3)
Clinical history		
No breastfeeding experience	1.0 (reference)	1.0 (reference)
Previous negative experience with breastfeeding	0.7 (0.2–2.2)	0.9 (0.2–2.8)
Previous positive experience with breastfeeding	3.1 (1.4–7.0)	3.0 (1.0–8.5)
Delivery and peripartum experiences		
Mode of delivery		
Eutocic delivery	1.0 (reference)	1.0 (reference)
Vacuum assisted delivery	2.4 (0.5–11.5)	1.9 (0.4–10.9)
Emergency cesarean delivery	0.4 (0.2–0.9)	0.8 (0.3–2.5)
Elective cesarean delivery	0.3 (0.2–0.8)	0.5 (0.2–1.5)
Twins		
Singleton	1.0 (reference)	1.0 (reference)
Twins	0.2 (0.1–0.4)	0.2 (0.1–0.5)
Skin-to-skin contact		
No skin-to-skin contact	1.0 (reference)	1.0 (reference)
Skin to skin contact	3.2 (0.7–15.2)	9.9 (0.8–119.0)
Rooming-in		
No rooming-in	1.0 (reference)	1.0 (reference)
Rooming-in	1.1 (0.4–3.1)	0.7 (0.2–2.6)
Lactation Factors		
Type of breastfeeding		
Scheduled breastfeeding	1.0 (reference)	1.0 (reference)
On demand	1.8 (0.9–3.3)	1.4 (0.6–2.9)
Latching		
No difficulties	1.0 (reference)	1.0 (reference)
Attachment difficulties	0.8 (0.5–1.3)	0.8 (0.5–1.2)
Pacifier		
Use of pacifier	1.0 (reference)	1.0 (reference)
No use of pacifiers	1.3 (0.9–1.7)	1.2 (0.7–2.0)
Milk supply		
No reduced milk supply	1.0 (reference)	1.0 (reference)
Feeling of reduced milk supply	0.4 (0.2–0.7)	0.3 (0.1–0.5)

* Each factor was adjusted for the others. Odds ratios were from univariate and multiple generalized estimation equation logistic regression models. OR: odds ratio; CI: confidence interval.

4. Discussion

Late preterms are increasing in number overall, adding substantially to the impact on health care services, both in the acute, and primary health care settings [2,12]. This study contributed to expanding the current body of knowledge by increasing awareness of how to best target support for mothers of late preterm infants.

Our data confirm that compared to infants born at term in the same hospital setting and in a similar sociodemographic context, late preterm infants were less likely to be exclusively breastfed in the hospital and after discharge, and required more time to acquire breastfeeding skills [13]. Accordingly, the breastfeeding rate in the late preterm population progressively increased to 40.3% at 15 days of life, whereas Colombo et al. reported the peak rate of exclusive breastfeeding to be 75.3% in term newborns at discharge [13]. The present study identified an increased maternal age, Italian ethnicity, low maternal education, lack of previous positive breastfeeding experiences, having twins, and the feeling of reduced milk supply as risk factors for the early discontinuation of exclusive breastfeeding.

Little is known about the effect of maternal age on breastfeeding rates for late preterm infants, and the results are conflicting when different social contexts are considered [14]. Nevertheless, the most developed regions have seen an increase in maternal age in the last two decades [15], and our data indicate that mothers aged 35 years or older are less likely to breastfeed. Accordingly, increased maternal age has been associated with a negative effect on breastfeeding among mothers of term infants in the same hospital setting with a similar sociodemographic context [13].

Italian mothers were less likely to breastfeed than were foreign mothers, unlike what was observed in a population of mothers of term newborns [13]. It can be hypothesized that the limited number of foreign mothers and the high percentage of Italian mothers older than 35 years could have affected this result.

Regarding the mode of delivery, the literature has shown that cesarean is negatively associated with breastfeeding [2,16,17]. Studies established a negative association between cesarean delivery, the onset of lactation, milk transfer and milk production [2,16,17]. Accordingly, Ayton et al. reported that late preterm infants delivered by cesarean section were 80% less likely to initiate breastfeeding within one hour of birth and identified the combination of cesarean delivery with prematurity as a synergic risk factor that creates a complex breastfeeding scenario [2]. In the univariate analysis, our data confirmed the known negative association between cesarean section and breastfeeding. However, the significance was lost in multivariate analysis, probably because of the influence of other variables; increased maternal age and/or having had an iterative elective cesarean section could have implied a previous maternal breastfeeding experience.

Rooming-in and skin-to-skin contact at least two hours after birth are well-known factors associated with successful breastfeeding [18]. Skin-to-skin contact encourages breastfeeding behavior, stimulates innate reflexes in newborns [19], accelerates neurophysiological development [20], and is positively associated with breastfeeding duration in preterm infants [19]. However, in our study, we could not find any significant associations among skin-to-skin contact, rooming-in and breastfeeding, probably due to the very small percentage of mothers who experienced one or both of these practices. The limited implementation of skin-to-skin contact and the partial implementation of rooming-in in our population may be attributable to the fact that late preterm infants frequently need an incubator for the first hours or possibly days of life.

The use of pacifiers could be justifiable in certain situations, particularly in a NICU setting and when the neonate is separated from the mother. The pacifier could support breastfeeding in low-birth-weight and premature infants by promoting the maintenance and maturation of the sucking reflex; it also helps to achieve a neurobehavioral organization and could relieve pain and decrease stress [21]. Other studies have reported that, both in term and preterm infants, the minimization of the use of a pacifier positively affected exclusive breastfeeding [13,19]. However, in our late preterm population in a well-baby nursery setting, avoiding the use of pacifiers was not found to be associated with breastfeeding.

Twin pregnancies were strongly correlated with the early cessation of breastfeeding in our population. Our possible explanation could be the greater maternal fatigue in simultaneously managing and feeding more than one premature infant. Few studies examining breastfeeding among preterm infants include or differentiate among multiple pregnancies. As reported by Giannì et al., having twins was reported by the mother's of late preterm infants to be a barrier to breastfeeding [8]. In contrast, Demirci et al. observed a higher rate of breastfeeding initiation among mothers of late preterm multiples than among mothers of singleton infants [14].

Maternal education was positively associated with breastfeeding. This finding was not surprising, and it was likewise previously described as a predictor of a longer duration of breastfeeding in both term [13] and late preterm infants [6,22]. With regard to lactation factors, the feeling of reduced milk supply and latching difficulties negatively affected breastfeeding, while breastfeeding on demand was strongly associated with the continuation of breastfeeding, according to the literature [6,23]. The maternal perception of inadequate milk supply, breastfeeding difficulties, and concerns that breast milk alone did not satisfy the infants were reported as the top three reasons for breastfeeding discontinuation in the study of Kair et al., which surveyed a total of 2530 mothers of late preterm infants [6]. Moreover, the same barriers were reported in two qualitative [9,24] studies that illustrated a common phenomenon of maternal frustration associated with breastfeeding difficulties.

Breastfeeding a late preterm infant could be challenging due to the peculiar characteristics of this population, such as relative hypotonia and consequent ineffective sucking [2] and immaturity in coordinating swallowing and breathing during breastfeeding [25]. In this scenario, the availability of expert lactation support is crucial [8,26] and affects mothers' self-efficacy, which could be crucial in the establishment of breastfeeding, even in late preterm populations [27,28]. We also believe that mothers' self-efficacy may be correlated with personal experiences. Previous encouraging breastfeeding experiences were strongly positively associated with breastfeeding initiation and duration, whereas a previous negative breastfeeding experience affected breastfeeding initiation and duration much more than having no experience at all. These findings are consistent with those concerning term infants [13] and reinforce the need to closely explore mothers' backgrounds to identify any possible breastfeeding issues and specific groups of mothers that will need extra help.

The present study has some limitations. First, the data were collected from a single institution where internal procedures are applied and thus it is not possible to generalize our findings. Moreover, the results were not stratified according to gestational age. However, it addressed a relatively large number of mothers who received the same modalities of support, and all infants were late preterm infants without comorbidities and with a low-risk birthweight, making the population homogenous and composed of infants with other risk factors, except being born as a late preterm.

5. Conclusions

Many studies have demonstrated that, even when considered healthy, this population is at risk of having issues typical of premature babies, with breastfeeding problems being the most predictable. Considering the importance of mothers' milk and its beneficial effects for both term and preterm infants, the main significance of our study was to underline the need for all health care professionals to be aware of the support required for breastfeeding late preterm infants. The implementation of specific and timely breastfeeding support measures for mothers (especially if old, having twins, with low education, with no previous positive breastfeeding experiences, or with the perception of reduced milk supply), could facilitate to give their preterm infants the best start in life.

Author Contributions: Conceptualization: L.C., M.E.B., L.Z., D.B., M.L.G. and F.M.; data curation: B.L.C., D.M., D.C., I.S., G.V. and A.C.; formal analysis: B.L.C. and D.C.; methodology: L.C.; resources: I.S., G.V. and A.C.; supervision: M.E.B., P.S., P.A.M., L.Z., P.R., L.P., D.B., S.Z., M.L.G. and F.M.; validation: D.C., M.E.B., P.S., P.A.M., L.Z., P.R., L.P., D.B., S.Z. and F.M.; visualization: M.E.B., P.S., P.A.M., L.Z., P.R., L.P., D.B. and S.Z.; writing of the original draft: B.L.C. and D.M.; writing, the review and editing: B.L.C., L.C., D.M. and M.L.C.

References

1. Kugelman, A.; Colin, A.A. Late Preterm Infants: Near Term but Still in a Critical Developmental Time Period. *Pediatrics* **2013**, *132*, 741–751. [CrossRef] [PubMed]
2. Ayton, J.; Hansen, E.; Quinn, S.; Nelson, M. Factors associated with initiation and exclusive breastfeeding at hospital discharge: Late preterm compared to 37 week gestation mother and infant cohort. *Int. Breastfeed. J.* **2012**, *7*, 16. [CrossRef] [PubMed]
3. Engle, W.A.; Tomashek, K.M.; Wallman, C. and the Committee on Fetus and Newborn. "Late Preterm" Infants: A Population at Risk. *Pediatrics* **2007**, *120*, 1390–1401. [CrossRef] [PubMed]
4. Dosani, A.; Hemraj, J.; Premji, S.S.; Currie, G.; Reilly, S.M.; Lodha, A.K.; Young, M.; Hall, M. Breastfeeding the late preterm infant: Experiences of mothers and perceptions of public health nurses. *Int. Breastfeed. J.* **2016**, *12*, 23. [CrossRef] [PubMed]
5. Meier, P.; Patel, A.L.; Wright, K.; Engstrom, J.L. Management of Breastfeeding During and After the Maternity Hospitalization for Late Preterm Infants. *Clin. Perinatol.* **2013**, *40*, 689–705. [CrossRef] [PubMed]
6. Kair, L.R.; Colaizy, T.T. Breastfeeding Continuation among Late Preterm Infants: Barriers, Facilitators, and Any Association with NICU Admission? *Hosp. Pediatr.* **2016**, *6*, 261–268. [CrossRef] [PubMed]
7. Victora, C.G.; Bahl, R.; Barros, A.J.D.; França, G.V.A.; Horton, S.; Krasevec, J.; Murch, S.; Sankar, M.J.; Walker, N.; Rollins, N.C. Lancet Breastfeeding Series Group Breastfeeding in the 21st century: Epidemiology, mechanisms, and lifelong effect. *Lancet* **2016**, *387*, 475–490. [CrossRef]
8. Giannì, M.L.; Bezze, E.; Sannino, P.; Stori, E.; Plevani, L.; Roggero, P.; Agosti, M.; Mosca, F. Facilitators and barriers of breastfeeding late preterm infants according to mothers' experiences. *BMC Pediatr.* **2016**, *16*, 1–8. [CrossRef]
9. Kair, L.R.; Flaherman, V.J.; Newby, K.A.; Colaizy, T.T. The Experience of Breastfeeding the Late Preterm Infant: A Qualitative Study. *Breastfeed. Med.* **2015**, *10*, 102–106. [CrossRef]
10. WHO. Baby-Friendly Hospital Initiative. Revised, Updated and Expanded for Integrated Care. Geneva. 2009. Available online: http://www.who.int/nutrition/topics/bfhi/en/ (accessed on 11 November 2018).
11. WHO. *WHO Indicators for Assessing Infant and Young Child Feeding Practices*; WHO: Geneva, Switzerland, 2010; pp. 1–19.
12. Moster, D.; Lie, R.T.; Markestad, T. Long-term medical and social consequences of preterm birth. *N. Engl. J. Med.* **2008**, *359*, 262–273. [CrossRef]
13. Colombo, L.; Crippa, B.L.; Consonni, D.; Bettinelli, M.E.; Agosti, V.; Mangino, G.; Bezze, E.N.; Mauri, P.A.; Zanotta, L.; Roggero, P.; et al. Breastfeeding determinants in healthy term newborns. *Nutrients* **2018**, *10*, 48. [CrossRef]
14. Demirci, J.R.; Sereika, S.M.; Bogen, D. Prevalence and Predictors of Early Breastfeeding among Late Preterm Mother-Infant Dyads. *Breastfeed. Med.* **2013**, *8*, 277–285. [CrossRef] [PubMed]
15. Kitano, N.; Nomura, K.; Kido, M.; Murakami, K.; Ohkubo, T.; Ueno, M.; Sugimoto, M. Combined effects of maternal age and parity on successful initiation of exclusive breastfeeding. *Prev. Med. Rep.* **2016**, *3*, 121–126. [CrossRef] [PubMed]
16. Dewey, K.G.; Nommsen-rivers, L.A.; Heinig, M.J.; Cohen, R.J. Onset of Lactation and Excess Neonatal Weight Loss. *Pediatrics* **2015**, *112*, 607–619. [CrossRef]
17. Scott, J.A.; Binns, C.W.; Oddy, W.H. Predictors of delayed onset of lactation. *Matern. Child Nutr.* **2007**, *3*, 186–193. [CrossRef]
18. Åkerström, S.; Asplund, I.; Norman, M. Successful breastfeeding after discharge of preterm and sick newborn infants. *Acta Paediatr. Int. J. Paediatr.* **2007**, *96*, 1450–1454. [CrossRef] [PubMed]
19. Maastrup, R.; Hansen, B.M.; Kronborg, H.; Bojesen, S.N.; Hallum, K.; Frandsen, A.; Kyhnaeb, A.; Svarer, I.; Hallström, I. Breastfeeding progression in preterm infants is influenced by factors in infants, mothers and clinical practice: The results of a national cohort study with high breastfeeding initiation rates. *PLoS ONE* **2014**, *9*, e108208. [CrossRef]
20. Scher, M.S.; Ludington-Hoe, S.; Kaffashi, F.; Johnson, M.W.; Holditch-Davis, D.; Kenneth, A.L. Neurophysiologic assessment of brain maturation after an eight-week trial of skin to skin contact on preterm infants. *Clin. Neurophysiol.* **2009**, *120*, 1812–1818. [CrossRef]
21. Lubbe, W.; ten Ham-Baloyi, W. When is the use of pacifiers justifiable in the baby-friendly hospital initiative context? A clinician's guide. *BMC Pregnancy Childbirth* **2017**, *17*, 1–10. [CrossRef]

22. Brown, C.R.L.; Dodds, L.; Attenborough, R.; Bryanton, J.; Rose, A.E.; Flowerdew, G.; Langille, D.; Lauzon, L.; Semenic, S. Rates and determinants of exclusive breastfeeding in first 6 months among women in Nova Scotia: A population-based cohort study. *CMAJ Open* **2013**, *1*, E9–E17. [CrossRef]
23. Callen, J.; Pinelli, J. A review of the literature examining the benefits and challenges, incidence and duration, and barriers to breastfeeding in preterm infants. *Adv. Neonatal Care* **2005**, *5*, 89–92. [CrossRef]
24. Demirci, R.J.; Happ, M.B.; Bogen, D.L.; Albrecht, S.A.; Cohen, S.M. Weighing worth against uncertain work: The interplay of exhaustion, ambiguity, hope and disappointment in mothers breastfeeding late preterm infants. *Matern. Child Nutr.* **2015**, *11*, 59–72. [CrossRef] [PubMed]
25. Santos, I.S.; Matijasevich, A.; Silveira, M.F.; Sclowitz, I.K.T.; Barros, A.J.D.; Victora, C.G.; Barros, F.C. Associated factors and consequences of late preterm births: Results from the 2004 Pelotas birth cohort. *Paediatr. Perinat. Epidemiol.* **2008**, *22*, 350–358. [CrossRef] [PubMed]
26. Rayfield, S.; Oakley, L.; Quigley, M.A. Association between breastfeeding support and breastfeeding rates in the UK: A comparison of late preterm and term infants. *BMJ Open* **2015**, *5*. [CrossRef] [PubMed]
27. Brockway, M.; Benzies, K.; Hayden, K.A. Interventions to Improve Breastfeeding Self-Efficacy and Resultant Breastfeeding Rates: A Systematic Review and Meta-Analysis. *J. Hum. Lact.* **2017**, *33*, 486–499. [CrossRef] [PubMed]
28. Brockway, M.; Benzies, K.M.; Carr, E.; Aziz, K. Breastfeeding self-efficacy and breastmilk feeding for moderate and late preterm infants in the Family Integrated Care trial: A mixed methods protocol. *Int. Breastfeed. J.* **2018**. [CrossRef] [PubMed]

13

Exclusive Breastfeeding Rates and Associated Factors in 13 "Economic Community of West African States" (ECOWAS) Countries

Kingsley Emwinyore Agho [1,2,*], Osita Kingsley Ezeh [1], Pramesh Raj Ghimire [1], Osuagwu Levi Uchechukwu [3], Garry John Stevens [4], Wadad Kathy Tannous [2,3,5], Catharine Fleming [1,2,3], Felix Akpojene Ogbo [2,6] and Global Maternal and Child Health Research collaboration (GloMACH) [†]

1. School of Science and Health, Western Sydney University, Locked Bag 1797, Penrith, NSW 2571, Australia; ezehosita@yahoo.com (O.K.E.); Prameshraj@hotmail.com (P.R.G.); Catharine.Fleming@westernsydney.edu.au (C.F.)
2. Translational Health Research Institute (THRI), School of Medicine, Western Sydney University, Campbelltown Campus, Locked Bag 1797, Penrith, NSW 2571, Australia; K.Tannous@westernsydney.edu.au (W.K.T.); F.Ogbo@westernsydney.edu.au (F.A.O.);
3. Diabetes, Obesity and Metabolism Translational Research Unit, Western Sydney University, Campbelltown, NSW 2560, Australia; L.osuagwu@westernsydney.edu.au
4. Humanitarian and Development Research Initiative (HADRI), School of Social sciences and Psychology, Western Sydney University, Locked Bag 1797, Penrith, NSW 2751, Australia; G.Stevens@westernsydney.edu.au
5. School of Business, Western Sydney University, Locked Bag 1797, Penrith, NSW 2751, Australia
6. General Practice Unit, Prescot Specialist Medical Centre, Welfare Quarters, Makurdi, Benue State 972261, Nigeria

* Correspondence: k.agho@westernsydney.edu.au

† Members are listed at the end of Acknowledgments.

Abstract: Exclusive breastfeeding (EBF) has important protective effects on child survival and also increases the growth and development of infants. This paper examined EBF rates and associated factors in 13 "Economic Community of West African States" (ECOWAS) countries. A weighted sample of 19,735 infants from the recent Demographic and Health Survey dataset in ECOWAS countries for the period of 2010–2018 was used. Survey logistic regression analyses that adjusted for clustering and sampling weights were used to determine the factors associated with EBF. In ECOWAS countries, EBF rates for infants 6 months or younger ranged from 13.0% in Côte d'Ivoire to 58.0% in Togo. EBF decreased significantly by 33% as the infant age (in months) increased. Multivariate analyses revealed that mothers with at least primary education, older mothers (35–49 years), and those who lived in rural areas were significantly more likely to engage in EBF. Mothers who made four or more antenatal visits (ANC) were significantly more likely to exclusively breastfeed their babies compared to those who had no ANC visits. Our study shows that EBF rates are still suboptimal in most ECOWAS countries. EBF policy interventions in ECOWAS countries should target mothers with no schooling and those who do not attend ANC. Higher rates of EBF are likely to decrease the burden of infant morbidity and mortality in ECOWAS countries due to non-exposure to contaminated water or other liquids.

Keywords: breastfeeding; Africa; antenatal care; infants; ECOWAS; mortality

1. Introduction

Exclusive breastfeeding (EBF) is the best source of nutrients for the healthy growth and development of newborns, as well as a natural immunity for protection against infectious (e.g., diarrhoea) [1–4] and long-term chronic diseases [4,5]. The World Health Organization and United Nations Children's Fund (WHO/UNICEF) recommends that nursing mothers should practice EBF, defined as providing the infant human breastmilk only, and oral rehydration solution, or drops/syrups of vitamins, minerals, or medicines, when required [6]. This is because EBF is strongly correlated with a reduced burden of infant and child morbidity and mortality [7]. A recently published report on EBF indicated that approximately 12% of deaths among children under five years old could be averted annually in low- and middle-income countries if all neonates were exclusively breastfed [8]. In sub-Saharan Africa, including Economic Community of West African States (ECOWAS), approximately 42% of diarrhoea-related deaths among children younger than five years of age could be attributed to prelacteal foods or unimproved water or liquids provided to newborns [9]. Mothers who exclusively breastfeed also have a reduced risk of developing type 2 diabetes mellitus and breast and ovarian cancers [4]. ECOWAS is a political and economic union of fifteen member countries in West Africa. The members include Benin, Burkina Faso, Cabo Verde, Côte d'Ivoire, The Gambia, Ghana, Guinea, Guinea-Bissau, Liberia, Mali, Niger, Nigeria, Senegal, Sierra Leone, and Togo. ECOWAS main aim is to promote socioeconomic integration among member countries in order to improve living standards and health outcomes of the population and promote the economic growth of member states [10].

Despite the numerous evidence showing the benefits of EBF for the mother–infant pair [1,4,11], EBF has remained low across ECOWAS countries and varies widely between and within countries [12–15]. Results from the recent Demographic and Health Survey (DHS) in ECOWAS countries between 2010 and 2018 revealed that many countries in the region had EBF rates that were well below the global target (50%) required to considerably reduce infant mortality [16,17]. This low rate of EBF indicates that a substantial proportion of newborns in ECOWAS countries are fed with water and/or prelacteal foods before the age of at least six months. This will, in turn, predispose the infant to gastrointestinal infections due to intake of contaminated prelacteal [18] or complementary foods [1,3,19]. In a recent study conducted in Nigeria, one of the ECOWAS countries with the largest population and economy [10], an estimated 22,371 diarrhoea-related deaths among children under five years could have been averted in 2016 if nursing mothers had strictly adhered to appropriate breastfeeding practices, particularly EBF [20].

In ECOWAS countries (Nigeria, Ghana, Mali, and Niger), past studies conducted based on data collected between 2006 and 2012 have elucidated some factors associated with appropriate EBF practice. The factors include place of residence and birthing [12], higher maternal and paternal education [14,21–23], higher household wealth index [21,23], child's birth order, frequent ($\geq$4) antenatal and postnatal visits [12,21,23], average size of newborns, vaginal birthing [12,24], assistance during delivery, maternal employment, and higher maternal age [12,14,21]. However, none of the previous studies had investigated EBF rates across ECOWAS countries or identified what acts as an enabler or barrier to appropriate EBF behaviours using the most recent country-specific and standardised data. Additionally, some of the previous studies were conducted at the subnational level in Nigeria and Ghana, where their findings may not inform national-level policy interventions [15,25]. Some of the previous nationwide studies used old datasets, which may not reflect the current sociodemographic and economic settings of those countries [12,23].

Understanding the current EBF rates and associated factors across ECOWAS countries is essential to key stakeholders in formulating integrated and effective health policy interventions. Furthermore, the study findings could offer credible information needed to prioritise cost-effective, evidence-based interventions that may rapidly improve EBF rates and subsequently reduce the high burden of under-five deaths in ECOWAS countries [26]. In the current United Nations Decade of Action on Nutrition (2016–2025) [16], the present study will provide policy-relevant data about EBF practice that would assist ministries of health, international agencies, and nongovernmental organizations to design programs that promote, protect, and support appropriate EBF practice in the region. This study aimed to examine EBF rates and the potential demographic, socioeconomic, and proximate factors that are associated with EBF in 13 ECOWAS countries using the combined dataset from 2010 to 2018.

2. Materials and Methods

The analyses were based on the most recent DHS dataset from 13 ECOWAS countries, which were obtained from a password-enabled Measure DHS website [27]. The DHS data were nationally representative and population-based surveys, collected by country-specific ministries of health or other relevant government-owned agencies, with technical support largely provided by Inner City Fund (ICF) International. These surveys were comparable, given the standardised nature of the data collection methods and instruments [28].

The DHS collects demographic data and population health status of people, including reproductive health, maternal and child health, mortality, nutrition, and self-reported health behaviour among adults [28]. Information was collected from eligible women, that is, all women aged 15–49 years who were either permanent residents in the households or visitors present in the households on the night before the survey. Child health information was collected from the mother based on the youngest child aged less than five years, with response rates that ranged from 96% to 99% [27]. Detailed information on the sampling design and questionnaire used is provided in the respective country-specific Measure DHS reports [27]. Our analyses were restricted to the last born child aged 0–5 months and living with the respondent, which yielded a weighted total of 19,735 infants for all 13 ECOWAS countries.

2.1. Outcome, Confounding and Exploratory Variables

EBF rate was estimated using the WHO/UNICEF definitions for assessing infant and young feeding practices in populations [29] and used by Measure DHS. EBF was measured as the proportion of infants 0–5 months of age who were fed exclusively with breast milk (but allows oral rehydration solution and drops or syrups of vitamins and medicines when required). Information on EBF was collected based on maternal recall on feeds provided to the infant in the last 24 h. EBF was categorized as "Yes" (1 = if the infant was exclusively breastfed) or "No" (0 = if the infant was not exclusively breastfed).

Previous studies conducted in sub-Saharan African countries that examined factors associated with EBF [23,30–33] played a vital role in determining the potential confounding variables for this study. The confounding variables were subdivided into four groups, and these were country and demographic factors, socioeconomic factors, access to media factors, and healthcare utilisation factors. The country variables were Benin, Burkina Faso, Côte d'Ivoire, The Gambia, Ghana, Guinea, Liberia, Mali, Niger, Nigeria, Senegal, Sierra Leone, and Togo. We considered Benin as the referenced category because it was the first country on the list of ECOWAS countries. The demographic variables were place of residence (urban or rural), mother's age, marital status, combined birth rank (the position of the youngest under-five child in the family), and birth interval (the interval between births; that is, whether there were no previous births, birth less 24 months prior, or birth more than or equal to 24 months prior), sex of baby, age of the child, and perceived size of the newborn by the mother. The socioeconomic level factors considered were maternal education, maternal work status, maternal literacy, and household wealth index variable. For the combined datasets, the household wealth index was constructed using the "hv271" variable. In the household wealth index categories, the bottom 20% of households was arbitrarily referred to as the poorest households, and the top 20% as the richest households, and was divided into poorest, poor, middle, rich, and richest. Access to media factors consists of the frequency of mothers listening to the radio, watching television, and reading newspapers or magazines. Healthcare utilisation factors were considered and included (birthplace, birth order, mode of delivery, delivery assistance, and antenatal clinic visits (ANC).

2.2. *Statistical Analysis*

Population-level weights were used for survey tabulation, which adjusts for a unique country-specific stratum, and clustering was used to determine the percentage, frequency count, and univariate and multivariate logistic regression of all selected characteristics. Country-specific weights were used for the Taylor series linearization method in the surveys when estimating 95% confidence intervals around the rate of EBF in each country.

For the combined dataset, sampling weight was denormalised, and a new population-level weight was created by dividing the sampling weights by the denormalised weight. We then created a unique country-specific cluster and strata because each country had individual clusters and strata in the DHS. This was done to account for the uneven country-specific population across the organisation and to avoid the effect of countries with a large population (such as Nigeria with over 175 million people in 2013) offsetting countries with a small population (such as The Gambia with about 1.8 million people in 2013) [10].

In the multivariate analyses, the factors associated were further tested by adjusted odds ratios (AOR) using hierarchical multiple logistic regression analyses as described in Table 1. The first stage (Model 1) included country and demographic factors. The second stage (Model 2) also included socioeconomic factors. The third stage (Model 3) added access to media covariates. The fourth and final stage (Model 4) added healthcare utilisation factors. The objective of this modelling strategy was to allow for a comparison of the relationship between each of the different sets of covariates in examining factors associated with EBF. All analyses were performed in Stata version 14.0 (Stata Corp, College Station, Texas, USA).

Table 1. Potential covariates used for hierarchical survey logistic regression model.

Model 1	Model 2	Model 3	Model 4
Country [1]	Country [1]	Country [1]	Country [1]
Demographic	Demographic	Demographic	Demographic
Residence	Socioeconomic	Socioeconomic	Socioeconomic
Mother's age	Household Wealth Index	Access to media	Access to media
Marital status	Work in the last 12 months	Frequency of reading newspaper or magazine	Healthcare utilization factors
Birth rank and birth interval	Maternal education	Frequency of listening to Radio	Place of delivery
Sex of baby	Maternal Literacy	Frequency of watching Television	Mode of delivery
Age of child			Type of delivery assistance
Size of baby			Antenatal Clinic visits

[1] Benin, Burkina Faso, Côte d'Ivoire, The Gambia, Ghana, Guinea, Liberia, Mali, Niger, Nigeria, Senegal, Sierra Leone or Togo.

3. Results

3.1. *Characteristics of the Sample and Unadjusted Analyses for EBF*

The overall EBF rate for all infants aged 0–5 months in the 13 ECOWAS countries was 31.0% between 2010 and 2018 (Figure 1). Higher EBF rates in ECOWAS countries ranged from 52.0% in Ghana to 58.0% in Togo, while Nigeria and Côte d'Ivoire had the lowest EBF rates of less than 20%. Table 2 illustrates the characteristics of the sample of infants aged 0–5 months and their unadjusted odds ratios. Overall, the number of mother–infant dyads included in our sample varied by country, with Nigeria contributing the most (20.0% of the study sample) and Togo the least (3.3%). Bivariate analyses revealed that Nigerian mothers were less likely to exclusively breastfeed their babies compared to those who resided in Benin (OR = 0.29, 95% CI: 0.22, 0.38).

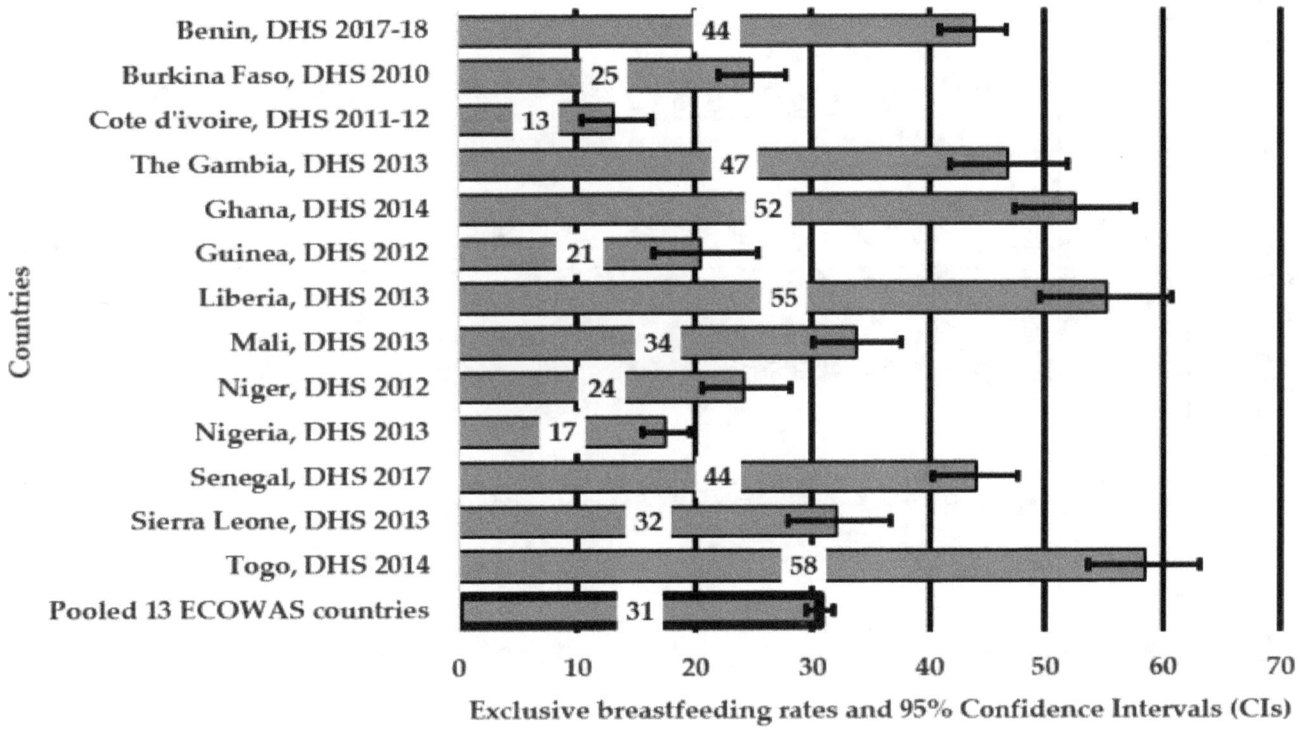

Figure 1. Exclusive breastfeeding rates of infants aged 0–5 months and corresponding 95% confidence intervals in 13 "Economic Community of West African States" (ECOWAS) countries.

Table 2. Individual, household, and community level characteristics and unadjusted odd ratios (OR) (95% CI) of exclusive breastfeeding (EBF) among infants aged 0–5 months in 13 ECOWAS countries.

Characteristic	*n* *	% *	%	EBF			
				OR	95% CI		*p*-Value
Demographic Factors							
Country							
Benin	1475	7.5	8.9	1.00			
Burkina Faso	1837	9.3	10.0	0.46	0.37	0.58	<0.001
Côte d'Ivoire	1110	5.6	5.3	0.17	0.12	0.26	<0.001
The Gambia	1422	7.2	6.6	0.99	0.64	1.52	0.946
Ghana	805	4.1	4.2	1.33	0.98	1.80	0.069
Guinea	981	5.0	4.9	0.42	0.26	0.68	<0.001
Liberia	927	4.7	4.9	1.50	1.02	2.21	0.040
Mali	1192	6.0	6.9	0.66	0.51	0.86	0.002
Niger	2196	11.1	9.0	0.46	0.32	0.64	<0.001
Nigeria	3996	20.2	20.2	0.29	0.22	0.38	<0.001
Senegal	1298	6.6	7.3	1.09	0.84	1.41	0.537
Sierra Leone	1842	9.3	7.7	0.55	0.39	0.78	0.001
Togo	655	3.3	4.2	1.81	1.37	2.39	<0.001
Residence							
Urban	6630	33.6	29.8	1.00			
Rural	13,106	66.4	70.2	0.79	0.66	0.94	0.008
Mother's age (in years)							
15–19	7215	36.6	36.3	1.00			
20–34	9267	47.0	46.0	1.01	0.88	1.17	0.876
35–49	3253	16.5	17.7	1.00	0.84	1.20	0.968
Marital status							
Currently married	18,357	93.0	93.3	1.00			
Formerly married ^	275	1.4	1.5	0.80	0.52	1.23	0.314
Never married	1103	5.6	5.1	1.10	0.79	1.53	0.574
Child Age (in months)	-	-	-	0.70	0.67	0.73	<0.001
Birth order							
First-born	3913	19.8	20.0	1.00			
2nd-4th	9579	48.5	46.6	0.93	0.79	1.09	0.355
5 or more	6243	31.6	33.4	0.70	0.59	0.83	<0.001
Preceding birth interval (n = 19,695)							
No previous birth	3913	19.8	19.7	1.00			
<24 months	1831	9.3	9.2	0.85	0.65	1.11	0.243
≥24 months	13,951	70.7	70.9	0.83	0.72	0.97	0.016

Table 2. *Cont.*

Characteristic	*n* *	% *	%	EBF			
				OR	95% CI		*p*-Value
Demographic Factors							
Combined Birth rank and birth interval							
1st birth rank	3913	19.8	19.7	1.00			
2nd/3rd birth rank, more than 2 years interval	8191	41.5	40.1	0.91	0.77	1.08	0.281
2nd/3rd birth rank, less than or equal to 2 years interval	1388	7.0	6.7	1.00	0.76	1.33	0.963
4th birth rank, more than 2 years interval	5432	27.5	29.2	0.71	0.60	0.85	<0.001
4th birth rank, less than or equal to 2 years interval	811	4.1	4.3	0.66	0.47	0.93	0.016
Sex of baby							
Male	9777	49.5	50.1	1.00			
Female	9958	50.5	49.9	1.09	0.95	1.24	0.206
Size of the baby (n = 19,584)							
Small	3701	18.8	18.5	1.00			
Average	8433	42.7	42.7	1.21	1.02	1.42	0.025
Large	7450	37.8	37.8	1.13	0.96	1.33	0.155
Socioeconomic factors							
Household Wealth Index							
Poorest	3252	16.5	20.2	1.00			
Poorer	3771	19.1	20.2	1.43	1.13	1.81	0.003
Middle	4071	20.6	20.4	1.45	1.16	1.82	0.001
Richer	3790	19.2	19.5	1.51	1.21	1.88	<0.001
Richest	4851	24.6	19.7	1.96	1.54	2.51	<0.001
Work in the last 12 months (n = 19,733)							
Not working	9252	46.9	44.2	1.00			
Working	10,481	53.1	55.8	0.92	0.80	1.07	0.288
Maternal education (n = 19,732)							
No formal education	12105	61.3	61.9	1.00			
Primary	3251	16.5	17.9	1.36	1.14	1.63	0.001
Secondary and above	4376	22.2	20.2	1.86	1.57	2.21	<0.001
Maternal Literacy (n = 19,603)							
Cannot read at all	14,935	75.7	77.6	1.00			
Able to read only part of sentences	4668	23.7	21.8	1.56	1.33	1.82	<0.001

Table 2. *Cont.*

Characteristic	n *	% *	%	EBF			
				OR	95% CI		p-Value
Access to media							
Frequency of reading a newspaper or magazine (n = 19,688)							
Not at all	17,770	90.0	91.6	1.00			
Less than once a week	998	5.1	4.4	1.63	1.22	2.19	0.001
At least once a week/almost every day	914	4.6	3.7	1.45	1.03	2.05	0.035
Frequency of listening to radio (n = 19,703)							
Not at all	6844	34.7	36.2	1.00			
Less than once a week	4957	25.1	25.2	1.18	1.00	1.41	0.054
At least once a week/almost every day	7734	39.2	37.6	1.35	1.16	1.58	<0.001
Frequency of watching television (n = 19,684)							
Not at all	11,558	58.6	61.0	1.00			
Less than once a week	2692	13.6	14.6	1.18	0.98	1.43	0.075
At least once a week/almost every day	5286	26.8	23.5	1.36	1.14	1.63	0.001
Healthcare utilization factors							
Place of delivery							
Home	8493	43.0	42.0	1.00			
Health facility	11,242	57.0	58.0	1.73	1.49	2.01	<0.001
Mode of delivery (n = 19,672)							
Noncaesarean	18,990	96.2	96.4	1.00			
Caesarean section	682	3.5	3.4	1.54	1.11	2.15	0.010
Type of delivery assistance (n = 15,940)							
Health professional	12,342	65.0	62.0	1.00			
Traditional birth attendant	476	2.4	2.7	0.65	0.48	0.89	0.007
Other untrained	1913	9.0	10.9	0.84	0.63	1.13	0.251
No one	1209	6.1	6.0	0.50	0.39	0.65	<0.001
Antenatal Clinic visits (n = 19,147)							
None	2446	12.4	12.8	1.00			
1–3	6485	32.9	34.4	2.12	1.65	2.71	<0.001
≥4	10,216	51.8	50.4	2.75	2.15	3.51	<0.001

* Weighted sample sizes and percentages; ^ divorced/separated/widowed.

Infants whose mothers were from the richer and richest households were significantly more likely to exclusively breastfeed compared to those from poor or poorer households (OR = 1.51, 95% CI: 1.21, 1.88 for richer and OR = 1.96, 95% CI: 1.54, 2.51 for richest). Mothers who watched television almost every day reported higher odds of EBF compared to those who did not watch television at all (OR = 5.44, 95% CI: 3.14, 9.43). This association was also observed among mothers who listened to the radio almost every day (OR = 3.98, 95% CI: 2.41, 6.58). Approximately 57.0% of mothers who delivered their babies in health facilities were significantly more likely to exclusively breastfeed their babies compared to those 43.0% who delivered at home (OR = 1.73, 95% CI: 1.49, 2.01).

Mothers who had caesarean delivery reported much lower proportions (3.5%) of EBF compared to those who had vaginal delivery (96.2%). More than half (51.8%) of mothers had four or more ANC visits, and those mothers who attended ANC visits reported a higher likelihood of EBF compared to those who did not attend any ANC visits (OR = 2.75, 95% CI: 2.15, 3.51) (Table 2).

3.2. *Factors Associated with Exclusive Breastfeeding in Multivariate (Adjusted) Analyses*

Table 3 illustrates the factors associated with EBF among infants aged 0–5 months in multivariate analyses. Among the 13 ECOWAS countries, mothers in Côte d'Ivoire and Nigeria showed the lowest likelihood to engage in EBF practice compared to those in Benin (OR = 0.18, 95% CI: 0.12, 0.28 for Côte d'Ivoire and OR = 0.33, 95% CI: 0.24, 0.45 for Nigeria). Mothers who resided in Burkina Faso, Guinea, Niger, and Sierra Leone were also less likely to engage in EBF compared to those in Benin (Model 4; OR = 0.49, 95% CI: 0.37, 0.64 for Burkina Faso, OR = 0.47, 95% CI: 0.26, 0.84 for Guinea, OR = 0.50, 95% CI: 0.32, 0.79 for Niger, and OR = 0.62, 95% CI: 0.40, 0.97 for Sierra Leone). Liberian and Togolese mothers were more likely to practice EBF compared to their counterparts in Benin (Model 4; OR = 1.65, 95% CI: 1.03, 2.66 for Liberia and OR = 1.52, 95% CI: 1.04, 2.21 for Togo) (Table 3).

Mothers who perceived their babies to be of average birth size were more likely to engage in EBF compared to those who perceived their babies to be of small birth size (OR = 1.22, 95% CI: 1.00, 1.50). Mothers who lived in rural areas and those who had female infants reported higher odds of EBF compared to their counterparts (OR = 1.25, 95% CI: 1.01, 1.55 for rural and OR = 1.17, 95% CI: 1.00, 1.37 for female infants) (Table 3).

Higher maternal age (35–49 years) and education (primary and above education) were associated with increased odds of EBF practice compared to young maternal age (15–19 years) and no maternal education, respectively (OR = 1.50, 95% CI: 1.12, 1.99 for maternal age, and OR = 1.32, 95% CI: 1.06, 1.65 for primary and OR = 1.83, 95% CI: 1.18, 2.82 for secondary and above education). Mothers who made ANC visits had higher odds of EBF practice compared to those who did not make any ANC visits (OR = 1.52, 95% CI: 1.14, 2.03 for 1–3 ANC visits and OR = 1.66, 95% CI: 1.24, 2.23 for four or more ANC visits) (Table 3).

Increasing age of the infant was the only common factor associated with a lower likelihood of EBF in ECOWAS countries (see Table 3) and across all ECOWAS countries (see Supplementary Tables S1 and S2).

Table 3. Adjusted OR (95% CI) of factors associated with exclusive breastfeeding among infants aged 0–5 months in 13 ECOWAS countries.

Characteristic	Model 1				Model 2				Model 3				Model 4			
	aOR	95% CI		*p*-Value	aOR	95% CI		*p*-Value	aOR	95% CI		*p*-Value	aOR	95% CI		*p*-Value
Demographic factors																
Benin	1.00				1.00				1.00				1.00			
Burkina Faso	0.46	0.36	0.58	<0.001	0.46	0.36	0.59	<0.001	0.46	0.35	0.59	<0.001	0.49	0.37	0.64	<0.001
Côte d'Ivoire	0.16	0.11	0.25	<0.001	0.17	0.11	0.26	<0.001	0.17	0.11	0.26	<0.001	0.18	0.12	0.28	<0.001
The Gambia	1.06	0.70	1.60	0.795	0.97	0.63	1.48	0.872	0.97	0.64	1.47	0.878	0.89	0.56	1.40	0.618
Ghana	1.43	1.01	2.04	0.047	1.17	0.77	1.77	0.462	1.16	0.76	1.78	0.493	1.15	0.73	1.80	0.557
Guinea	0.39	0.25	0.61	<0.001	0.40	0.24	0.65	<0.001	0.40	0.24	0.65	<0.001	0.47	0.26	0.84	0.010
Liberia	1.76	1.19	2.61	0.005	1.72	1.15	2.57	0.008	1.73	1.15	2.59	0.008	1.65	1.03	2.66	0.039
Mali	0.64	0.49	0.85	0.002	0.76	0.55	1.04	0.083	0.76	0.55	1.04	0.086	0.81	0.57	1.13	0.211
Niger	0.46	0.32	0.67	<0.001	0.45	0.31	0.66	<0.001	0.45	0.31	0.65	<0.001	0.50	0.32	0.79	0.003
Nigeria	0.28	0.22	0.37	<0.001	0.26	0.20	0.34	<0.001	0.26	0.20	0.34	<0.001	0.33	0.24	0.45	<0.001
Senegal	1.17	0.88	1.56	0.279	1.11	0.81	1.51	0.518	1.12	0.81	1.54	0.497	1.08	0.77	1.52	0.665
Sierra Leone	0.56	0.38	0.83	0.004	0.53	0.36	0.78	0.001	0.54	0.37	0.78	0.001	0.62	0.40	0.97	0.037
Togo	2.00	1.48	2.68	<0.001	1.82	1.34	2.47	<0.001	1.58	1.12	2.23	0.009	1.52	1.04	2.21	0.031
Residence																
Urban	1.00				1.00				1.00				1.00			
Rural	0.98	0.81	1.18	0.838	1.24	1.01	1.51	0.035	1.24	1.01	1.51	0.037	1.25	1.01	1.55	0.042
Mother's age																
15–19 years	1.00				1.00				1.00				1.00			
20–34 years	1.23	1.03	1.48	0.022	1.20	1.00	1.45	0.051	1.22	1.01	1.46	0.041	1.17	0.96	1.42	0.121
35–49 years	1.50	1.15	1.95	0.003	1.46	1.12	1.90	0.005	1.47	1.13	1.92	0.004	1.50	1.12	1.99	0.006
Marital status																
Currently married	1.00				1.00				1.00				1.00			
Formerly married ^	0.80	0.50	1.30	0.370	0.82	0.51	1.33	0.427	0.83	0.51	1.34	0.441	0.78	0.45	1.36	0.386
Never married	0.81	0.56	1.17	0.260	0.72	0.49	1.06	0.096	0.73	0.50	1.07	0.111	0.75	0.50	1.13	0.167
Combined Birth rank and birth interval																
1st birth rank	1.00				1.00				1.00				1.00			
2nd/3rd birth rank, more than 2 years interval	0.88	0.73	1.06	0.186	0.96	0.78	1.17	0.688	0.95	0.78	1.17	0.651	0.93	0.75	1.16	0.542
2nd/3rd birth rank, less than or equal to 2 years interval	0.97	0.71	1.32	0.843	1.03	0.76	1.40	0.858	1.03	0.76	1.39	0.861	0.85	0.60	1.20	0.361
4th birth rank, more than 2 years interval	0.61	0.48	0.78	<0.001	0.75	0.57	0.97	0.031	0.74	057	0.97	0.030	0.76	0.56	1.03	0.074
4th birth rank, less than or equal to 2 years interval	0.64	0.44	0.93	0.019	0.75	0.50	1.01	0.146	0.74	0.50	1.10	0.141	0.81	0.52	1.28	0.358
Sex of baby																
Male	1.00				1.00				1.00				1.00			
Female	1.12	0.98	1.29	0.102	1.13	0.98	1.30	0.094	1.13	0.98	1.31	0.082	1.17	1.00	1.37	0.046
Child Age (in months)	0.67	0.64	0.69	<0.001	0.66	0.64	0.69	<0.001	0.66	0.64	0.69	<0.001	0.67	0.64	0.71	<0.001
Size of the baby																
Small	1.00				1.00				1.00				1.00			
Average	1.26	1.05	1.51	0.013	1.23	1.02	1.48	0.032	1.23	1.02	1.48	0.030	1.22	1.00	1.50	0.050
Large	1.22	1.01	1.47	0.039	1.18	0.98	1.43	0.081	1.19	0.98	1.43	0.078	1.18	0.95	1.45	0.135

Table 3. *Cont.*

Characteristic	Model 1			Model 2			Model 3			Model 4		
	aOR	95% CI	*p*-Value	aOR	95% CI	*p*-Value	aOR	95% CI	*p*-Value	aOR	95% CI	*p*-Value
Socioeconomic factors												
Household Wealth Index												
Poorest				1.00			1.00			1.00		
Poorer				1.39	1.04 1.84	0.024	1.39	1.04 1.85	0.026	1.34	0.99 1.80	0.056
Middle				1.35	1.04 1.75	0.025	1.35	1.04 1.76	0.026	1.13	0.86 1.50	0.369
Richer				1.32	1.03 1.68	0.027	1.31	1.02 1.68	0.035	1.14	0.87 1.48	0.340
Richest				1.46	1.09 1.95	0.010	1.44	1.05 1.99	0.025	1.20	0.86 1.68	0.272
Work in the last 12 months												
Not working				1.00			1.00			1.00		
Working				1.00	0.85 1.17	0.962	0.99	0.84 1.16	0.911	1.01	0.85 1.20	0.899
Maternal education												
No education				1.00			1.00			1.00		
Primary				1.22	0.99 1.51	0.058	1.22	0.99 1.51	0.058	1.32	1.06 1.65	0.015
Secondary and above				1.79	1.12 2.86	0.014	1.84	1.15 2.93	0.011	1.83	1.18 2.82	0.006
Maternal Literacy												
Cannot read at all				1.00			1.00			1.00		
Able to read only part of sentences				0.97	0.64 1.47	0.873	0.95	0.62 1.46	0.826	1.00	0.67 1.48	0.983
Access to media												
Frequency of reading newspaper or magazine												
Not at all							1.00					
Less than once a week							1.08	0.76 1.53	0.655	1.03	0.73 1.46	0.860
At least once a week/Almost every day							0.83	0.53 1.30	0.404	0.83	0.53 1.31	0.420
Frequency of listening to Radio												
Not at all							1.00					
Less than once a week							0.99	0.82 1.19	0.878	0.91	0.75 1.11	0.362
At least once a week/Almost every day							1.01	0.84 1.22	0.916	0.98	0.81 1.19	0.846
Frequency of watching Television												
Not at all							1.00					
Less than once a week							1.03	0.83 1.27	0.800	1.02	0.81 1.28	0.883
At least once a week/Almost every day							1.02	0.83 1.27	0.543	0.93	0.74 1.17	0.551

Table 3. *Cont.*

Characteristic	Model 1			Model 2			Model 3			Model 4		
	aOR	95% CI	*p*-Value	aOR	95% CI	*p*-Value	aOR	95% CI	*p*-Value	aOR	95% CI	*p*-Value
					Healthcare utilization factors							
Place of delivery												
Home										1.00		
Health facility										1.09	0.84 1.43	0.508
Mode of delivery												
Non-caesarean										1.00		
Caesarean section										1.24	0.84 1.83	0.270
Type of delivery assistance												
Health professional										1.00		
Traditional birth attendant.										0.80	0.53 1.21	0.285
Other untrained										1.00	0.71 1.41	0.993
No one										0.81	0.59 1.10	0.178
Antenatal Clinic visits												
None										1.00		
1–3										1.52	1.14 2.03	0.004
≥4										1.66	1.24 2.23	0.001

^ Divorce/separated/widowed.

4. Discussion

Our study indicated that the overall rate of EBF among infants aged 0–5 months of life in 13 ECOWAS countries was at a suboptimum level between 2010 and 2018 compared to the global target of 50% by 2025 [17]. There is a need for further improvement in order to gain the full benefits of EBF as 10 out of the 13 ECOWAS countries had EBF rates between 13% and 47%. This study found that place of residence (rural), maternal education (primary or secondary), mother's age (35–49 years), and antenatal care visit (1–3 or ≥4), increased the likelihood of EBF in 13 ECOWAS countries. Baby size at birth (average) and child's gender (female) were associated with EBF.

The present study showed that nursing mothers who resided in rural areas were more likely to exclusively breastfeed their newborns for less than six months compared with their urban counterparts. This finding is consistent with previous studies conducted in Ethiopia [34], Egypt [35], Malaysia [36], and Lebanon [37]. This finding, however, contradicts earlier reports from Nigeria [30] and Bangladesh [38], which indicated a negative association between rural residence and EBF. An increased likelihood of the association between EBF and rural residence noted in the current study (even after accounting for maternal employment status) could be attributed to a high number of nonworking rural women (rural: 68% vs. urban: 32%). This can, in turn, allow unlimited time for nonworking rural women to breastfed their babies exclusively. Most working nursing mothers reside in urban areas, and labour law concerning maternity leave duration in most ECOWAS countries remains a serious challenge for promotion, protection, and support of EBF practice [13,39]. Fewer than six months of maternity leave are granted to nursing mothers in many ECOWAS countries; for example, in Ghana (12 weeks) [40], Nigeria (16 weeks) [39], and Senegal (14 weeks) [41]. This often leads to early weaning of EBF among working nursing mothers. In addition to the short duration of maternity leave, inadequate facilities and unallocated official time for breastfeeding in the workplace also limit EBF [42]. Urban regions (e.g., urban slums) with potentially disadvantaged communities may deserve special focus with targeted interventions for improving EBF practice in these ECOWAS countries.

The odds of EBF practice were higher among nursing mothers who had primary or higher education, in comparison to their counterparts who had no formal education. This is contrary to previous studies conducted in Ethiopia [34] and Bangladesh [38], where mothers who had no formal education were more likely to report EBF practice. Nevertheless, other studies conducted in sub-Saharan African countries [21,23,33] have also suggested that higher maternal education was significantly associated with EBF practice. Educated mothers are more knowledgeable in utilizing maternal health care services appropriately, including ANC [43], postnatal care (PNC) [44], and institutional delivery [45], which remains an important initiative to scale up EBF participation [46]. To add, past studies have suggested that no formal education among mothers was associated with both underutilization of ANC [47,48] and PNC [49] services.

Furthermore, older mothers (≥35 years) reported a higher likelihood of EBF practice compared with younger mothers. This result is not consistent with previous studies [35,36,50], which indicated that younger mothers were more likely to maintain EBF practice than older mothers. The difference in outcomes may be linked to maternal age classification, characteristics adjusted for, and diverse populations. However, our finding is in line with previous studies conducted in Bangladesh [38] and six low- and middle-income countries [51] that used similar data and maternal age limits. An explanation for the higher odds of EBF noted among older mothers may be their experience in child-rearing, better knowledge of breastfeeding, and being well informed of the benefits of breastfeeding to both newborns and mothers. Additionally, older mothers may also have more time for EBF due to decreased paid job opportunities compared with younger mothers.

Mothers who had one or more ANC visits to the health institution prior to childbirth showed higher odds of EBF practice compared to those who did not attend any ANC visits. This finding is similar to cross-sectional studies carried out in sub-Saharan Africa [23,30] and Bangladesh [38]. The increased odds of EBF in the current study may be attributed to breastfeeding counselling received through the Baby-Friendly Hospital Initiative (BFHI) program during the ANC visits, which may have improved mothers' knowledge and benefits of EBF practice. This is supported by previous evidence from regional Egypt and Ethiopia [35,52], which showed that breastfeeding counselling during ANC was positively related to EBF practice.

This study found that female infants were also associated with higher EBF rates, and this finding is similar to the research conducted in Nigeria, which found that female infants were 2.13 times more likely to be exclusively breastfed than male infants [30]. A study conducted by Johns Hopkins Children's Center revealed that the protective effect of EBF was higher in female infants than male infants [53]. Even though our result on female babies was positively related to EBF practice, caution needs to be exercised in concluding this finding and would warrant further investigation to better understand the impact of gender on EBF in ECOWAS countries. Furthermore, our study also showed that increasing infant age was the only common factor associated with a lower likelihood of EBF in all ECOWAS countries. This finding has been reported in India, where EBF practice decreases faster with increasing infant age in Indian regions with higher socioeconomic status women [54]. Country-specific decline in EBF associated with increasing infant age has not been well studied in ECOWAS countries, and thus, would need further assessment to inform targeted interventions. Reasons why other factors were not significant across the ECOWAS countries varied, including methodological (e.g., sample size) and/or qualitative factors (e.g., cultural norms).

Babies perceived by their mothers to be of average size at birth had an increased likelihood of EBF practice compared to babies perceived by their mothers to be of small size at birth. This finding was similar to a cross-sectional study carried out in Timor-Leste in 2014, which showed that babies perceived to be of a small size at birth by their mothers were less likely to be EBF [55]. Furthermore, a cross-sectional study done in the United States in 2011 reported that very low birth weight (a proxy for babies perceived to be of a small size at birth) was significantly related to a lower likelihood of EBF practice compared to babies born at normal or above-normal birth weights [56]. The significantly lower chance of EBF practice for newborns perceived to be of a small size by their mothers in ECOWAS countries may be attributed to obstacles related to breastfeeding small-sized babies, such as poor sucking and illness (e.g., hypoglycaemia), leading to babies being kept away from their mothers [57], resulting in early introduction of complementary foods and drinks. Although caesarean birthing was associated with non-EBF practice in the bivariate analyses, this association was not significant in multivariate analyses. The possible reasons why caesarean birth was related to non-EBF have been described elsewhere [12,24,58], including a limited number of BFHI-certified maternal health centres, or health practitioners' limited knowledge of appropriate EBF immediately post-birth [59,60]. The BFHI was introduced in 1990 by WHO/UNICEF to promote, protect, and support breastfeeding [61] and has been shown to be successful in increasing EBF participation worldwide [62,63].

The main strengths of our study were the nationally representative sample [27], the comprehensive data on standard infant feeding indicators, and the appropriate adjustments for sampling design in the analysis. There are five limitations of note in this study: Firstly, the subjectivity of information in recalling the time of EBF, especially among mothers who have older infants. Secondly, measurement error and recall bias by mothers may have underestimated or overestimated our effect sizes because information concerning some of the study variables was obtained from mothers whose youngest child may have been up to five years of age. Thirdly, findings in the study cannot be regarded as causal because they were obtained with a cross-sectional design. Fourthly, the study was unable to account for other study and confounding factors, including information on the health status of mothers, partner support, smoking status and alcohol intake, and prenatal breastfeeding intention as documented elsewhere [59,60]. Lastly, the 24 h recall approach was used for EBF investigation, and it is possible that day-to-day variability in nutritional intake may have affected EBF estimates.

5. Conclusions

In summary, the rates of EBF in 10 out of the 13 ECOWAS countries were below the WHO global nutrition target of 50% for breastfeeding. The low rates of EBF in ECOWAS countries may be contributing to higher infant and child morbidity and mortality in each country, given that it is a strong indicator for infant and child growth and survival. At the community level, "baby-friendly" initiative needs to be implemented as a trial in order to empower the community for better nutrition and health improvement of children, as well as to test its effectiveness. At the individual level, the practice of giving water and other liquids is a significant contributor to the decrease in EBF in Africa [18,64]. Awareness must be spread to inform mothers that their babies do not require water and liquids until the completion of the recommended time of six months. These are crucial messages that could be spread by community-level campaigns, including peer support community intervention for young mothers who are vulnerable and have lower rates of EBF. However, further improvement is needed in order to gain the full benefits of breastfeeding practices. Our results suggest that breastfeeding interventions should target urban residents, working mothers, mothers who do attend antennal care, those who give birth to male infants, and mothers who perceive their babies to be small at birth.

Author Contributions: Conceptualization, K.E.A. and F.A.O.; methodology, K.E.A. and O.K.E.; software, K.E.A.; validation, O.L.U., F.A.O., and O.K.E.; formal analysis, K.E.A. and P.R.G.; investigation, O.K.E. and P.R.G.; resources, W.K.T. and C.F.; data curation, F.A.O., P.R.G., and O.L.U.; writing—original draft preparation, K.E.A. and O.K.E.; writing—review and editing, O.L.U., W.K.T., and C.F.; visualization, G.J.S. and O.L.U.; supervision, K.E.A., W.K.T., and G.J.S.; project administration, F.A.O., P.R.G., and K.E.A.

Acknowledgments: The authors are grateful to Measure DHS, ICF International, Rockville, Marylands, USA for providing the data for this study. GloMACH: Members are Kingsley E Agho, Felix A Ogbo, Thierno Diallo, Osita K. Ezeh, Osuagwu L Uchechukwu, Pramesh R Ghimire, Blessing Akombi, Paschal Ogeleka, Tanvir Abir, Abukari I Issaka, Kedir Yimam Ahmed, Rose Victor, Deborah Charwe, Abdon Gregory Rwabilimbo, Daarwin Subramanee, Mehak Mehak, Nilu Nagdev and Mansi Dhami.

References

1. Ogbo, F.A.; Agho, K.; Ogeleka, P.; Woolfenden, S.; Page, A.; Eastwood, J.; Global Child Health Research Interest Group. Infant feeding practices and diarrhoea in sub-Saharan African countries with high diarrhoea mortality. *PLoS ONE* **2017**, *12*, e0171792. [CrossRef] [PubMed]
2. Ogbo, F.A.; Page, A.; Idoko, J.; Claudio, F.; Agho, K.E. Diarrhoea and suboptimal feeding practices in Nigeria: Evidence from the national household surveys. *Paediatr. Perinat. Epidemiol.* **2016**, *30*, 346–355. [CrossRef] [PubMed]
3. Ogbo, F.A.; Nguyen, H.; Naz, S.; Agho, K.E.; Page, A. The association between infant and young child feeding practices and diarrhoea in Tanzanian children. *Trop. Med. Health* **2018**, *46*, 2. [CrossRef] [PubMed]
4. Victora, C.G.; Bahl, R.; Barros, A.J.D.; França, G.V.A.; Horton, S.; Krasevec, J.; Murch, S.; Sankar, M.J.; Walker, N.; Rollins, N.C.; et al. Breastfeeding in the 21st century: Epidemiology, mechanisms, and lifelong effect. *Lancet* **2016**, *387*, 475–490. [CrossRef]
5. Mannan, H. Early Infant Feeding of Formula or Solid Foods and Risk of Childhood Overweight or Obesity in a Socioeconomically Disadvantaged Region of Australia: A Longitudinal Cohort Analysis. *Int. J. Environ. Res. Public Health* **2018**, *15*, 1685. [CrossRef] [PubMed]
6. WHO. *Indicators for Assessing Infant and Young Child Feeding Practices I*; World Health Organization: Geneva, Switzerland, 2008.
7. Black, R.E.; Victora, C.G.; Walker, S.P.; Bhutta, Z.A.; Christian, P.; de Onis, M.; Ezzati, M.; Grantham-McGregor, S.; Katz, J.; Martorell, R.; et al. Maternal and child undernutrition and overweight in low-income and middle-income countries. *Lancet* **2013**, *382*, 427–451. [CrossRef]

8. Debes, A.K.; Kohli, A.; Walker, N.; Edmond, K.; Mullany, L.C. Time to initiation of breastfeeding and neonatal mortality and morbidity: A systematic review. *BMC Public Health* **2013**, *13*, S19. [CrossRef]
9. Wardlaw, T.; Salama, P.; Brocklehurst, C.; Chopra, M.; Mason, E. Diarrhoea: Why children are still dying and what can be done. *Lancet* **2010**, *375*, 870–872. [CrossRef]
10. Economic Community of West African States (ECOWAS). 2019. Available online: https://www.ecowas.int/ (accessed on 23 October 2019).
11. Lamberti, L.M.; Walker, C.L.F.; Noiman, A.; Victora, C.; Black, R.E. Breastfeeding and the risk for diarrhea morbidity and mortality. *BMC Public Health* **2011**, *11*, S15. [CrossRef]
12. Ogbo, F.A.; Agho, K.E.; Page, A. Determinants of suboptimal breastfeeding practices in Nigeria: Evidence from the 2008 demographic and health survey. *BMC Public Health* **2015**, *15*, 259. [CrossRef]
13. Ogbo, F.A.; Page, A.; Idoko, J.; Claudio, F.; Agho, K.E. Have policy responses in Nigeria resulted in improvements in infant and young child feeding practices in Nigeria? *Int. Breastfeed. J.* **2017**, *12*, 9. [CrossRef] [PubMed]
14. Otoo, G.E.; Lartey, A.A.; Pérez-Escamilla, R. Perceived incentives and barriers to exclusive breastfeeding among Periurban Ghanaian women. *J. Hum. Lact.* **2009**, *25*, 34–41. [CrossRef] [PubMed]
15. Agunbiade, O.M.; Ogunleye, O.V. Constraints to exclusive breastfeeding practice among breastfeeding mothers in Southwest Nigeria: Implications for scaling up. *Int. Breastfeed. J.* **2012**, *7*, 5. [CrossRef] [PubMed]
16. United Nations General Assembly. *The UN Decade of Action on Nutrition: Working together to Implement the Outcomes of the Second International Conference on Nutrition*; United Nations: New York, NY, USA, 2016.
17. World Health Organisation. *Global Nutrition Targets 2025: Policy Brief Series (WHO/NMH/NHD/14.2)*; World Health Organisation: Geneva, Switzerland, 2014.
18. Agho, K.E.; Ogeleka, P.; Ogbo, F.A.; Ezeh, O.K.; Eastwood, J.; Page, A. Trends and predictors of prelacteal feeding practices in Nigeria (2003–2013). *Nutrients* **2016**, *8*, 462. [CrossRef]
19. Dhami, M.V.; Ogbo, F.A.; Osuagwu, U.L.; Ugboma, Z.; Agho, K.E. Stunting and severe stunting among infants in India: The role of delayed introduction of complementary foods and community and household factors. *Glob. Health Action* **2019**, *12*, 1638020. [CrossRef]
20. Ogbo, F.A.; Okoro, A.; Olusanya, B.O.; Olusanya, J.; Ifegwu, I.K.; Awosemo, A.O.; Ogeleka, P.; Page, A. Diarrhoea deaths and disability-adjusted life years attributable to suboptimal breastfeeding practices in Nigeria: Findings from the global burden of disease study 2016. *Int. Breastfeed. J.* **2019**, *14*, 4. [CrossRef]
21. Ogbo, F.A.; Eastwood, J.; Page, A.; Efe-Aluta, O.; Anago-Amanze, C.; Kadiri, E.A.; Ifegwu, I.K.; Woolfenden, S.; Agho, K.E. The impact of sociodemographic and health-service factors on breast-feeding in sub-Saharan African countries with high diarrhoea mortality. *Public Health Nutr.* **2017**, *20*, 3109–3119. [CrossRef]
22. Ogunlesi, T.A. Maternal socio-demographic factors influencing the initiation and exclusivity of breastfeeding in a Nigerian semi-urban setting. *Matern. Child Health J.* **2010**, *14*, 459–465. [CrossRef]
23. Yalçin, S.S.; Berde, A.S.; Yalçin, S. Determinants of Exclusive Breast Feeding in sub-Saharan Africa: A Multilevel Approach. *Paediatr. Perinat. Epidemiol.* **2016**, *30*, 439–449. [CrossRef]
24. Ogbo, F.A.; Page, A.; Agho, K.E.; Claudio, F. Determinants of trends in breast-feeding indicators in Nigeria, 1999–2013. *Public Health Nutr.* **2015**, *18*, 3287–3299. [CrossRef]
25. Maduforo, A.N.; Ubah, N.C.; Obiakor-okeke, P.N. The practice of exclusive breastfeeding by lactating women in Owerri metropolis, Imo State, Nigeria. *Glob. Adv. Res. J. Med. Med. Sci.* **2013**, *2*, 13–19.
26. Haidong, W.; Abajobir, A.A.; Abate, K.H.; Abbafati, C.; Abbas, K.M.; Abd-Allah, F.; Abera, S.F.; Abraha, H.N.; Abu-Raddad, L.J.; Abu-Rmeileh, N.M.E.; et al. Global, regional, and national under-5 mortality, adult mortality, age-specific mortality, and life expectancy, 1970–2016: A systematic analysis for the Global Burden of Disease Study 2016. *Lancet* **2017**, *390*, 1084–1150.
27. Measure DHS. The Demographic and Health Survey Program. 2019. Available online: https://dhsprogram.com/publications/index.cfm (accessed on 26 October 2019).
28. Corsi, D.J.; Neuman, M.; Finlay, J.E.; Subramanian, S.V. Demographic and health surveys: A profile. *Int. J. Epidemiol.* **2012**, *41*, 1602–1613. [CrossRef] [PubMed]
29. WHO; UNICEF, USAID, AED, UCDAVIS, IFPRI. *Indicators for Assessing Infant and Young Child Feeding Practices Part 2*; World Health Organization: Geneva, Switzerland, 2008.
30. Agho, K.E.; Dibley, M.J.; Odiase, J.I.; Ogbonmwan, S.M. Determinants of exclusive breastfeeding in Nigeria. *BMC Pregnancy Childbirth* **2011**, *11*, 2. [CrossRef]

31. Victor, R.; Baines, S.K.; Agho, K.E.; Dibley, M.J. Determinants of breastfeeding indicators among children less than 24 months of age in Tanzania: A secondary analysis of the 2010 Tanzania Demographic and Health Survey. *BMJ Open* **2013**, *3*, e001529. [CrossRef]
32. Aidam, B.A.; Pérez-Escamilla, R.; Lartey, A.; Aidam, J. Factors associated with exclusive breastfeeding in Accra, Ghana. *Eur. J. Clin. Nutr.* **2005**, *59*, 789–796. [CrossRef]
33. Tariku, A.; Alemu, K.; Gizaw, Z.; Muchie, K.F.; Derso, T.; Abebe, S.M.; Yitayal, M.; Fekadu, A.; Ayele, T.A.; Alemayehu, G.A.; et al. Mothers' education and ANC visit improved exclusive breastfeeding in Dabat Health and Demographic Surveillance System Site, northwest Ethiopia. *PLoS ONE* **2017**, *12*, e0179056. [CrossRef]
34. Asfaw, M.M.; Argaw, M.D.; Kefene, Z.K. Factors associated with exclusive breastfeeding practices in Debre Berhan District, Central Ethiopia: A cross sectional community based study. *Int. Breastfeed. J.* **2015**, *10*, 23. [CrossRef]
35. El Shafei, A.M.H.; Labib, J.R. Determinants of exclusive breastfeeding and introduction of complementary foods in rural Egyptian communities. *Glob. J. Health Sci.* **2014**, *6*, 236. [CrossRef]
36. Tan, K.L. Factors associated with exclusive breastfeeding among infants under six months of age in peninsular Malaysia. *Int. Breastfeed. J.* **2011**, *6*, 2. [CrossRef]
37. Batal, M.; Boulghourjian, C.; Abdallah, A.; Afifi, R. Breast-feeding and feeding practices of infants in a developing country: A national survey in Lebanon. *Public Health Nutr.* **2006**, *9*, 313–319. [CrossRef]
38. Hossain, M.; Islam, A.; Kamarul, T.; Hossain, G. Exclusive breastfeeding practice during first six months of an infant's life in Bangladesh: A country based cross-sectional study. *BMC Pediatr.* **2018**, *18*, 93. [CrossRef] [PubMed]
39. Ogbo, F.A. *Infant and Young Child Feeding Practices in Nigeria: Epidemiology and Policy Implications*; Centre for Health Research, School of Medicine, Western Sydney University: Sydney, Australia, 2016.
40. Stumbitz, B.; Kyei, A.; Lewis, S.; Lyon, F. *Maternity Protection and Workers with Family Responsibilities in the Formal and Informal Economy of Ghana Practices, Gaps and Measures for Improvement*; International Labour Organization: Geneva, Switzerland, 2017.
41. International Labour Organization. Senegal—Maternity Protection-2011. Available online: https://www.ilo.org/dyn/travail/travmain.sectionReport1?p_lang=en&p_structure=3&p_year=2011&p_start=1&p_increment=10&p_sc_id=2000&p_countries=SN&p_print=Y (accessed on 26 October 2019).
42. Atabay, E.; Moreno, G.; Nandi, A.; Kranz, G.; Vincent, I.; Assi, Ti.; Winfrey, E.M.V.; Earle, A.; Raub, A.; Heymann, S.J. Facilitating working mothers' ability to breastfeed: Global trends in guaranteeing breastfeeding breaks at work, 1995–2014. *J. Hum. Lact.* **2015**, *31*, 81–88. [CrossRef] [PubMed]
43. Ogbo, F.A.; Dhami, M.V.; Ude, E.M.; Senanayake, P.; Osuagwu, U.L.; Awosemo, A.O.; Ogeleka, P.; Akombi, B.J.; Ezeh, O.K.; Agho, K.E. Enablers and Barriers to the Utilization of Antenatal Care Services in India. *Int. J. Environ. Res. Public Health* **2019**, *16*, 3152. [CrossRef] [PubMed]
44. Agho, K.E.; Ezeh, O.K.; Issaka, A.I.; Enoma, A.I.; Baines, S.; Renzaho, A.M.N. Population attributable risk estimates for factors associated with non-use of postnatal care services among women in Nigeria. *BMJ Open* **2016**, *6*, e010493. [CrossRef]
45. Moyer, C.A.; Mustafa, A. Drivers and deterrents of facility delivery in sub-Saharan Africa: A systematic review. *Reprod. Health* **2013**, *10*, 1. [CrossRef]
46. Ogbo, F.A.; Page, A.; Idoko, J.; Agho, K.E. Population attributable risk of key modifiable risk factors associated with non-exclusive breastfeeding in Nigeria. *BMC Public Health* **2018**, *18*, 247. [CrossRef]
47. Agho, K.E.; Ezeh, O.K.; Ogbo, F.A.; Enoma, A.I.; Raynes-Greenow, C. Factors associated with inadequate receipt of components and use of antenatal care services in Nigeria: A population-based study. *Int. Health* **2018**, *10*, 172–181. [CrossRef]
48. Joshi, C.; Torvaldsen, S.; Hodgson, R.; Hayen, A. Factors associated with the use and quality of antenatal care in Nepal: A population-based study using the demographic and health survey data. *BMC Pregnancy Childbirth* **2014**, *14*, 1. [CrossRef]
49. Neupane, S.; Doku, D.T. Determinants of time of start of prenatal care and number of prenatal care visits during pregnancy among Nepalese women. *J. Community Health* **2012**, *37*, 865–873. [CrossRef]
50. Seid, A.M.; Yesuf, M.E.; Koye, D.N. Prevalence of Exclusive Breastfeeding Practices and associated factors among mothers in Bahir Dar city, Northwest Ethiopia: A community based cross-sectional study. *Int. Breastfeed. J.* **2013**, *8*, 14. [CrossRef] [PubMed]

51. Patel, A.; Bucher, S.; Pusdekar, Y.; Esamai, F.; Krebs, N.F.; Goudar, S.S.; Chomba, E.; Garces, A.; Pasha, O.; Saleem, S.; et al. Rates and determinants of early initiation of breastfeeding and exclusive breast feeding at 42 days postnatal in six low and middle-income countries: A prospective cohort study. *Reprod. Health* **2015**, *12*, S10. [CrossRef] [PubMed]
52. Mekuria, G.; Edris, M. Exclusive breastfeeding and associated factors among mothers in Debre Markos, Northwest Ethiopia: A cross-sectional study. *Int. Breastfeed. J.* **2015**, *10*, 1. [CrossRef] [PubMed]
53. More Girls than Boys Benefit from Breastfeeding, Hopkins Children's Research Shows. Available online: https://www.eurekalert.org/pub_releases/2008-06/jhmi-mgt052908.php (accessed on 15 February 2015).
54. Ogbo, F.A.; Dhami, M.V.; Awosemo, A.O.; Olusanya, B.O.; Olusanya, J.; Osuagwu, U.L.; Ghimire, P.R.; Page, A.; Agho, K.E. Regional prevalence and determinants of exclusive breastfeeding in India. *Int. Breastfeed. J.* **2019**, *14*, 20. [CrossRef] [PubMed]
55. Khanal, V.; da Cruz, J.L.N.B.; Karkee, R.; Lee, H.A. Factors associated with exclusive breastfeeding in Timor-Leste: Findings from demographic and health survey 2009–2010. *J. Nutr.* **2014**, *6*, 1691–1700. [CrossRef] [PubMed]
56. Jones, J.R.; Kogan, M.D.; Singh, G.K.; Dee, D.L.; Grummer-Strawn, L.M. Factors associated with exclusive breastfeeding in the United States. *Pediatrics* **2011**, *128*, 1117–1125. [CrossRef]
57. Mulready-Ward, C.; Sackoff, J. Outcomes and factors associated with breastfeeding for <8 weeks among preterm infants: Findings from 6 states and NYC, 2004–2007. *Matern. Child Health J.* **2013**, *17*, 1648–1657. [CrossRef]
58. Tawiah-Agyemang, C.; Kirkwood, B.R.; Edmond, K.; Bazzano, A.; Hill, Z. Early initiation of breast-feeding in Ghana: Barriers and facilitators. *J. Perinatol.* **2008**, *28*, 46–52. [CrossRef]
59. Ogbo, F.A.; Eastwood, J.; Page, A.; Arora, A.; McKenzie, A.; Jalaludin, B.; Tennant, E.; Miller, E.; Kohlhoff, J.; Noble, J.; et al. Prevalence and determinants of cessation of exclusive breastfeeding in the early postnatal period in Sydney, Australia. *Int. Breastfeed. J.* **2017**, *12*, 16. [CrossRef]
60. Ogbo, F.A.; Ezeh, O.K.; Khanlari, S.; Naz, S.; Senanayake, P.; Ahmed, K.Y.; McKenzie, A.; Ogunsiji, O.; Agho, K.; Page, A.; et al. Determinants of exclusive breastfeeding cessation in the early postnatal period among culturally and linguistically diverse (CALD) Australian mothers. *Nutrients* **2019**, *11*, 1611. [CrossRef]
61. World Health Organisation; United Nation Childen Education Fund. *Baby-Friendly Hospital Initiative Revised, Updated and Expanded for Integrated Care*; WHO Document Production Services: Geneva, Switzerland, 2009.
62. Pérez-Escamilla, R. Evidence based breast-feeding promotion: The Baby-Friendly Hospital Initiative. *J. Nutr.* **2007**, *137*, 484–487. [CrossRef] [PubMed]
63. Abrahams, S.W.; Labbok, M.H. Exploring the impact of the Baby-Friendly Hospital Initiative on trends in exclusive breastfeeding. *Int. Breastfeed. J.* **2009**, *4*, 1. [CrossRef] [PubMed]
64. Khanal, V.; Adhikari, M.; Sauer, K.; Zhao, Y. Factors associated with the introduction of prelacteal feeds in Nepal: Findings from the Nepal Demographic and Health Survey 2011. *Int. Breastfeed. J.* **2013**, *8*, 9. [CrossRef] [PubMed]

14

Comparison of Human Milk Immunoglobulin Survival during Gastric Digestion between Preterm and Term Infants

Veronique Demers-Mathieu [1], Mark A. Underwood [2], Robert L. Beverly [1], Søren D. Nielsen [1] and David C. Dallas [1,*]

[1] Nutrition Program, School of Biological and Population Health Sciences, College of Public Health and Human Sciences, Oregon State University, Corvallis, OR 97331, USA; Veronique.Demers-Mathieu@oregonstate.edu (V.D.-M.); beverlyr@oregonstate.edu (R.L.B.); sodn@food.au.dk (S.D.N.)

[2] Department of Pediatrics, University of California, Davis, Sacramento, CA 95817, USA; munderwood@ucdavis.edu

* Correspondence: Dave.Dallas@oregonstate.edu

Abstract: Human milk provides immunoglobulins (Igs) that supplement the passive immune system of neonates; however, the extent of survival of these Igs during gastric digestion and whether this differs between preterm and term infants remains unknown. Human milk, and infant gastric samples at 2 h post-ingestion were collected from 15 preterm (23–32 week gestational age (GA)) mother-infant pairs and from 8 term (38–40 week of GA) mother-infant pairs within 7–98 days postnatal age. Samples were analyzed via ELISA for concentration of total IgA (secretory IgA (SIgA)/IgA), total secretory component (SC/SIgA/SIgM), total IgM (SIgM/IgM), and IgG as well as peptidomics. Total IgA concentration decreased by 60% from human milk to the preterm infant stomach and decreased by 48% in the term infant stomach. Total IgM and IgG concentrations decreased by 33% and 77%, respectively, from human milk to the term infant stomach but were stable in the preterm infant stomach. Release of peptides from all Ig isotypes in the term infant stomach was higher than in the preterm stomach. Overall, the stability of human milk Igs during gastric digestion is higher in preterm infant than in term infants, which could be beneficial for assisting the preterm infants' immature immune system.

Keywords: passive immunity; antibodies; lactation; peptidomics; prematurity; proteolysis; breast milk

1. Introduction

Immunoglobulins (Igs) are important effectors of the adaptive immune system [1]. During the third trimester, the mother's placenta transports IgG to the fetus via a neonatal Fc receptor. These maternal IgG antibodies protect the infant during the first 6 months of postnatal age while the infant's own immune system is developing [2]. After birth, human milk provides another form of protection against pathogens for infants, as it contains an array of Igs, including IgA, secretory IgA (SIgA), IgM, secretory IgM (SIgM), and IgG [3,4]. Indeed, feeding mother's milk reduces risks of infectious diseases in the respiratory and gastrointestinal tract in infancy [5]. Though human milk provides different Ig isotypes, milk SIgA is thought to be the most important in the infant gut as it neutralizes bacterial and viral pathogens by binding to them, thus reducing their ability to interact with epithelial cells and infect [6,7]. The presence of SIgA in human milk temporarily replaces the normal intestinal SIgA secretion that is lacking in the infant until 4 weeks of postnatal age [8].

SIgA is the first line of defense in protecting the intestinal epithelium from pathogens by immune exclusion [9]. Though SIgA is the most well-known and abundant Ig of intestinal secretions [10], IgG and IgM are also secreted by plasma cells in neonatal intestinal mucosa [11,12]. IgG may have function in the gut: passive administration of virus-neutralizing IgG prevented mucosal immunodeficiency virus transmission from mother to infant in macaques [13], suggesting potential transmission of these IgG in the gut. However, the ability of IgG to bind to viruses to prevent attachment to the mucosal surface or trap pathogens in mucus appears to be inefficient compared with SIgA [13]. Human neonatal Fc receptor (FcRn) may be able to transport IgG (alone or bound to an antigen) across the intestinal epithelial barrier into the lamina propria [11]. Though IgM-secreting cells have been identified in the infant gut [12] and IgM was shown to be synthesized in amounts similar to IgA in pig small intestinal mucosal explants [14,15], no study has determined the extent to which IgM plays a role in the adult or infant intestinal mucosal immune defense.

In order to function in immunoprotection in the gut, IgA and potentially the other Ig must resist proteolytic degradation and remain intact and able to bind to pathogens through the digestive system. Though the provision of milk Igs to the infant is known to reduce infection risk, the degree to which Igs survive in the gastrointestinal tract remains unknown. Few studies have investigated the stability of Igs in digestion. Two oral supplementation studies (in adults fed bovine colostrum SIgA/IgA, IgM and IgG [16] and in preterm infants fed serum IgA and IgG [17]) demonstrated that IgG and IgM survive intact to the stool, whereas SIgA/IgA does not. However, some studies have demonstrated that human milk-derived SIgA survived intact to the infant stool and urine [8,18,19].

Our previous study demonstrated that preterm infants had lower gastric digestion capacity for human milk proteins than term infants [20]. This difference in digestion capacity could affect the survival of immunoglobulins. Our recent studies demonstrated that preterm infants partially degrade IgA but not IgG and IgM in the stomach [21,22]. Whether differences in preterm and term infant gastric digestion result in differences in Ig survival remain unknown. The aim of the present study was to determine whether preterm infant Ig survival in the stomach is higher than in term infants.

As preterm infants are born early and miss some of the placenta-fetal IgG transfer [23], produce less diverse of antibodies in their gut in comparison with term infants [24], and are at higher risk for bacterial [25] and viral infections [26] than term infants, the presence of Ig in human milk may be even more critically important to their health outcomes than for term infants. Therefore, milk-provided Ig may be even more critically important than for term infants. Increased survival of milk Igs in the preterm infant stomach due to lower protein digestion capacity could provide increased direct support of their naïve immune systems through immune exclusion.

2. Materials and Methods

2.1. Participants and Sample Collection

This study was approved by the Institutional Review Board of the University of California, Davis (UC Davis) and Oregon State University (OSU). Inclusion criteria included inpatient admission to the neonatal intensive care unit (NICU), an indwelling nasogastric or orogastric feeding tube and tolerance of full enteral feeding. Most of the enrolled infants required a feeding tube because of uncoordinated or immature capacity to suck and swallow. Exclusion criteria were anatomic or functional gastrointestinal disorders. Enrolled infants had a variety of medical conditions, including respiratory distress syndrome, chronic lung disease, apnea of prematurity, and Dandy–Walker malformation in the premature infants and cleft palate, respiratory distress syndrome, hypoxic-ischemic encephalopathy, and congenital diaphragmatic hernia in the term infants, but no overt gastrointestinal tract issues. Respiratory distress syndrome and congenital diaphragmatic hernia can delay gastric emptying in preterm infants [27,28]; however, the other medical conditions in this cohort have not been associated with an effect on gastric emptying or digestion capacity. Hypoxic-ischemic encephalopathy may result in gastrointestinal tissue damage [29]; however, the effects on gastric emptying and protein digestion are unknown. The infants with hypoxic ischemic encephalopathy were fasted and underwent whole body cooling for 72 h starting shortly after birth, however this treatment was completed and the infants advanced to full enteral feeding prior to enrollment. The infant with congenital diaphragmatic hernia had the defect repaired and was advanced to full enteral feeding prior to enrollment. Gastroesophageal reflux is almost universal in this population; however, none of the infants sampled received medications known to affect gastric pH or gastric digestion capacity, including prokinetics, H2 blockers/antagonists or proton-pump inhibitors. The enrolled infants were clinically stable at the time of sample collection (not on mechanical ventilation, stable vital signs). Samples were collected from 15 premature-delivering mother-infant pairs ranging in gestational age (GA) at birth from 23 to 32 weeks and 8 term-delivering mother-infant pairs ranging in GA at birth from 38 to 40 weeks (Table 1) over 7–98 days of postnatal age at the UC Davis Children's Hospital NICU in Sacramento, California. Enrolled infants had a variety of medical conditions, but no overt gastrointestinal tract issues or other medical conditions that have been associated with an effect on gastric emptying or digestion capacity. The enrolled infants were clinically stable at the time of sample collection (not on mechanical ventilation, stable vital signs). Human milk samples were collected as described in our previous study [30]. The preterm infants were fed their mother's milk (raw, not pasteurized) with fortifier (Similac Human Milk Fortifier Powder, Abbott Park, IL). The powdered fortifier contained intact bovine milk proteins and its protein composition was designed to match the whey:casein of human milk (60:40) using non-fat milk and whey protein concentrate. Each 25 mL of human milk was fortified with 0.25 g of bovine milk proteins (adding 10 mg protein/mL). Term infants were fed their mother's milk (raw, not pasteurized) without fortification. The human milk feedings were delivered via the nasogastric tubes over 30 min. Two hours after the initiation of feeding, 2 mL of each preterm and term infant's gastric contents were collected in a syringe back through the feeding tube via suction as previously described in our studies [21]. Gastric samples were aspirated at 2 h postprandial to obtain samples that represented a compromise between when adequate sample remained recoverable from the stomach and a maximum feasible length of gastric digestion time had passed based on gastric emptying times [31]. Human milk and gastric samples were placed into sterile vials and stored at −20 °C and were transported to OSU on dry ice and stored at −80 °C.

Table 1. Demographics of preterm- and term-delivering mother-infant pairs sampled for human milk and gastric contents at 2 h postprandial.

Demographics	Preterm-Delivering Mother Infant Pairs [1–2]	Term-Delivering Mother-Infant Pairs [1–2]
GA, weeks	27 ± 3 (23−32)	38.9 ± 0.5 (38−40)
Postnatal age, day	39 ± 28 (7−98)	23 ± 11 (16−42)
Postmenstrual age, day	32 ± 2 (30−37)	42 ± 2 (41−45)
Birth weight, kg	1.0 ± 0.4 (0.5−1.6)	3.5 ± 0.3 (3.0−3.8)
Infant sex	13 females; 2 males	6 females; 2 males
Mother's age, year	35 ± 3 (32−39)	24 ± 10 (17−42)

[1] Values are mean ± SD (range); [2] Number of paired milk and gastric samples from preterm and term infants is n = 15 and n = 8, respectively.

2.2. Sample Reparation and ELISAs

Samples were thawed at 4 °C, pH was determined, and samples were centrifuged at 4226× g for 10 min at 4 °C. The infranate was collected, separated into aliquots and stored at −80 °C. The pH of the samples was measured with an S220 SevenCompact pH/Ion meter (Mettler-Toledo, Columbus, OH, USA) equipped with a combined sealed glass electrode.

The spectrophotometric ELISAs were recorded with a microplate reader (Spectramax M2, Molecular Devices, Sunnyvale, CA, USA) with two replicates of blanks, standards, and samples. SoftMax Pro 7.0 Microplate Data Analysis Software (Molecular Devices) was used to create a standard curve with a Four Parameters Logistic curve fit. ELISAs were performed according to the methods described by the manufacturers with some modifications as described (Table S1). The specific

Ig concentrations in the samples were determined with antibody specificities as follows: human anti-alpha-chain antibody for total IgA (SIgA/IgA), anti-SC antibody for total SC (SC/SIgA/SIgM), gamma-chain antibody for IgG and mu-chain antibody for total IgM (SIgM/IgM). Concentrations of total IgA, total SC, total IgM and IgG were determined in human milk and gastric samples as well as in the fortifier alone.

For a separate test of the effect of the gastric pH change on Igs, ELISA were performed on standard Igs (total IgA, total SC, total IgM and IgG) in milk before and after incubation at pH 4.5 for 1 h at 37 °C. HCl (10 mM) was used to adjust the pH to 4.5.

2.3. Peptidomic Analysis

Peptide extraction from human milk and gastric samples was performed as described previously [32]. Mass spectrometric parameters were as described previously [33]. Spectra were analyzed by database searching in Thermo Proteome Discoverer (v2.1.0.81) using an in-house human milk protein sequence database. The tandem spectra were used to determine the counts and abundance of Ig alpha-chain (from IgA or SIgA), Ig gamma-chain (from IgG), Ig mu-chain (from IgM or SIgM), Ig J-chain (from IgA, SIgA, IgM or SIgM), Ig kappa-chain and Ig lambda-chain (from IgA, SIgA, IgM, SIgM or IgG), SC (f19–603 of total polymeric immunoglobulin receptor (PIgR)), and neonatal Fc receptors (FcRn). Only peptides identified with high confidence ($p < 0.01$) were included, and peptide sequences with multiple modifications were grouped into a single peptide for counts. Peptide counts measured the number of unique peptides identified in a sample whereas peptide abundance measured the ion intensity of the peak in a sample.

2.4. Statistical Analyses

Wilcoxon matched-pairs signed-rank test for paired sample comparisons (across milk and gastric samples within the same infant) and Mann–Whitney tests for unpaired sample comparisons (preterm versus term infants) were applied using GraphPad Prism software (version 7.03). All tests were nonparametric as some of the values did not pass the D 'Agostino & Pearson normality test. Linear regression models were applied to determine if the concentrations of total IgA, total SC, total IgM and IgG in human milk and in gastric samples in both infant groups changed across postnatal age, GA, postmenstrual age (PMA), body weight at birth (BW_b), body weight at sampling (BW_s), and feed volume. Differences were designated significant at $p < 0.05$. Pearson correlation coefficients (r) were determined when $p < 0.1$. The sample size of preterm ($n = 15$) and term ($n = 8$) paired milk and gastric samples was selected based on our previous study [20] and proved to be adequately powered to detect differences based on the results.

3. Results

3.1. Infant Demographics

Demographic details for the preterm- and term-delivering mother–infant pairs are presented in Table 1.

3.2. Ig Concentrations

3.2.1. Total IgA Concentration

Total IgA (SIgA/IgA) concentration decreased 60% ($p = 0.001$, Figure 1A) from human milk to the preterm infant stomach, and 47.8% from human milk to the term infant stomach ($p = 0.016$, Figure 1B). Total IgA concentration was similar between preterm and term milks and between preterm and term gastric contents ($p > 0.05$, Table S2). Total IgA concentration in preterm milk and gastric samples decreased with increased postnatal age, PMA, and BW_s ($p < 0.05$) but did not change in term samples ($p > 0.05$) (Table S3). Total IgA concentration in human milk or gastric contents did not change across GA and feed volume within preterm and term infants ($p > 0.05$, Table S3). When human milk was incubated under in vitro acidic conditions (pH 4.5) to match stomach conditions but without the proteases, there was no decrease in IgA concentration. No IgA was detected in the fortifier.

3.2.2. Total SC Concentration

Human milk total SC (SC/SIgA/SIgM) concentration significantly decreased 62% ($p = 0.031$, Figure 1D) from human milk to the term stomach but did not change in the preterm infant stomach ($p = 0.33$, Figure 1C). Total SC concentration did not differ between human milk from preterm- and term-delivering mothers ($p = 0.22$), nor between preterm and term gastric contents ($p = 0.11$). Total SC concentration in milk and gastric samples in term and preterm infants did not change across GA, postnatal age, or PMA ($p > 0.05$, Table S3). No total SC was detected in the fortifier.

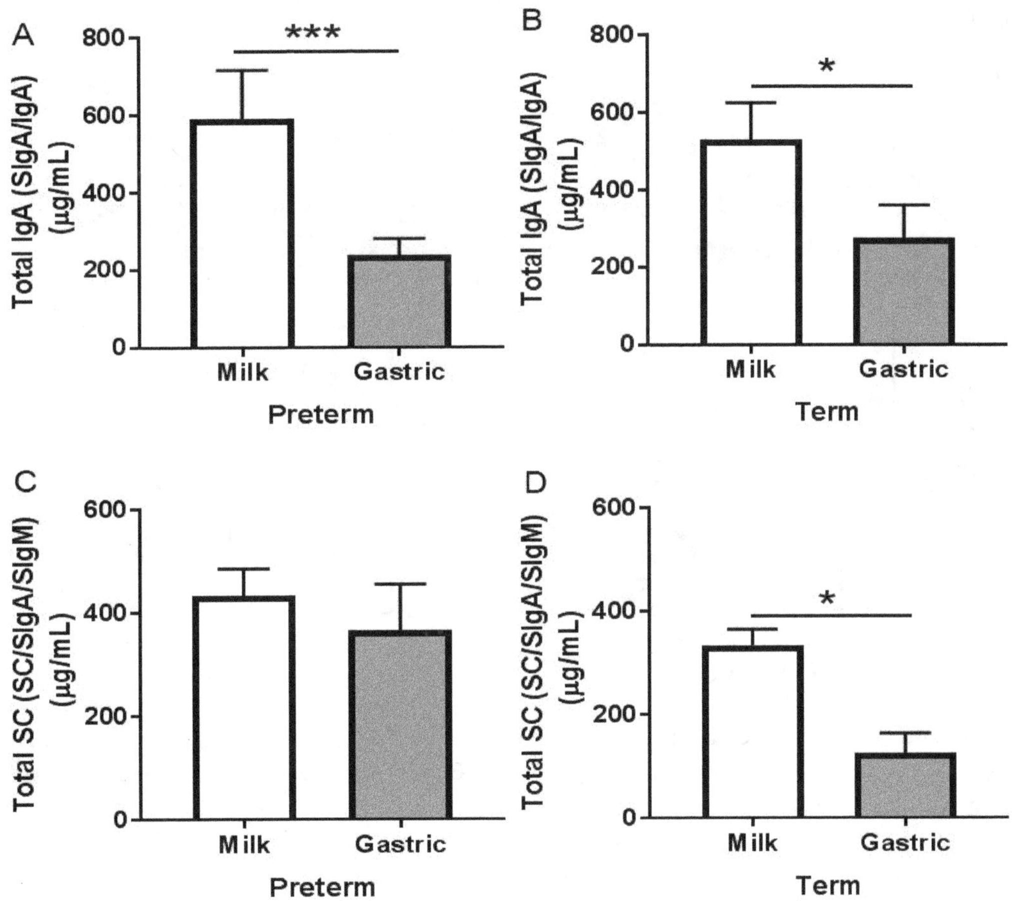

Figure 1. Immunoglobulin concentrations in human milk and gastric samples at 2 h postprandial time from paired mother-infant delivered prematurely (23–32 week of gestational age (GA), 7–98 days of postnatal age) and at term (38–40 week of GA, 16–42 days of postnatal age). Concentration of total IgA (SIgA/IgA) (**A**) in preterm infant samples and (**B**) in term infant samples; Concentration of total secretory component (SC/SIgA/SIgM) (**C**) in preterm infant samples and (**D**) in term infant samples. Values are mean ± SEM, $n = 15$ for preterm infants and $n = 8$ for term infants. Asterisks show statistical significant differences between variables (*** $p < 0.001$; * $p < 0.05$) using the Wilcoxon matched-pairs signed-rank test.

3.2.3. Total IgM Concentration

Total IgM (SIgM/IgM) concentration decreased significantly ($p = 0.016$, Figure 2B) 33% from human milk to the term infant stomach but did not change in the preterm infant stomach ($p = 0.54$, Figure 2A). Total IgM concentration in human milk from preterm-delivering mothers was 77% lower than in milks from term-delivering mothers ($p < 0.001$, Figure S1A) but did not differ in the gastric contents between preterm and term infants ($p = 0.56$). Total IgM concentration in either milk or gastric samples did not change across postnatal age, GA, PMA, or BW_b for term or preterm infants ($p > 0.05$, Table S3). Total IgM concentration decreased in preterm milk with increasing postnatal age or BW_s ($p < 0.05$) but did not change in term milk or in either preterm or term stomach samples ($p > 0.05$, Table S3). Total IgM concentration increased with increasing feed volume in preterm milk and gastric samples but did not change in term samples. No total IgM was detected in the fortifier.

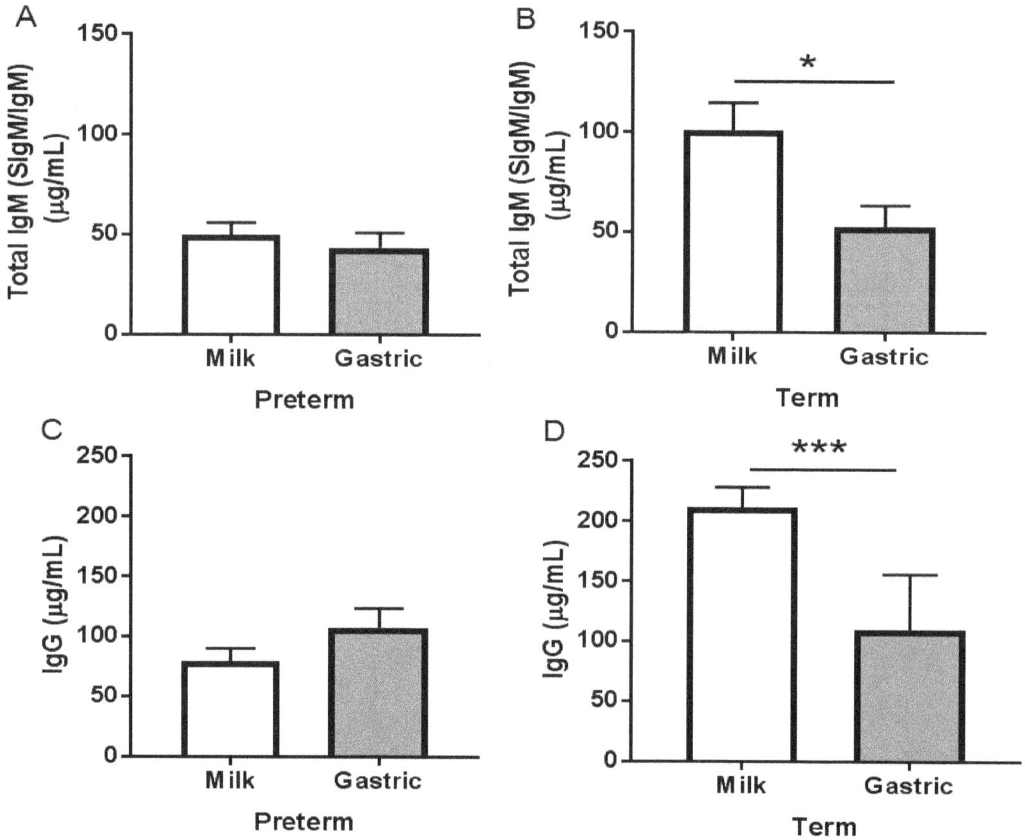

Figure 2. Immunoglobulin concentrations in human milk and gastric samples at 2 h postprandial time from paired mother-infant delivered prematurely (23–32 week of gestational age (GA), 7–98 days of postnatal age) and at term (38–40 week of GA, 16–42 days of postnatal age). Concentration of total IgM (SIgM/IgM) (**A**) in preterm infant samples and (**B**) in term infant samples; Concentration of IgG (**C**) in preterm infant samples and (**D**) in term infant samples. Values are mean ± SEM, $n = 15$ for preterm infants and $n = 8$ for term infants. Asterisks show statistical significant differences between variables (*** $p < 0.001$; * $p < 0.05$) using the Wilcoxon matched-pairs signed-rank test.

3.2.4. IgG Concentration

IgG concentration decreased significantly (48%, $p = 0.026$, Figure 2D) from human milk to the term infant stomach but did not change in the preterm infant stomach ($p = 0.11$, Figure 2C). IgG concentration in human milk from preterm-delivering mothers was 97% lower than in milks from term-delivering mothers ($p < 0.001$, Figure S1B) but did not differ in the gastric contents between preterm and term infants ($p = 0.58$). IgG concentration in preterm and term milk did not change across postnatal age, GA, PMA, BW_b, or feed volume ($p > 0.05$, Table S3). IgG concentration in preterm gastric samples decreased with increasing PMA or BW_s and increased with increasing BW_b in term stomach but did not change across GA or feed volume. No IgG was detected in the fortifier.

3.3. Peptidomic Results

No peptides (counts or abundance) for Ig alpha-chain, Ig gamma-chain, Ig mu-chain, Ig J-chain, Ig lambda-chain, and Ig kappa-chain were detected in human milk from either the mothers who delivered prematurely or at term, but peptides from each of these proteins appeared in the gastric samples from both preterm and term infants (Figures S2–S4). Peptides from SC (f19–603 of PIgR) was detected in both milk and gastric samples from both preterm and term infants.

Ig alpha-chain peptide counts in gastric samples were 1.2-fold lower in preterm infants than in term infants (not significant, but a tendency: $p = 0.081$, Figure 3A). Ig alpha-chain peptide abundance in gastric contents was 16-fold lower in preterm infants than in term infants ($p = 0.038$, Figure 3D). Ig mu-chain peptide counts and abundance in gastric contents were 2.3- ($p = 0.032$, Figure 3B) and 13-fold ($p = 0.010$, Figure 3E), respectively, lower in preterm infants than in term infants. Ig gamma-chain peptide counts and abundance in gastric contents were 1.9- ($p = 0.002$, Figure 3C) and 34-fold ($p < 0.001$, Figure 3F), respectively, lower in preterm infants than in term infants. Peptide counts and abundance of Ig J-chain, lambda-chain and Ig kappa-chain did not differ between preterm and term infant gastric samples ($p > 0.05$, Table S2). Peptide counts of SC (f19–603 of PIgR) decreased 37% and 56% from human milk to the stomach for preterm and term infants, respectively ($p < 0.05$, Figure 4A,B). Peptide abundance of SC decreased 89% and 68% from human milk to the stomach for preterm and term infants, respectively ($p < 0.05$, Figure 4C,D).

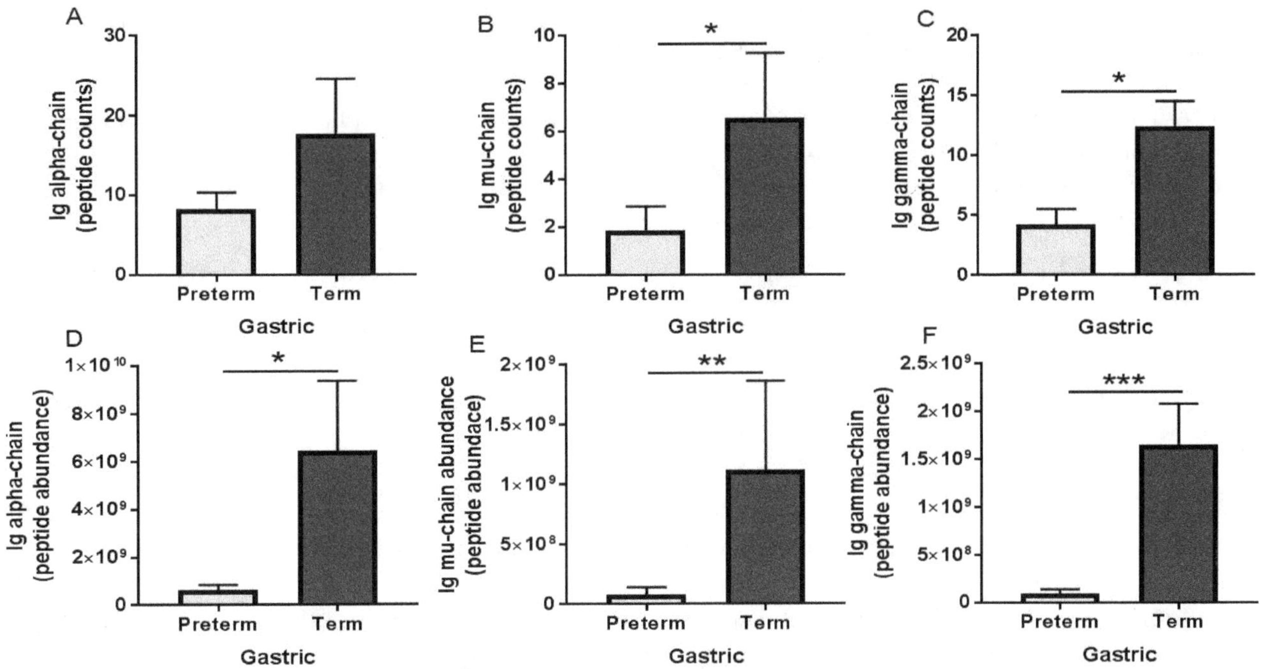

Figure 3. Peptide counts and abundance of human immunoglobulin fragments in human milk and gastric samples at 2 h postprandial time from paired mother-infant delivered prematurely (23–32 week of gestational age (GA), 7–98 days of postnatal age) and at term (38–40 week of GA, 16–42 days of postnatal age). (**A**,**D**) Ig alpha-chain (from SIgA/IgA) and (**B**,**E**) Ig mu-chain (from SIgM/IgM); (**C**,**F**) Ig gamma-chain (from IgG). Values are mean ± SEM, $n = 15$ for preterm infants and $n = 8$ for term infants. Asterisks show statistical significant differences between variables (*** $p < 0.001$; ** $p < 0.01$; * $p < 0.05$) using the Mann–Whitney test (unpaired samples).

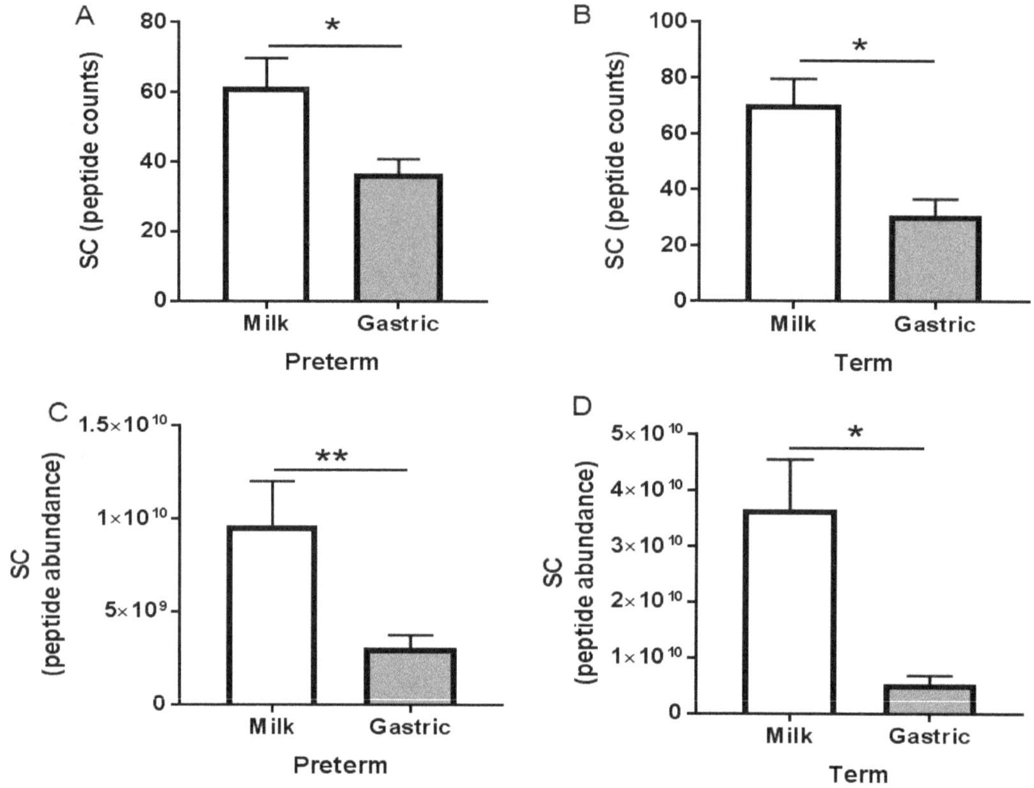

Figure 4. Peptides counts and abundance of SC (f19–603 of PIgR) in human milk and gastric samples from mother–infant pairs with preterm delivery (23–32 week of gestational age (GA), 7–98 days of postnatal age) and term delivery (38–40 week of GA, 16–42 days of postnatal age. Peptides counts of SC (**A**) in preterm infant samples; (**B**) in term infant samples. Peptide abundance of SC (**C**) in preterm infant samples and (**D**) in term infant samples. Values are mean ± SEM, $n = 15$ for preterm infants and $n = 8$ for term infants. Asterisks show statistical significant differences between variables (** $p < 0.01$; * $p < 0.05$) using the Wilcoxon matched-pairs signed-rank test.

3.4. *pH*

For preterm and term mother-infant samples, pH values in gastric samples were lower than those in human milk ($p < 0.001$, Figure S5). Neither milk nor gastric sample pH differed between preterm and term mother-infant pairs ($p > 0.05$, Table S2).

4. Discussion

The Ig concentrations in milk from preterm- and term-delivering mothers have been previously studied [34–37]. No study has compared the survival of Igs in the stomach or intestine between preterm and term infants. Our recent studies demonstrated that preterm infants partially degrade IgA but not IgG and IgM in the stomach [21,22]. A few studies have measured the survival of milk Igs to infant stool [17,38]. However, measuring Igs in infant stool samples does not accurately represent the biologically relevant survival of Igs within the upper GI tract, as Igs are exposed to proteases from the infant gastrointestinal tract as well as protein-fermenting colonic bacteria, which can degrade them before they are identified in stool [39]. To begin to address this lack of knowledge, the present study examined the stability of human milk Igs—total IgA (SIgA/IgA), total IgM (SIgM/IgM), IgG, and total SC (SC/SIgA/SIgM)—during gastric digestion in preterm and term infants.

Concentrations of Igs in human milk from mothers delivering prematurely and at term were congruent with those found in previous studies [36,37,40,41]. Concentrations of total IgA or total SC did not differ between preterm and term milk, which matches with the observation in a previous study [34] that milk total IgA did not differ between preterm and term milk (3.2 mg/mL) from 6 to

28 days postnatal age. Ballabio et al. [34] observed a higher concentration of total IgA than measured in this present study and did not detect IgM or IgG in preterm and term milk (we detected IgM and IgG). This difference could be due to their use of an immunoelectrophoretic technique (SDS-PAGE and immunoblotting) to determine the concentration of Igs in their milk samples. ELISA is more quantitative (lower detection limit) than SDS-PAGE and immunoblotting. We found that total IgA concentration decreased with increasing postnatal age, PMA, and BW_S in preterm milk, which matches with this same previous study [34] (total IgA concentration decreased from colostrum to mature milk from preterm-delivering mothers). A few studies found higher amounts of total IgA in colostrum from preterm-delivering mothers compared with colostrum from term-delivering mothers [3,34,35,42]; however, as no colostrum was collected in the present study, we cannot compare our results to that data. Another study found that preterm milk IgA concentration was 1.1- to 1.4-fold higher than in term milk from 3 to 15 days but found no differences in concentration from 28 to 56 days of postnatal age [3]. Thus, the observed lack of difference for total IgA concentration between preterm and term milk in the present study is likely due to the older postnatal age (average: 39 days for preterm and 23 days for term infants) for milk collection.

The concentration of total SC (mostly SIgA but can include SC and SIgM) represented 73.5% of total IgA in preterm milk and 63.6% of total IgA in term milk. These percentages are somewhat lower than the observations reported by Goldman et al. [4] that total SC (called "SIgA" by the authors but actually representing total SC, as an anti-SC primary antibody was used) concentration represented 90% of the total IgA in term milk.

The concentration of IgG and total IgM were lower in human milk from preterm-delivering mothers than term-delivering mothers. Previous studies observed IgG and IgM concentrations in human milk that were similar between mothers delivering prematurely and at term [36,41]. On the other hand, Chandra et al. [3] found that IgM and IgG concentrations were 1.5-fold higher in preterm milk than in term milk from 14 to 28 days of postnatal age.

The total IgA concentration decreased from human milk to the preterm and term infant stomach. The stability of SC/SIgA/SIgM during gastric digestion in preterm suggests that SC remains intact and detectable by the anti-SC even if it is released from the SIgA complex. Unlike in preterm infant, total SC concentration decreased in the term infant stomach. The reduction of total IgA (SIgA/IgA) was likely due to degradation by proteases (pepsin and/or milk proteases [21]) and not acid-induced structural deterioration in the stomach, as incubation of standard IgA in acid conditions did not decrease its concentration (Figure S6). If we consider that 74% of total IgA in preterm milk is SIgA—we could not distinguish between SC/SIgA/SIgM, the decrease of total IgA likely derived from preterm gastric digestion of partly IgA and partly SIgA. We found higher peptide abundance of Ig alpha-chain (which could derive from either IgA or SIgA) in term infant gastric contents than in preterm infants, which suggests that IgA/SIgA is more digested by term infants than preterm infants.

We also observed that human milk total IgM decreased and IgG tended to decrease in the term stomach (48% and 49% reduction, respectively) but were stable in the preterm stomach. We found higher peptide counts and abundance of Ig mu (which could derive from either IgM or SIgM) and Ig gamma (which derive from IgG) in term infant gastric infants than preterm infants, which suggests that SIgM/IgM and IgG is more digested by term infants than preterm infants. This decrease of Igs is unlikely to relate to gastric pH as preterm and term infants' gastric pH did not differ. We also observed that pH 4.5 had no effect on the stability of Igs (Figure S2). Gastric proteases are likely responsible for observed differences, as we previously demonstrated that gastric pepsin activity and proteolysis were higher in term infants than in preterm infants [20].

We observed that the stability of IgG and total IgM during gastric preterm digestion was higher than total IgA. No previous study evaluated the digestibility of Igs in the preterm or term infant stomach or small intestine, but a previous study [17] found a greater reduction of IgA compared with IgG or IgM in preterm infant stools. When preterm infants (1–28 days of postnatal age (GA unknown) 0.8–2 kg BW) were fed only infant formula or infant formula plus pasteurized pooled human milk supplemented with 600 mg daily of serum-derived human IgA (73%) and IgG (26%), the stool samples collected contained 1–10 mg IgG per g of dried feces (percentage reduction not calculated) and no IgA [17]. We showed that IgG was decreased in the term infant stomach but stable in the preterm infant stomach.

Using peptidomics, we demonstrated partial digestion (demonstrated by an increase in peptide counts and abundances from milk to the stomach) of Ig alpha-chain (from IgA and SIgA), Ig gamma-chain (from IgG), Ig mu-chain (from IgM or SIgM), and Ig J-chain (from IgA, SIgA, IgM or SIgM), Ig kappa-chain and Ig lambda-chain (from all Igs) in both preterm and term infants. Dallas et al. [43] also observed that alpha-1-chain (named IGHA1) was not detected in term milk but was detected in the term stomach. SC peptide counts decreased in both preterm and term gastric samples, suggesting that SIgA or SIgM were partially digested in the stomach from both infants. We found a decrease in peptide counts and abundance of SC (which could derive from either SIgA or SIgM) in both preterm and term infant gastric samples, suggesting a digestion of these Igs in the infant stomach.

A limitation of this study is the small number of samples for preterm and term infants. Another limitation is that we did not measure Ig concentrations in the infant intestine contents. Therefore, we plan to examine how human milk Ig concentrations change in the stomach and intestine in a future study with a larger number of preterm and term infants. The infants in our study had conditions that required a naso-gastric tube, which could affect Ig digestion. However, we included only infants with conditions that are not expected to interfere with protein digestion. Ideally, the study would include healthier infants; however, placing a feeding tube in infants that do not require them is very challenging from an ethical and patient enrollment perspective. Development of non-invasive techniques to collect digestive samples from fragile infants would be highly beneficial to this field. The placement of the nasogastric tube in these infants could also modify the gastric microbiome, which could influence Ig digestion. However, as we currently have no technique to assess gastric digestion in infants without a feeding tube, we cannot assess this potential impact.

5. Conclusions

The present study revealed that total IgA (SIgA/IgA) was digested in the preterm and term infant stomach. Human milk total SC (SC/SIgA/SIgM), IgM, and IgG were stable in the preterm stomach but were digested in the term stomach. Ig-derived peptides from all different Ig isotypes were in higher amounts in the gastric contents of term infants than in preterm infants, demonstrating a higher overall gastric Ig digestion in term infants. Therefore, human milk Igs are less digested in the preterm infant stomach than the term infant stomach. As the stomach represents only the beginning of the digestive system, the concentrations of human milk Igs in intestinal samples from preterm and term infants need to be determined to clarify their potential survival during infant digestion. The longer that milk Igs survive through the digestive system, the longer they can act as passive immune system components, which is particularly important in the context of the immune system immaturity of the early postnatal period in preterm and term infants.

Supplementary Materials:
Table S1: Details for the assays performed in human milk and gastric samples; Table S2: Statistical results (*p*-values) for Wilcoxon matched-pairs signed rank test to compare immunoglobulin concentrations (ELISA) and peptides (peptidomics) in human milk and gastric samples in preterm and term infants (PM vs. PG or TM vs. TG); Table S3: Statistical results (*p*-value) from the linear regression of the pH and the concentration of total IgA (SIgA/IgA), total SC (SC/SIgA/SIgM), IgG and total IgM (SIgM/IgM) across postnatal age (P), gestational age at birth (GA), postmenstrual age (PMA), BW_b, BW_s and feed volume (FV) in human milk and in gastric contents at 1, 2 and 3 h postprandial from preterm infants (23–32 week of gestational age, 7–98 days of postnatal age) and term infants (38–40 week of GA, 16–42 days of postnatal age); Figure S1: Immunoglobulin concentrations of (A) total IgM (SIgM/IgM) and (B) IgG in mother's milks delivering prematurely (23–32 week of gestational age (GA), 7–98 days of postnatal age) and at term (38–40 week of GA, 16–42 days of postnatal age). Figures S2–S4: Peptide counts and abundance of human immunoglobulin fragments in human milk and gastric samples at 2 h postprandial time from paired mother-infant delivered prematurely (23–32 week of gestational age (GA), 7–98 days of postnatal age) and at term (38–40 week of GA, 16–42 days of postnatal age). Figure S5: The pH in human milk and gastric

samples in human milk and gastric samples at 2 h postprandial time from paired (A) mother-infant delivered prematurely (23–32 week of gestational age (GA), 7–98 days of postnatal age) and (B) at term (38–40 week of GA, 16–42 days of postnatal age). Figure S6: Stability of standard immunoglobulins (Igs) before and after the incubation at pH 4.5.

Author Contributions: V.D.-M. conducted the ELISA analyses, analyzed data and conducted the statistical analysis. M.A.U. provided milk and gastric samples. R.L.B. and S.D.N. conducted the peptidomic analyses. V.D.-M. and D.C.D. designed the study and drafted the manuscript. V.D.-M. and D.C.D. have primary responsibility for the final content.

Acknowledgments: The authors acknowledge the Mass Spectrometry Center at Oregon State University, which is supported in part by the National Institute of Health grant S10OD020111. This study was supported by the K99/R00 Pathway to Independence Career Award, Eunice Kennedy Shriver Institute of Child Health & Development of the National Institutes of Health (R00HD079561) (D.C.D.) and The Gerber Foundation.

References

1. Tha-In, T.; Bayry, J.; Metselaar, H.J.; Kaveri, S.V.; Kwekkeboom, J. Modulation of the cellular immune system by intravenous immunoglobulin. *Trends Immunol.* **2008**, *29*, 608–615. [CrossRef] [PubMed]
2. Palmeira, P.; Quinello, C.; Silveira-Lessa, A.L.; Zago, C.A.; Carneiro-Sampaio, M. IgG placental transfer in healthy and pathological pregnancies. *Clin. Dev. Immunol.* **2011**, *2012*, 985646. [CrossRef] [PubMed]
3. Chandra, R. Immunoglobulin and protein levels in breast milk produced by mothers of preterm infants. *Nutr. Res.* **1982**, *2*, 27–30. [CrossRef]
4. Goldman, A.S.; Garza, C.; Nichols, B.L.; Goldblum, R.M. Immunologic factors in human milk during the first year of lactation. *J. Pediatr.* **1982**, *100*, 563–567. [CrossRef]
5. Duijts, L.; Jaddoe, V.W.; Hofman, A.; Moll, H.A. Prolonged and exclusive breastfeeding reduces the risk of infectious diseases in infancy. *Pediatrics* **2010**, *126*, e18. [CrossRef] [PubMed]
6. Janeway, C.A., Jr.; Travers, P.; Walport, M.; Shlomchik, M.J. The distribution and functions of immunoglobulin isotypes. In *Immunobiology, the Immune System in Health and Disease*, 5th ed.; Garland Science: New York, NY, USA, 2001.
7. Melis, J.P.; Strumane, K.; Ruuls, S.R.; Beurskens, F.J.; Schuurman, J.; Parren, P.W. Complement in therapy and Disease: Regulating the complement system with antibody-based therapeutics. *Mol. Immunol.* **2015**, *67*, 117–130. [CrossRef] [PubMed]
8. Bakker-Zierikzee, A.; Tol, E.; Kroes, H.; Alles, M.; Kok, F.; Bindels, J. Faecal SIgA secretion in infants fed on pre-or probiotic infant formula. *Pediatr. Allergy Immunol.* **2006**, *17*, 134–140. [CrossRef] [PubMed]
9. Mantis, N.J.; Rol, N.; Corthésy, B. Secretory IgA's complex roles in immunity and mucosal homeostasis in the gut. *Mucosal Immunol.* **2011**, *4*, 603. [CrossRef] [PubMed]
10. Macpherson, A.J.; Hunziker, L.; McCoy, K.; Lamarre, A. IgA responses in the intestinal mucosa against pathogenic and non-pathogenic microorganisms. *Microbes Infect.* **2001**, *3*, 1021–1035. [CrossRef]
11. Yoshida, M.; Claypool, S.M.; Wagner, J.S.; Mizoguchi, E.; Mizoguchi, A.; Roopenian, D.C.; Lencer, W.I.; Blumberg, R.S. Human neonatal Fc receptor mediates transport of IgG into luminal secretions for delivery of antigens to mucosal dendritic cells. *Immunity* **2004**, *20*, 769–783. [CrossRef] [PubMed]
12. Perkkiö, M.; Savilahti, E. Time of appearance of immunoglobulin-containing cells in the mucosa of the neonatal intestine. *Pediatr. Res.* **1980**, *14*, 953. [CrossRef] [PubMed]
13. Robert-Guroff, M. IgG surfaces as an important component in mucosal protection. *Nat. Med.* **2000**, *6*, 129. [CrossRef] [PubMed]
14. Hansen, G.H.; Niels-Christiansen, L.-L.; Immerdal, L.; Danielsen, E.M. Antibodies in the small Intestine: Mucosal synthesis and deposition of anti-glycosyl IgA, IgM, and IgG in the enterocyte brush border. *Am. J. Physiol. Gastrointest. Liver Physiol.* **2006**, *291*, G82–G90. [CrossRef] [PubMed]
15. Hansen, G.H.; Pedersen, E.D.; Immerdal, L.; Niels-Christiansen, L.-L.; Danielsen, E.M. Anti-glycosyl antibodies in lipid rafts of the enterocyte brush Border: A possible host defense against pathogens. *Am. J. Physiol. Gastrointest. Liver Physiol.* **2005**, *289*, G1100–G1107. [CrossRef] [PubMed]
16. Roos, N.; Mahe, S.; Benamouzig, R.; Sick, H.; Rautureau, J.; Tome, D. 15N-labeled immunoglobulins from bovine colostrum are partially resistant to digestion in human intestine. *J. Nutr.* **1995**, *125*, 1238–1244. [PubMed]

17. Eibl, M.M.; Wolf, H.M.; Fürnkranz, H.; Rosenkranz, A. Prevention of necrotizing enterocolitis in low-birth-weight infants by IgA–IgG feeding. *N. Engl. J. Med.* **1988**, *319*, 1–7. [CrossRef] [PubMed]
18. Schanler, R.J.; Goldblum, R.M.; Garza, C.; Goldman, A.S. Enhanced fecal excretion of selected immune factors in very low birth weight infants fed fortified human milk. *Pediatr. Res.* **1986**, *20*, 711. [CrossRef] [PubMed]
19. Goldblum, R.M.; Schanler, R.J.; Garza, C.; Goldman, A.S. Human milk feeding enhances the urinary excretion of immunologic factors in low birth weight infants. *Pediatr. Res.* **1989**, *25*, 184. [CrossRef] [PubMed]
20. Demers-Mathieu, V.; Qu, Y.; Underwood, M.; Borghese, R.; Dallas, D. Premature infants have lower gastric digestion capacity for human milk proteins than term infants. *J. Pediatr. Gastroenterol. Nutr.* **2018**, *66*, 816–821. [CrossRef] [PubMed]
21. Demers-Mathieu, V.; Nielsen, S.D.; Underwood, M.A.; Borghese, R.; Dallas, D.C. Changes in proteases, antiproteases and bioactive proteins from mother's breast milk to the premature infant stomach. *J. Pediatr. Gastroenterol. Nutr.* **2017**, *66*, 318–324. [CrossRef] [PubMed]
22. Demers-Mathieu, V.; Underwood, M.A.; Beverly, R.L.; David, D.C. Survival of immunoglobulins from human milk to preterm infant gastric samples at 1, 2, and 3 hours postprandial. *Neonatology* **2018**, in press.
23. Malek, A.; Sager, R.; Kuhn, P.; Nicolaides, K.H.; Schneider, H. Evolution of maternofetal transport of immunoglobulins during human pregnancy. *Am. J. Reprod. Immunol.* **1996**, *36*, 248–255. [CrossRef] [PubMed]
24. Zemlin, M.; Hoersch, G.; Zemlin, C.; Pohl-Schickinger, A.; Hummel, M.; Berek, C.; Maier, R.F.; Bauer, K. The postnatal maturation of the immunoglobulin heavy chain IgG repertoire in human preterm neonates is slower than in term neonates. *J. Immunol.* **2007**, *178*, 1180–1188. [CrossRef] [PubMed]
25. Langkamp, D.L.; Davis, J.P. Increased risk of reported pertussis and hospitalization associated with pertussis in low birth weight children. *J. Pediatr.* **1996**, *128*, 654–659. [CrossRef]
26. Groothuis, J.R.; Simoes, E.A.; Hemming, V.G. Respiratory syncytial virus (RSV) infection in preterm infants and the protective effects of RSV immune globulin (RSVIG). *J. Pediatr.* **1995**, *95*, 463–467.
27. Victor, Y. Effect of body position on gastric emptying in the neonate. *Arch. Dis. Child.* **1975**, *50*, 500–504. [CrossRef] [PubMed]
28. Arena, F.; Romeo, C.; Baldari, S.; Arena, S.; Antonuccio, P.; Campennì, A.; Zuccarello, B.; Romeo, G. Gastrointestinal sequelae in survivors of congenital diaphragmatic hernia. *Pediatr. Int.* **2008**, *50*, 76–80. [CrossRef] [PubMed]
29. Faingold, R.; Cassia, G.; Prempunpong, C.; Morneault, L.; Sant'Anna, G.M. Intestinal ultrasonography in infants with moderate or severe hypoxic-ischemic encephalopathy receiving hypothermia. *Pediatr. Radiol.* **2016**, *46*, 87–95. [CrossRef] [PubMed]
30. Demers-Mathieu, V.; Nielsen, S.D.; Underwood, M.A.; Borghese, R.; Dallas, D.C. Analysis of milk from mothers who delivered prematurely reveals few changes in proteases and protease inhibitors across gestational age at birth and infant postnatal age. *J. Nutr.* **2017**, *147*, 1152–1159. [CrossRef] [PubMed]
31. Siegel, M.; Lebenthal, E.; Topper, W.; Krantz, B.; Li, P.K. Gastric emptying in prematures of isocaloric feedings with differing osmolalities. *Pediatr. Res.* **1982**, *16*, 141–147. [CrossRef] [PubMed]
32. Nielsen, S.D.; Beverly, R.L.; Dallas, D.C. Peptides released from foremilk and hindmilk proteins by breastmilk proteases are highly similar. *Front. Nutr.* **2017**, *4*, 54. [CrossRef] [PubMed]
33. Nielsen, S.D.; Beverly, R.L.; Dallas, D.C. Milk proteins are human mammary gland. *J. Mammary Gland. Biol. Neoplasia* **2017**, *22*, 251–261. [CrossRef] [PubMed]
34. Ballabio, C.; Bertino, E.; Coscia, A.; Fabris, C.; Fuggetta, D.; Molfino, S.; Testa, T.; Sgarrella, M.; Sabatino, G.; Restani, P. Immunoglobulin-A profile in breast milk from mothers delivering full term and preterm infants. *Int. J. Immunopathol. Pharmacol.* **2007**, *20*, 119–128. [CrossRef] [PubMed]
35. Montagne, P.; Cuillière, M.L.; Molé, C.; Béné, M.C.; Faure, G. Immunological and nutritional composition of human milk in relation to prematurity and mothers' parity during the first 2 weeks of lactation. *J. Pediatr. Gastroenterol. Nutr.* **1999**, *29*, 75–80. [CrossRef] [PubMed]
36. Gross, S.J.; Buckley, R.H.; Wakil, S.S.; McAllister, D.C.; David, R.J.; Faix, R.G. Elevated IgA concentration in milk produced by mothers delivered of preterm infants. *J. Pediatr.* **1981**, *99*, 389–393. [CrossRef]
37. Castellote, C.; Casillas, R.; Ramírez-Santana, C.; Pérez-Cano, F.J.; Castell, M.; Moretones, M.G.; López-Sabater, M.C.; Franch, À. Premature delivery influences the immunological composition of colostrum and transitional and mature human milk. *J. Nutr.* **2011**, *141*, 1181–1187. [CrossRef] [PubMed]

38. Blum, P.M.; Phelps, D.L.; Ank, B.J.; Krantman, H.J.; Stiehm, E.R. Survival of oral human immune serum globulin in the gastrointestinal tract of low birth weight infants. *Pediatr. Res.* **1981**, *15*, 1256–1260. [CrossRef] [PubMed]
39. Dallas, D.C.; Sanctuary, M.R.; Qu, Y.; Khajavi, S.H.; Van Zandt, A.E.; Dyandra, M.; Frese, S.A.; Barile, D.; German, J.B. Personalizing protein nourishment. *Crit. Rev. Food Sci. Nutr.* **2017**, *57*, 3313–3331. [CrossRef] [PubMed]
40. Evans, T.; Ryley, H.; Neale, L.; Dodge, J.; Lewarne, V. Effect of storage and heat on antimicrobial proteins in human milk. *Arch. Dis. Child.* **1978**, *53*, 239–241. [CrossRef] [PubMed]
41. Koenig, Á.; Diniz, E.M.d.A.; Barbosa, S.F.C.; Vaz, F.A.C. Immunologic factors in human Milk: The effects of gestational age and pasteurization. *J. Hum. Lact.* **2005**, *21*, 439–443. [CrossRef] [PubMed]
42. Araújo, E.D.; Gonçalves, A.K.; Cornetta, M.d.C.; Cunha, H.; Cardoso, M.L.; Morais, S.S.; Giraldo, P.C. Evaluation of the secretory immunoglobulin A levels in the colostrum and milk of mothers of term and pre-trerm newborns. *Braz. J. Infect. Dis.* **2005**, *9*, 357–362. [CrossRef] [PubMed]
43. Dallas, D.C.; Guerrero, A.; Khaldi, N.; Borghese, R.; Bhandari, A.; Underwood, M.A.; Lebrilla, C.B.; German, J.B.; Barile, D. A peptidomic analysis of human milk digestion in the infant stomach reveals protein-specific degradation patterns. *J. Nutr.* **2014**, *144*, 815–820. [CrossRef] [PubMed]

15

Antenatal Influenza A-Specific IgA, IgM and IgG Antibodies in Mother's Own Breast Milk and Donor Breast Milk and Gastric Contents and Stools from Preterm Infants

Veronique Demers-Mathieu [1], Robert K. Huston [2], Andi M. Markell [2], Elizabeth A. McCulley [2], Rachel L. Martin [2] and David C. Dallas [1,*]

[1] Nutrition Program, School of Biological and Population Health Sciences, College of Public Health and Human Sciences, Oregon State University, Corvallis, OR 97331, USA
[2] Department of Pediatrics, Randall Children's Hospital at Legacy Emanuel, Portland, OR 97227, USA
* Correspondence: Dave.Dallas@oregonstate.edu

Abstract: Antenatal milk anti-influenza antibodies may provide additional protection to newborns until they are able to produce their own antibodies. To evaluate the relative abundance of milk, we studied the antibodies specific to influenza A in feeds and gastric contents and stools from preterm infants fed mother's own breast milk (MBM) and donor breast milk (DBM). Feed (MBM or DBM) and gastric contents (MBM or DBM at 1 h post-ingestion) and stool samples (MBM/DBM at 24 h post-ingestion) were collected, respectively, from 20 preterm (26–36 weeks gestational age) mother-infant pairs at 8–9 days and 21–22 days of postnatal age. Samples were analyzed via ELISA for anti-H1N1 hemagglutinin (anti-H1N1 HA) and anti-H3N2 neuraminidase (anti-H3N2 NA) specificity across immunoglobulin A (IgA), immunoglobulin M (IgM), and immunoglobulin G (IgG) isotypes. The relative abundance of influenza A-specific IgA in feeds and gastric contents were higher in MBM than DBM at 8–9 days of postnatal age but did not differ at 21–22 days. Anti-influenza A-specific IgM was higher in MBM than in DBM at both postnatal times in feed and gastric samples. At both postnatal times, anti-influenza A-specific IgG was higher in MBM than DBM but did not differ in gastric contents. Gastric digestion reduced anti-H3N2 NA IgG from MBM at 21–22 days and from DBM at 8–9 days of lactation, whereas other anti-influenza A antibodies were not digested at either postnatal times. Supplementation of anti-influenza A-specific antibodies in DBM may help reduce the risk of influenza virus infection. However, the effective antibody dose required to induce a significant protective effect remains unknown.

Keywords: passive immunization; maternal immunoglobulins; lactation; prematurity; flu vaccine; human milk

---

1. Introduction

Infants are susceptible to influenza infections and cannot be vaccinated before six months of age [1,2]. Therefore, the Centers for Disease Control and Prevention recommends that all pregnant women receive the inactivated influenza virus vaccine during the second or third trimester [3]. Antenatal vaccination helps protect the infant against influenza infection [4–7]. Part of that protection stems from the vaccine-stimulated increased maternal blood influenza-specific immunoglobulin G (IgG), which allows increased transfer of influenza-specific IgG across the placenta and leads to increased persistence of these antibodies in the infant bloodstream post-birth [8]. In addition to the changes in blood, antenatal vaccination increases secretion of influenza-specific antibodies into breast milk [9]. Milk anti-influenza antibodies may provide additional protection to newborns until they are able to produce antibodies against the virus [9]. Regardless of whether a mother was recently vaccinated, their breast milk typically contains some influenza-specific Ig as they were likely exposed to the virus or vaccinated in the past [10]. These milk antibodies may be protective against influenza infection [9].

The site of action for milk antibodies is mainly thought to be within the gastrointestinal tract, whereas influenza A infects within the lung mucosal tissue. Thus, the relevance of human milk antibodies to influenza protection in unclear. However, milk influenza A-specific antibodies can be studied as a model for other milk antibodies to enteric pathogens for which the gut is their site of action. To neutralize enteric pathogens throughout the infant gastrointestinal tract, milk antibodies must survive the digestive protease actions. No oral supplementation studies have determined the percentage of remaining relative abundance of anti-influenza A IgA, IgM, and IgG during infant digestion.

In neonatal intensive care units (NICU), very preterm infants are often fed donor breast milk (DBM) to supplement an insufficient maternal supply of mother's own breast milk (MBM) [11,12]. Whether MBM and DBM differ in milk anti-influenza A antibody relative abundance is unknown. DBM typical processing includes pooling milks from different mothers, pasteurizing (Holder pasteurization, 62.5 °C for 30 min) and freezing and thawing at least twice, which could reduce the antibody abundance. Our previous study demonstrated that total IgA, secretory IgA (SIgA), total IgM, and IgG concentrations were higher in MBM than DBM and higher in gastric contents (1 h post-ingestion) when preterm infants were fed with MBM than when infants were fed DBM [13]. A previous study demonstrated that IgA survived intact after Holder pasteurization in non-centrifuged MBM (0% loss) whereas IgG concentration was reduced (34.3% loss) (IgM was not measured) [14]. In another study, IgA from centrifuged MBM was reduced 22% after Holder pasteurization whereas IgM concentration was completely destroyed [15].

The remaining relative abundance of milk antibodies specific to influenza A virus from MBM or DBM during gastric digestion is unknown and a comparison of mother's milk and donor milk have not been determined. The aim of this study was to determine the difference of antenatal influenza A-specific IgA, IgM, and IgG antibodies in MBM and DBM, and gastric contents and stools from preterm infants. Milk anti-influenza A neutralizing antibodies can be specific to subtypes of HA or NA [3]. In this study, we examined anti-H1N1 HA and anti-H3N2 NA antibodies.

2. Materials and Methods

2.1. Participants and Sample Collection

2.1.1. Participants and Enrollment

This study was approved by the Institutional Review Boards of The Legacy Health and Oregon State University (1402–2016, first approved on 05/03/17). Samples were collected from 20 premature-delivering mother-infant pairs ranging in gestational age (GA) at birth from 26 weeks to 36 weeks (Table S1) in the NICU. Parents of all eligible infants in the NICU were approached for participation and informed consent. Clinical data were collected for each mother-infant pair, including GA and postnatal age for both type of feeding (see Table S1). Eligibility criteria included having an indwelling naso/orogastric feeding tube, bolus feeding (<60 min infusion tolerated), feeding volumes of at least four milliliter, and mothers who could produce a volume of MBM adequate for one full-volume feed per day. Exclusion criteria included neonates with diagnoses that were incompatible with life, gastrointestinal system anomalies, major gastrointestinal surgery, severe genitourinary anomalies and significant metabolic, or endocrine diseases.

2.1.2. Feeding and Sampling

To compare the effects of DBM and MBM, two separate feedings of DBM and MBM without fortification were given to infants. Milk and gastric samples (2 mL) were collected on 8–9 and

21–22 days of postnatal age (Figure 1). At both sample time periods, each infant received two of the normal eight daily feedings as unfortified MBM or DBM on alternate days (randomized order). The order of feeding MBM and DBM was randomized to control for any potential effect of infant day of life on antibody digestion. The pool of DBM was acquired from two batches at Northwest Mother's Milk Bank. Three-liter batches were pasteurized and frozen in 50 mL doses so that only a small fraction was thawed for each infant feeding. The power analysis based in our previous study indicated that at least 15 infants were required to compare DBM and MBM-fed infants [16].

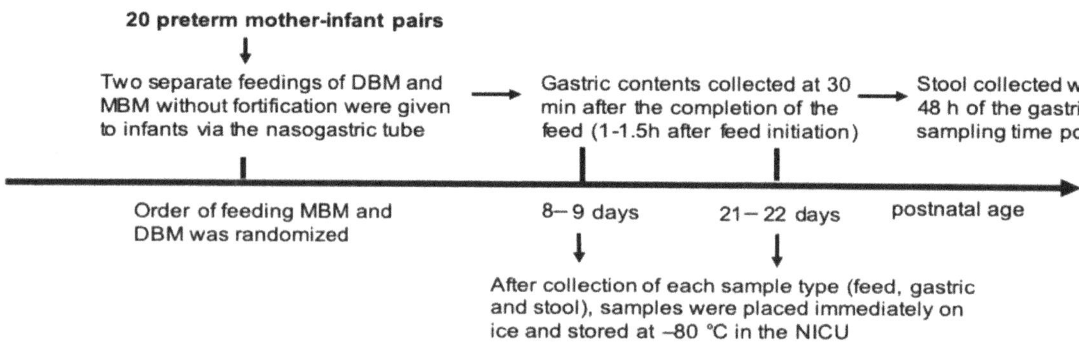

Figure 1. Schema of study design to determine the difference of antenatal influenza-specific antibodies in mother's breast milk (MBM) and donor breast milk (DBM) in gastric contents and stool samples from preterm infants.

The protocol of feeding is described in our previous study [13]. Milk (either MBM or DBM) was fed to the infant via the nasogastric tube with a feeding pump set to deliver the entire bolus over 30–60 min. A sample of the gastric fluid was collected 30 min after the completion of the feed (1–1.5 h after feed initiation). Stool (1 g) was collected within 48 h of the gastric sampling time point and was recovered from the diaper and scraped into a sterile jar. Stool sample collection was not specific to DBM/MBM and thus represents stools deriving from a mixture of DBM and MBM feeding. After collection of each sample type (feed, gastric and stool), samples were placed immediately on ice and stored at −80 °C in the NICU. Samples were transported on dry ice to the Dallas laboratory at Oregon State University for sample analysis.

2.2. Sample Preparation and ELISAs

Feed (MBM and DBM) and gastric samples were thawed at 4 °C, pH was determined and samples (1 mL) were centrifuged at 3500× *g* for 30 min at 4 °C. The infranate was collected, separated into aliquots (100 µL) and stored at −80 °C. Frozen stool samples (0.1 g) were diluted in 700 µL of phosphate-buffered saline pH 7.4 (Thermo Fisher Scientific, MA, USA) with 0.05% Tween-20 (Bio-Rad Laboratories, Irvine, CA, USA) (PBST) and 3% fraction V bovine serum albumin solution (Innovative Research, Novi, MI, USA). Diluted stool samples were mixed by vortex for 2 min and the vials were centrifuged at 3500× *g* for 20 min at 4 °C. The supernatant was collected, separated into aliquots (100 µL) and stored at −80 °C. Sample pH and protein concentration measurements were performed and results were published previously [13].

The spectrophotometric ELISAs were recorded with a microplate reader (Spectramax M2, Molecular Devices, Sunnyvale, CA, USA) with two replicates of blanks, standards and samples. Clear flat-bottom 96-well plates (Thermo Fisher Scientific, Waltham, MA, USA) were coated with 0.75 µg/mL (100 µL) of influenza A/Hong Kong/4801/2014 H3N2 neuraminidase (H3N2 NA) or influenza A/California/07/2009 H1N1 hemagglutinin (H1N1 HA) (Sino Biological US Inc., Wayne, PA, USA). These antigens were chosen based on the strains present in the vaccine (Flucelvax Quadrivalent, 2017–2018 formula, Seqirus, Holly Springs, NC, USA, Table S2) that mothers received for 2017–2018 when samples were collected. Plates were incubated overnight at 4 °C. After incubation, plates were washed three times with PBST. Blocking buffer (100 µL PBST with 3% fraction V bovine serum albumin solution) was added in all wells and incubated for 1 h at room temperature. Standards were prepared using human serum from a female adult that received the influenza vaccine (Flucelvax Quadrivalent, 2017–2018 formula, Seqirus, Holly Springs, NC, USA, Table S2) four months prior. Blood was collected into six BD vacutainer serum separation tubes (SSTTM) (Becton Dickinson, Franklin Lakes, NJ, USA), incubated at room temperature for 5 min, and centrifuged at 3900× *g* for 5 min. Serum was aliquoted into several vials and stored at −80 °C until used. The relative abundance of influenza A antibodies was derived by interpolation from the standard curve generated from human serum with the assigned quantity of anti-influenza A antibodies expressed in ELISA units/mL (EU/mL) (non-diluted serum (1x) = 50,000 arbitrary EU/mL). The standard curves were prepared using a dilution series of standard human serum in blocking buffer and the final concentration covered a range from 12.5× (4000 EU/mL) to 25,600× (1.95 EU/mL). Feed (MBM or DBM) and gastric samples were diluted 10× with blocking buffer for anti-influenza IgA, IgM, and IgG measurements whereas a 2× dilution was used for the prediluted stool samples. For each step (addition of 100 µL standards/samples and secondary antibodies at 1 µg/mL), washing and incubation for 1 h at room temperature were performed. The detection antibodies were goat anti-human IgA alpha-chain: horseradish peroxidase (HRP) for anti-influenza IgA, goat anti-human IgM mu-chain:HRP for anti-influenza IgM and goat anti-human IgG gamma-chain:HRP for anti-influenza IgG (Bio-Rad Laboratories). The substrate 3, 3′, 5, 5′-tetramethylbenzidine (Thermo Fisher Scientific) (1×, 100 µL) was added for 5 min at room temperature followed by addition of 2 N sulfuric acid (100 µL) to stop the reaction. Optical density was measured at 450 nm.

2.3. Pasteurization Effect on Antibodies Specific to Influenza A

To examine the effects of pasteurization directly, a breast milk sample was collected from one mother who was vaccinated with the 2017–2018 influenza vaccine at 25 weeks of pregnancy and gave birth at term. At 12 days of lactation, the mother pumped and collected 150 mL of milk into a sterile plastic bag. Six 1 mL aliquots were centrifuged at 4000× *g* for 30 min, 4 °C and infranates were collected (skim). Three of these aliquots were used for the control raw human milk (RHM) and 3 others were pasteurized at 62.5 °C for 30 min, referred to as the pasteurized skimmed human milk (PSHM). Three other 1-mL aliquots were pasteurized whole (referred to as pasteurized whole human milk, PWHM) and centrifuged at 4000× *g* for 30 min at 4 °C prior to ELISA.

2.4. Statistical Analyses

Wilcoxon matched-pairs signed-rank test in GraphPad Prism software (version 8) was used to compare relative abundance of each anti-influenza antibody isotype (EU/mL) in milk and in gastric contents between MBM and DBM (type of feeding) within the same mother-infant pairs at 8–9 days and 21–22 days of postnatal age. Student's t-tests were used to evaluate the effect of whether or not infants received antibiotics in gastric and stool samples from both feeding types (MBM and DBM) (Table S3). One-way ANOVA followed by Dunnett's multiple comparisons test was performed to compare RHM to PSHM and PWHM. Differences were designated significant at $p < 0.05$. Geometric mean relative abundances (GMRA) of these antibodies in samples at 8–9 days and 21–22 days of postnatal age were also calculated.

3. Results

3.1. Infant Demographics

Demographic details for the preterm-delivering mother-infant pairs are presented in Table S1.

3.2. Anti-Influenza Antibody Relative Abundance in Feeds

The relative abundance of H1N1 HA- (Figure 2) and H3N2 NA-specific IgA (Figure 2) were 3.6- and 2-fold higher, respectively, in MBM than DBM feeds given at 8–9 days of postnatal age but did not differ at 21–22 days. H1N1 HA- (10- and 3-fold) and H3N2 NA-specific IgM (13- and 8-fold) were higher in MBM than in DBM feeds given at 8–9 days and 21–22 days of postnatal age, respectively. H1N1 HA-specific IgG was 2-fold higher in MBM than DBM feeds given at 8–9 days and 21–22 days of postnatal age. H3N2 NA-specific IgG was 30% higher in MBM than DBM feeds given at 8–9 days but did not differ at 21–22 days. The GMRA of each anti-influenza isotype are summarized in Table S4.

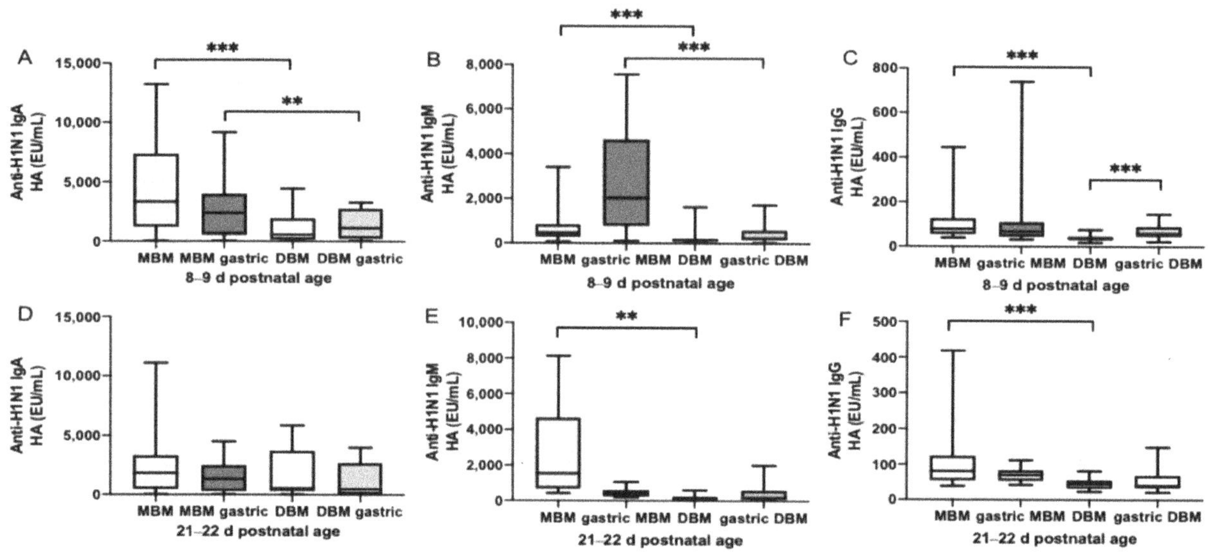

Figure 2. Milk antibodies specific to anti-H1N1 hemagglutinin (anti-H1N1 HA) in mother's own breast milk (MBM) and donor breast milk (DBM) feeds, and gastric samples from preterm infants fed MBM and DBM (26–36 wk of GA). Relative abundance of (**A**) anti-H1N1 HA IgA, (**B**) anti-H1N1 HA IgM, and (**C**) anti-H1N1 HA IgG at 8–9 days of postnatal age. Relative abundance (EU/mL) of (**D**) anti-H1N1 HA IgA, (**E**) anti-H1N1 HA IgM, and (**F**) anti-H1N1 HA IgG at 21–22 days of postnatal age. Values are min, max, and median, $n = 20$ for 8–9 days and $n = 16$ for 21–22 days of postnatal age. Asterisks show statistically significant differences between variables (*** $p < 0.001$; ** $p < 0.01$) using the Wilcoxon matched-pairs signed-rank test.

3.3. Anti-Influenza Antibody Relative Abundance in Gastric Contents

At 8–9 days of postnatal age, relative abundance of H1N1 HA- (Figure 2) and H3N2 NA-specific IgA (Figure 2) were 4- and 7-fold higher in gastric contents from infants fed MBM than those fed DBM. At 21–22 days, H3N2 NA-specific IgA was 4-fold higher in gastric contents after feeding MBM than after feeding DBM but did not differ for H1N1 HA-specific IgA. H1N1 HA- and H3N2 NA-specific IgM were 6- and 11-fold higher in gastric contents from infants fed MBM than those fed DBM at 8–9 days. At 21–22 days, H3N2 NA-specific IgM was 5-fold higher in MBM than DBM but did not differ for H1N1 HA-specific IgM. H1N1 HA- and H3N2 NA-specific IgG in gastric contents did not differ after feeding infants MBM and those fed DBM. The GMRA of each anti-influenza isotype are summarized in Table S5.

3.4. Gastric Digestion of Anti-Influenza Antibody from MBM and DBM

Relative abundance of H1N1 HA- (Figure 1) and H3N2 NA-specific IgA and IgM (Figure 3) did not significantly decrease from feed to gastric contents in infants fed MBM or DBM at 8–9 days or 21–22 days of postnatal age. H1N1 HA-specific IgG from MBM did not change from feed to gastric contents at 8–9 days or 21–22 days, whereas H1N1 HA-specific IgG from DBM slightly increased in gastric contents at 8–9 days but did not differ at 21–22 days of postnatal age. H3N2 NA-specific IgG from DBM decreased in the gastric contents at 8–9 days but did not differ at 21–22 days. H3N2 NA-specific IgG from MBM decreased in gastric contents at 21–22 days but not at 8–9 days. The GMRA abundances of each anti-influenza isotype are summarized in Table S6.

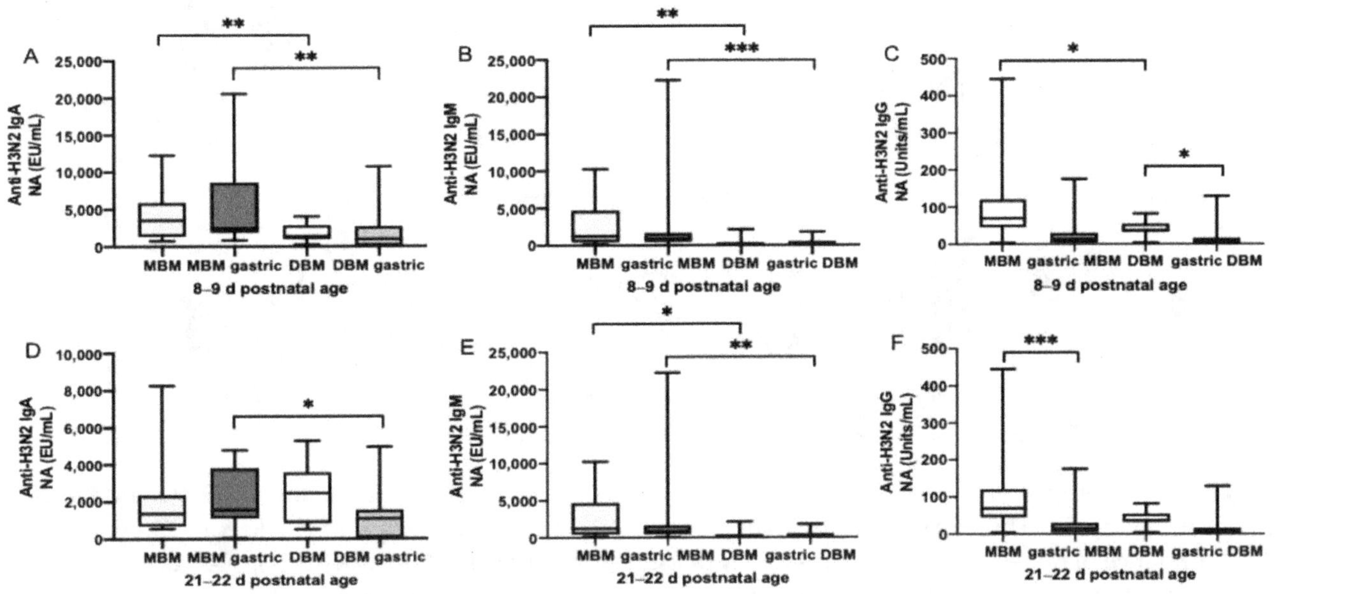

Figure 3. Milk antibodies specific to anti-H3N2 neuraminidase (anti-H3N2 NA) in mother's own breast milk (MBM) and donor breast milk (DBM) feeds, and gastric samples from preterm infants fed MBM and DBM (26–36 wk of GA). Relative abundance of (**A**) anti-H3N2 NA IgA, (**B**) anti-H3N2 NA IgM, and (**C**) anti-H3N2 NA IgG at 8–9 d postnatal age. Relative abundance (EU/mL) of (**D**) anti-H3N2 NA IgA, (**E**) anti-H3N2 NA IgM, and (**F**) anti-H3N2 NA IgG at 21–22 days of postnatal age. Values are min, max, and median, $n = 20$ for 8–9 days and $n = 16$ for 21–22 days of postnatal age. Asterisks show statistically significant differences between variables (*** $p < 0.001$; ** $p < 0.01$; * $p < 0.05$) using the Wilcoxon matched-pairs signed-rank test.

3.5. Postnatal Age Effects on Anti-Influenza A Antibodies in Preterm Infant Stools Derived from Mixed MBM/DBM

The relative abundance of H1N1 HA- and H3N2 NA-specific IgA, IgM and IgG in infant stools did not differ between 8–9 days and 21–22 days of postnatal age (Table S7).

3.6. Pasteurization Effects on Human Milk Anti-Influenza A Antibodies

The anti-influenza antibodies in RHM to PWHM and PSHM were compared to determine the effect of Holder pasteurization on them. Whole and skim breast milk were pasteurized because previous literature reported different results with and without delipidation before pasteurization [14,15]. The relative abundance of anti-H1N1 HA IgA, anti-H3N2 NA IgA, and anti-H1N1 HA IgG did not differ between RHM and PWHM or PSHM (Figure 4). Anti-H1N1 HA IgM, anti-H3N2 NA IgM, and anti-H3N2 NA IgG in RHM were 2.5-, 23-, and 2-fold higher than in PSHM. Anti-H3N2 NA IgM in RHM was 3-fold higher than in PWHM. Anti-H1N1 HA IgM, anti-H3N2 NA IgM, and anti-H3N2 NA IgG in PWHM were 2.5-, 7.3-, and 1.5-fold higher than PSHM but did not differ for other antibodies.

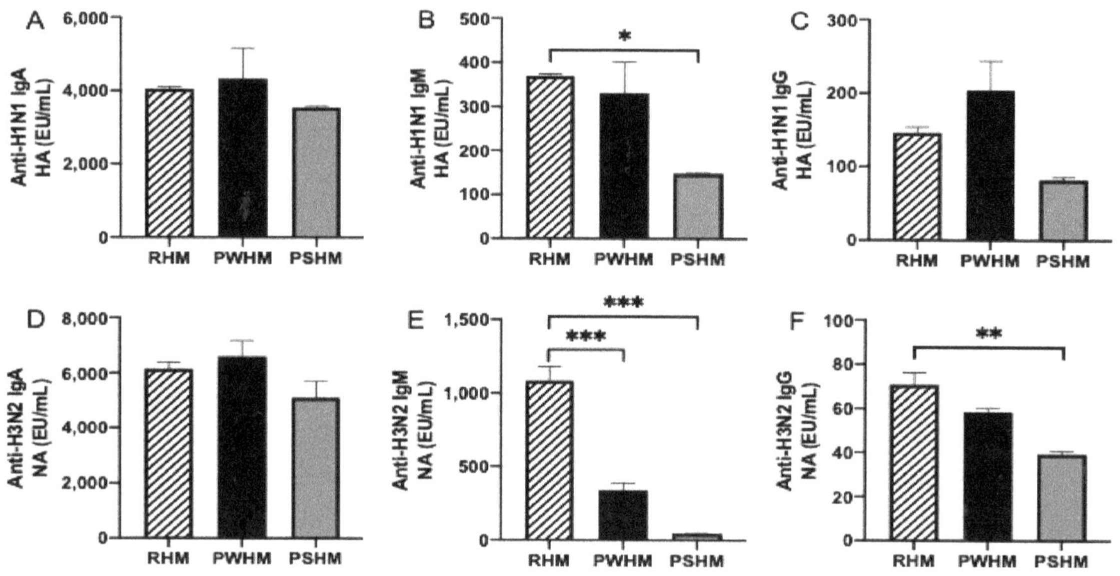

Figure 4. Comparison of immunoglobulin relative abundance between raw human milk (RHM) and pasteurized whole human milk (PWHM) or pasteurized skimmed human milk (PSHM) ($n = 3$). Relative abundance of anti-H1N1 HA (**A**) IgA, (**B**) IgM, (**C**) IgG, and of anti-H3N2 NA. (**D**) IgA, (**E**) IgM, and (**F**) IgG in mother's milk. Milk samples were from one mother who delivered one term infant at 38 wk of GA and collected milk at 12 days of postnatal age. Asterisks show statistically significant differences between variables (*** $p < 0.001$; ** $p < 0.01$; * $p < 0.05$) using one-way ANOVA followed by Dunnett's multiple comparisons test.

4. Discussion

This study aimed to determine whether the relative abundance of maternal milk anti-influenza A antibodies differed between MBM and DBM and across their digestion in gastric contents and in stool of preterm infants. Influenza A viruses vary based on their hemagglutinin (HA) and neuraminidase (NA) subtypes; each influenza A virus has a specific combination of an HA and an NA subtype [3]. Milk anti-influenza A neutralizing antibodies can be specific to subtypes of HA or NA. In this study, we examined anti-H1N1 HA and anti-H3N2 NA antibodies. Anti-influenza IgA level was previously evaluated in human milk via ELISA [9]. The anti-H1N1 HA IgA relative abundance measured herein was higher than those measured previously in term-delivering influenza-vaccinated mothers by Schlaudecker et al. [9]. However, abundance values of milk antibodies cannot be compared with those reported in other studies because different human serums were used to prepare the standard curve for each anti-influenza antibody isotype. No commercial standard exists for anti-influenza IgA, IgM, and IgG; therefore, determining absolute concentrations was not possible in this study. This research is the first to determine the anti-influenza A IgM and IgG relative abundance in breast milk.

Anti-influenza A H1N1 HA and H3N2 NA IgA in MBM were higher than in DBM during the first week of postnatal age for both feeds and gastric contents from preterm infants but did not differ during the third week for either feed or gastric contents. Neither anti-influenza A H1N1 HA nor H3N2 NA IgA was reduced by pasteurization of whole or skim breast milk. Therefore, we speculate that high relative abundance of anti-influenza IgA in MBM is related to early GA and early postnatal age of infants when mothers delivered prematurely. DBM is donated from mothers delivering mostly term infants and milk is usually collected later than three months of lactation, which could have different milk antibody levels compared with those from preterm-delivering mothers at early lactation times. Our recent clinical study demonstrated that antibody concentrations (total IgA and SIgA) were higher in MBM than DBM in feeds and gastric samples (1 h post-feeding) from preterm infants [13]. A previous study found that IgA concentration in preterm milk was higher than in term milk from 3 to 15 days of lactation time [17]. Total IgA concentration in colostrum from preterm-delivering mothers was higher than colostrum (1–3 days of lactation time) from term-delivering mothers in several studies [17–19]. However, our previous study showed that total IgA did not differ between preterm milk and term milk from 6 days to 28 days of lactation time [16]. No study has previously evaluated the difference in relative abundance of milk anti-influenza IgA antibodies between preterm- and term-delivering mothers or between early and late lactation time. Our results suggest that the provision of passive immune protection with milk anti-influenza A IgA was highest when infants are fed MBM during their first week of postnatal age.

Anti-influenza A H1N1 HA and H3N2 NA IgM in MBM were higher than in DBM during the first and third week of postnatal age in both feeds and in infant gastric samples. Among isotypes, anti-influenza IgM relative abundance differed most between DBM and MBM. Anti-H1N1 HA IgM was reduced when skim milk was pasteurized but not when whole breast milk was pasteurized. On the other hand, anti-H3N2 NA IgM was decreased by pasteurizing whole and skim milk. We hypothesize that the lower relative abundance of anti-influenza A IgM in DBM compared with MBM was due to the pasteurization of pooled donor milk after fat loss during freezing and thawing. The reduction of anti-influenza IgM was not likely due to the difference of GA or lactation time between MBM (preterm-delivering mothers) and DBM (term-delivering mothers). Anti-influenza IgM did not change across lactation time (1 weeks to 3 weeks) in milk from preterm-delivering mothers. Our recent clinical study demonstrated that total IgM concentration was higher in MBM than DBM in feeds and gastric samples (1 h post-feeding) from preterm infants [13]. Previous studies showed that IgM concentration in preterm-delivering mothers was lower than [16], higher than [17] or similar to [20,21] term-delivering mothers, suggesting a high variability of IgM concentration between mothers. A strong variation of anti-H3N2 NA IgM in MBM from preterm-delivering mothers (0 EU/mL to 4301 EU/mL at 1 week; 0–900 EU/mL at 3 weeks) was observed, which could be due to the time of vaccination during pregnancy and the mother's immune response to the vaccine.

Anti-H1N1 HA IgG was higher in MBM than in DBM fed during the first and third week of postnatal age. Pasteurization did not affect anti-H1N1 HA IgG in whole or skim breast milk. The higher relative abundance of anti-H1N1 HA IgG in MBM could be due to the difference of GA and lactation time between preterm-delivering mothers and term-delivering mothers (DBM). Anti-influenza A H1N1 HA and H3N2 NA IgG did not differ in gastric contents of infants fed MBM and DBM either at 1 week or 3 weeks of postnatal age. Interestingly, anti-H3N2 NA IgG was higher in MBM than in DBM during the first week but did not differ at third week of MBM lactation. Anti-H3N2 NA IgG relative abundance in skimmed milk but not whole milk was reduced by pasteurization. We speculate that anti-H3N2 NA IgG was low in DBM due to the time of lactation. Our recent clinical study demonstrated that total IgG concentration was higher in MBM than DBM in feed and gastric samples (1 h post-feeding) from preterm infants [13].

Gastric digestion reduced anti-H3N2 NA IgG from MBM at 21–22 days and from DBM at 8–9 days of postnatal age, but the other anti-influenza A antibodies were not digested in the gastric contents of preterm infants. A slight increase of anti-H3N2 NA IgG from DBM in gastric contents at 8–9 days of postnatal age was observed, which could be due to contamination of the gastric contents with residual from previous feeds based on MBM.

All influenza A antibodies most likely resisted preterm infant overall digestion to some extent as all were detected in stools 24 h post-feeding. Antibodies detected in stool samples could derive from the MBM and/or DBM feeding or potentially be generated by the infant. Anti-H1N1 and anti-H3N2 antibodies in stool samples did not differ between the first and third week of postnatal age.

Five infants among twenty received antibiotics (Table S1). Provision of antibiotics could change the microbiome and alter the survival of maternal influenza antibodies to the stool. However, no differences were detected in their survival in the gastric contents and stools between infants with and without antibiotics (Table S3).

Schlaudecker et al. [9] demonstrated that anti-influenza IgA level in breast milk correlated inversely with frequency of respiratory illness with fever in term infants. The authors hypothesized that orally ingested milk antibodies may contribute to immune protection within airways against respiratory infections [9]. However, this high protection effect could also be due to the high anti-influenza antibody concentration (IgG) in mother's blood that was transmitted to the infant across the placenta.

The function of milk anti-influenza antibodies may be to neutralize viruses in breast milk or in the gastrointestinal or respiratory tracts. Small amounts of breast milk can reach the infant respiratory tract as a result of regurgitation and inhalation of breast milk during and after feeding [22]. Therefore, milk influenza-specific antibodies may reach the respiratory tract through regurgitation and inhalation of breast milk and protect the mucosa of the respiratory tract against influenza A viruses, as previously hypothesized for milk anti-respiratory syncytial virus-specific Ig [23]. Nutritional intervention studies are needed to confirm whether the milk antibodies specific to influenza A can contribute to protection against respiratory pathogens.

Milk antibodies may also interact with immune cells within the infant intestinal lumen to protect against pathogens. Maternal milk-derived SIgA2 and IgA2 (but not IgA1, IgG or IgM) can adhere to the apical surfaces of mice intestinal M cells and be transported across the epithelial cell layer [24]. IgA1 has a heavily O-glycosylated hinge region, whereas the smaller IgA2 hinge region is not glycosylated. The investigators speculated that the extended hinge of IgA1 may interfere with binding to the M cell receptor [24]. A hypothetical IgA receptor on M cells could mediate the delivery of SIgA2 from the intestinal lumen to the mucosa-associated lymphoid tissues. SIgA2-antigen complexes absorbed across M cells could be sampled by subepithelial B lymphocytes and dendritic cells [25]. Indeed, SIgA was detected on the apical surface of M cells in the infant ileum, suggesting that they may be able to endocytose SIgA. Therefore, milk anti-influenza antibodies complexed with influenza antigens could hypothetically be absorbed by M cells, sampled by leukocytes and lead to altered mucosal immune response in the respiratory tract.

A limitation in our study was the absence of information on vaccination (vaccinated or not and dates) from recruited mothers in order to demonstrate a positive correlation between vaccinated mothers and anti-influenza antibody level in breast milk. However, this association was already demonstrated in previous a study for anti-influenza IgA in breast milk [9].

Another study limitation is that too few subjects were included to detect many differences between MBM and DBM feeds and gastric contents when grouped by GA (26–27 weeks, 30–31 weeks, and 35–36 weeks).

5. Conclusions

The present study suggests that passive immunization with milk anti-influenza A IgA may have been highest when infants were fed MBM rather than DBM during the first week of postnatal age. Anti-influenza A IgM was higher in MBM than in DBM during the first and third week of postnatal age in both type of samples (feeds and gastric samples). Anti-influenza IgM differed most between DBM and MBM, likely due to its sensitivity to pasteurization. Anti-influenza IgG relative abundance was higher in MBM than DBM feeds but did not differ in gastric contents at first and third week of postnatal age. Passive immune protection with maternal anti-influenza antibodies from MBM may provide infant protection. Milk antibodies could neutralize viruses within the mammary gland, in the infant mouth and after entering their respiratory system. Supplementing DBM with additional influenza A-specific antibodies could benefit infants.

Supplementary Materials:
Table S1. Demographics of preterm-delivering mother-infant pairs sampled for MBM and DBM feeds, gastric contents (1-h postprandial time) and stools (24-h post-feeding); Table S2. Description of influenza vaccine (Flucelvax Quadrivalent 2017-2018 Formula) given to mothers during pregnancy; Table S3. Statistical results (p-values) for Student's t-tests comparing antibody concentration between infants that received antibiotics ($n = 5$ at 8–9 days and $n = 5$ at 21–22 days of postnatal age) and infants that did not receive antibiotics ($n = 15$ at 8–9 days and

n = 11 at 21–22 days) in gastric and stool samples. G, gastric contents; S, stool; Table S4. GMRA of anti-influenza A IgA, IgM and IgG (H1N1 HA and H3N2 NA) in MBM and DBM at 8–9 days and for 21–22 days of postnatal age. MBM samples were from 20 preterm-delivering mothers (26–36 wk of GA). P-values were calculated using the Wilcoxon matched-pairs signed-rank test; Table S5. GMRA of anti-influenza IgA, IgM, and IgG (H1N1 HA and H3N2 NA) in gastric contents fed MBM and DBM feeds. Gastric contents from infants fed MBM or DBM were from 20 mother-preterm pairs (26–36 wk of GA at 8–9 days and for 21–22 days of postnatal age. p-values were calculated using the Wilcoxon matched-pairs signed-rank test; Table S6. p-value for the difference between MBM and gastric MBM or between DBM and gastric DBM on anti-influenza IgA, IgM, and IgG reactivities (H1N1 HA and H3N2 NA). Feed and gastric samples were from 20 mother-preterm pairs (26–36 wk of GA). p-values were calculated using the Wilcoxon matched-pairs signed-rank test; Table S7. GMRA for anti-influenza IgA, IgM and IgG antibodies (H1N1 HA and H3N2 NA) in stools from preterm infants. Stool samples were from 20 preterm infants at 26–36 wk of GA. p-values were calculated using the Wilcoxon matched-pairs signed-rank test between 8–9 days and 21–22 days of postnatal age.

Author Contributions: V.D.-M. conducted the ELISA analyses, analyzed data and conducted the statistical analysis. R.K.H., A.M.M., E.A.M., and R.L.M. provided milk and gastric samples. V.D.-M, D.C.D., R.K.H., A.M.M., E.A.M., and R.L.M. designed the clinical study. V.D.-M. designed the study and drafted the manuscript. V.D.-M. and D.C.D. have primary responsibility for the final content.

Acknowledgments: We thank the Northwest Mother's Milk Bank for providing DBM for this study.

References

1. Glezen, W.P.; Taber, L.H.; Frank, A.L.; Gruber, W.C.; Piedra, P.A. Influenza virus infections in infants. *Pediatr. Infect. Dis. J.* **1997**, *16*, 1065–1068. [CrossRef] [PubMed]
2. Louie, J.K.; Schechter, R.; Honarmand, S.; Guevara, H.F.; Shoemaker, T.R.; Madrigal, N.Y.; Woodfill, C.J.; Backer, H.D.; Glaser, C.A. Severe pediatric influenza in California, 2003–2005: Implications for immunization recommendations. *Pediatrics* **2006**, *2005*, 1373. [CrossRef] [PubMed]
3. Cox, R.J.; Brokstad, K.A.; Ogra, P.L. Influenza virus: Immunity and vaccination strategies. Comparison of the immune response to inactivated and live, attenuated influenza vaccines. *Scand. J. Immunol.* **2004**, *59*, 1–15. [CrossRef] [PubMed]
4. Salam, R.A.; Das, J.K.; Soeandy, C.D.; Lassi, Z.S.; Bhutta, Z.A. Impact of Haemophilus influenzae type B (Hib) and viral influenza vaccinations in pregnancy for improving maternal, neonatal and infant health outcomes. *Cochrane Datab. Syst. Rev.* **2015**, *6*, 1–41. [CrossRef] [PubMed]
5. Omer, S.B.; Clark, D.R.; Aqil, A.R.; Tapia, M.D.; Nunes, M.C.; Kozuki, N.; Steinhoff, M.C.; Madhi, S.A.; Wairagkar, N. Maternal influenza immunization and prevention of severe clinical pneumonia in young infants. *Pediatr. Infect. Dis. J.* **2018**, *37*, 436–440. [CrossRef] [PubMed]
6. Zaman, K.; Roy, E.; Arifeen, S.E.; Rahman, M.; Raqib, R.; Wilson, E.; Omer, S.B.; Shahid, N.S.; Breiman, R.F.; Steinhoff, M.C. Effectiveness of maternal influenza immunization in mothers and infants. *N. Engl. J. Med.* **2008**, *359*, 1555–1564. [CrossRef] [PubMed]
7. Eick, A.A.; Uyeki, T.M.; Klimov, A.; Hall, H.; Reid, R.; Santosham, M.; O'Brien, K.L. Maternal influenza vaccination and effect on influenza virus infection in young infants. *Arch. Pediatr. Adolesc. Med.* **2011**, *165*, 104–111. [CrossRef]
8. Niewiesk, S. Maternal Antibodies: Clinical Significance, Mechanism of interference with immune responses, and possible vaccination strategies. *Front. Immunol.* **2014**, *5*, 446. [CrossRef]
9. Schlaudecker, E.P.; Steinhoff, M.C.; Omer, S.B.; McNeal, M.M.; Roy, E.; Arifeen, S.E.; Dodd, C.N.; Raqib, R.; Breiman, R.F.; Zaman, K. IgA and neutralizing antibodies to influenza A virus in human milk: A randomized trial of antenatal influenza immunization. *PLoS ONE* **2013**, *8*, e70867. [CrossRef]
10. Finn, A. *Clinical Trials of Influenza Vaccines: Special Challenges*; Humana Press: New York, NY, USA, 2019; pp. 567–573.
11. Sagrera, X.; Ginovart, G.; Raspall, F.; Rabella, N.; Sala, P.; Sierra, M.; Demestre, X.; Vila, C. Outbreaks of influenza A virus infection in neonatal intensive care units. *Pediatr. Infect. Dis. J.* **2002**, *21*, 196–200. [CrossRef]
12. Carroll, K.; Herrmann, K.R. The cost of using donor human milk in the NICU to achieve exclusively human milk feeding through 32 weeks postmenstrual age. *Breastfeed. Med.* **2013**, *8*, 286–290. [CrossRef] [PubMed]
13. Demers-Mathieu, V.; Huston, R.K.; Markell, A.M.; McCulley, E.A.; Martin, R.L.; Spooner, M.; Dallas, D.C. Differences in maternal immunoglobulins within mother's own breast milk and donor breast milk and across digestion in preterm infants. *Nutrients* **2019**, *11*, 920. [CrossRef] [PubMed]

14. Evans, T.J.; Ryley, H.C.; Neale, L.M.; Dodge, J.A.; Lewarne, V.M. Effect of storage and heat on antimicrobial proteins in human milk. *Arch. Dis. Child.* **1978**, *53*, 239–241. [CrossRef] [PubMed]
15. Ford, J.E.; Law, B.A.; Marshall, V.M.; Reiter, B. Influence of the heat treatment of human milk on some of its protective constituents. *J. Pediatr.* **1977**, *90*, 29–35. [CrossRef]
16. Demers-Mathieu, V.; Underwood, M.A.; Beverly, R.L.; Nielsen, S.D.; Dallas, D.C. Comparison of human milk immunoglobulin survival during gastric digestion between preterm and term infants. *Nutrients* **2018**, *10*, 631. [CrossRef] [PubMed]
17. Chandra, R.K. Immunoglobulin and protein levels in breast milk produced by mothers of preterm infants. *Nutr. Res.* **1982**, *2*, 27–30. [CrossRef]
18. Ballabio, C.; Bertino, E.; Coscia, A.; Fabris, C.; Fuggetta, D.; Molfino, S.; Testa, T.; Sgarrella, M.; Sabatino, G.; Restani, P. Immunoglobulin—A profile in breast milk from mothers delivering full term and preterm infants. *Int. J. Immunopathol. Pharmacol.* **2007**, *20*, 119–128. [CrossRef] [PubMed]
19. Montagne, P.; Cuillière, M.L.; Molé, C.; Béné, M.C.; Faure, G. Immunological and nutritional composition of human milk in relation to prematurity and mothers' parity during the first 2 weeks of lactation. *J. Pediatr. Gastroenterol. Nutr.* **1999**, *29*, 75–80. [CrossRef]
20. Gross, S.J.; Buckley, R.H.; Wakil, S.S.; McAllister, D.C.; David, R.J.; Faix, R.G. Elevated IgA concentration in milk produced by mothers delivered of preterm infants. *J. Pediatr.* **1981**, *99*, 389–393. [CrossRef]
21. Koenig, Á.; Diniz, E.M.D.A.; Barbosa, S.F.C.; Vaz, F.A.C. Immunologic factors in human milk: The effects of gestational age and pasteurization. *J. Hum. Lact.* **2005**, *21*, 439–443. [CrossRef]
22. Decarlo, J.O.; Tramer, A.; Startzman, H.N. Iodized oil aspiration in the newborn. *Arch. Pediatr. Adolesc. Med.* **1952**, *84*, 442–445. [CrossRef]
23. Laegreid, A.; OTNÆSS, A.B.K.; Ørstavik, I.; Carlsen, K.H. Neutralizing activity in human milk fractions against respiratory syncytial virus. *Acta Paediatr.* **1986**, *75*, 696–701. [CrossRef]
24. Mantis, N.J.; Cheung, M.C.; Chintalacharuvu, K.R.; Rey, J.; Corthésy, B.; Neutra, M.R. Selective adherence of IgA to murine Peyer's patch M cells: Evidence for a novel IgA receptor. *J. Immunol.* **2002**, *169*, 1844–1851. [CrossRef] [PubMed]
25. Iwasaki, A.; Kelsall, B.L. Unique functions of CD11b+, CD8α+, and double-negative Peyer's patch dendritic cells. *J. Immunol.* **2001**, *166*, 4884–4890. [CrossRef] [PubMed]

16

The Impact of Maternal Diet during Pregnancy and Lactation on the Fatty Acid Composition of Erythrocytes and Breast Milk of Chilean Women

Cynthia Barrera [1], Rodrigo Valenzuela [1,2,*], Rodrigo Chamorro [1], Karla Bascuñán [1], Jorge Sandoval [2,3], Natalia Sabag [1], Francesca Valenzuela [1], María-Paz Valencia [1], Claudia Puigrredon [2,3] and Alfonso Valenzuela [2]

1. Department of Nutrition, Faculty of Medicine, University of Chile, Av. Independencia 1027, Independencia, Casilla 70000, Santiago 8380453, Chile; cynthia.barrera@gmail.com (C.B.); rodrigochamorro@med.uchile.cl (R.C.); kbascunan@med.uchile.cl (K.B.); n.sabag.c@gmail.com (N.S.); francesca.valenzuelar@gmail.com (F.V.); mpvalencia@ug.uchile.cl (M.-P.V.)
2. Lipid Center, Institute of Nutrition and Food Technology (INTA), University of Chile, Av. El Líbano 5524, Macul, Santiago 8380453, Chile; jsandoval@hcuch.cl (J.S.); cpuigrredon@hcuch.cl (C.P.); avalenzu@inta.uchile.cl (A.V.)
3. Obstetrics and Gynecology Department, Clinical Hospital of the University of Chile, Av. Santos Dumont 999, Independencia, Santiago 8380453, Chile

* Correspondence: rvalenzuelab@med.uchile.cl

Abstract: Maternal diet during pregnancy is relevant for fatty acid supply during fetal life and lactation. Arachidonic (AA) and docosahexaenoic (DHA) acids are also relevant for the normal growth and development of brain and visual system. AA and DHA provided by the mother to the fetus and infant are directly associated with maternal dietary intake and body stores. Our aim was to evaluate the impact of maternal diet, specially referring to the quality of fatty acid intake, in a sample of Chilean women during last stage of pregnancy and across the lactation period. Fifty healthy pregnant women (age range 20–33 years) were studied from the 6th month of pregnancy and followed until 6th month of lactation period. Diet characteristics were evaluated through food frequency questionnaires. Fatty acids composition of erythrocyte phospholipids and breast milk samples was assessed by gas-liquid chromatography. Overall, women had high saturated fatty acids intake with sufficient intake of mono- and polyunsaturated fatty acids (PUFA). Diet was high in *n*-6 PUFA and low in *n*-3 PUFA (mainly DHA), with imbalanced *n*-6/*n*-3 PUFA ratio. Erythrocytes and breast milk DHA concentration was significantly reduced during lactation compared to pregnancy, a pattern not observed for AA. We concluded that is necessary to increase the intake of *n*-3 PUFA during pregnancy and lactation by improving the quality of consumed foods with particular emphasis on its DHA content.

Keywords: pregnancy; breast milk; lactation; maternal diet; *n*-6 and *n*-3 polyunsaturated fatty acid; docosahexaenoic acid

---

1. Introduction

Arachidonic acid (C20:4*n*-6, AA) and docosahexaenoic acid (C22:6*n*-3, DHA) are long chain polyunsaturated fatty acids (LCPUFA) that have a relevant role in different metabolic and physiological process during embryonic and fetal development, and the first years of life [1]. Highest concentrations of AA and DHA are found in nervous system, particularly in brain and retina, specifically in the phospholipids of cell membranes [2,3]. AA and DHA have an active role in brain development during neurogenesis, synaptogenesis, neuronal migration, neuronal differentiation, and also in gene expression and in the general metabolic energy status [4]. AA is formed from the precursor linoleic acid (C18:2*n*-6 LA) and DHA from the precursor alpha-linolenic acid (C18:3*n*-3, ALA) [5]. Humans can synthesize AA and DHA, mainly in the liver, through a complex metabolic process that includes different enzymatically catalyzed desaturations and elongations of their respective metabolic precursors (LA and ALA); Δ-5 and Δ-6 desaturases are the most relevant enzymes participating in these processes [6].

Hepatic synthesis of AA and DHA is a fundamental metabolic process necessary to ensure the constant supply of these LCPUFA to other tissues [7]. Synthesis of AA and DHA in women is more efficient than in men due the active positive control of estrogens over desaturase activities [8]. Women, in addition, can store LCPUFA during pregnancy and lactation to ensure an adequate flow of AA and DHA to the fetus and newborn [9]. During pregnancy, the transport of AA and DHA from the mother to embryo and fetus is facilitated by specific transporter proteins that enhance the transfer of these fatty acids through the placenta [10]. During this period, women can also incorporate AA and DHA in their diet by eating eggs and meat (as sources of preformed AA) and fatty fish (i.e., tuna, mackerel, and salmon, among others) as a sources of preformed DHA [11]). However, in western countries DHA intake from fish consumption is very low compared to the intake of LA (from vegetable oils) and AA (from eggs and meat) [11]. In addition to the high dietary intake of *n*-6 fatty acids, the synthesis of AA from LA when this fatty acid is highly consumed is more efficient than the synthesis of DHA from ALA [12].

Several studies have established the relevance of the fatty acid composition of breast milk and its direct association with the diet of the mother during pregnancy and lactation [13–15]. The aim of our research was to evaluate the impact of maternal diet, with specific reference to the quality of fatty acids intake, in a sample of Chilean women during the last stage of pregnancy and across the lactation period. The fatty acid composition of erythrocyte phospholipids (during pregnancy and lactation) and of breast milk (during the first sixth months of lactation) were assessed as analytical criteria for *n*-6 and *n*-3 LCPUFA availability.

2. Materials and Methods

2.1. Study Design and Subjects

Pregnant women ($n = 50$) who attended the Obstetrical and Gynecology Health Service of the Clinical Hospital, University of Chile, Santiago, Chile were included in the study. Inclusion criteria were women between 20 and 33 years; gestational age at least 22 and up to 25 weeks according to the date of the last menstrual period and confirmed by ultrasound; and history of successful lactation. Exclusion criteria were women with history of drug or alcohol consumption; with current consumption of *n*-6 and/or *n*-3 LCPUFA supplements; who were underweight (as defined by the Chilean chart for pregnant women [16]); who had a history of twins; who had been diagnosed with chronic diseases such as diabetes, arterial hypertension, or other illnesses that could affect fetal growth. Recruited women mainly belonged to the low and middle socioeconomic status according to the European Society for Opinion and Marketing Research (ESOMAR) [17]. All women were of Hispanic origin.

At the time of recruitment, all women who fulfilled the inclusion criteria were given general information about the study, and a dietitian explained the objectives and main characteristics of the research. The protocol was reviewed and approved by the Institutional Review Board of the Faculty of Medicine, University of Chile (Protocol #073-2011), and by the Ethics Committee of the Clinical Hospital, University of Chile (Protocol #507/11). All information regarding the study was given to each participant who voluntarily agreed to participate and signed the informed consent.

2.2. Clinical and Nutritional Assessment

Participants were subject to a clinical evaluation when incorporated into the study. A physician and a nurse assessed each woman regarding her health by following the standard clinical approach for pregnant women. Anthropometric data of weight (kg) and height (m) were assessed to determine body-mass index (BMI, kg/m^2), which was then used to establish the maternal nutritional status according to gestational week following the Chilean reference [17]. Energy and nutrient requirements were established according to WHO criteria [18] and recommended dietary intakes according to the American Institute of Medicine, 2001 [19].

2.3. Dietary Intake

All women were interviewed by trained dietitians at the enrollment of the study and asked to report all groups of foods consumed at the first week after delivery and during the six-month of lactation, using a food frequency questionnaire. In addition to this questionnaire and in order to improve the estimation of eaten foods, dietitians used a photographic atlas of commonly consumed foods in Chile [20], which is a validated graphic instrument that helps to estimate the amount of each food/beverage consumed. Food intake data were checked by contrasting the energy/nutrient intake data composition with dietary questionnaires, identifying potential under- or over-reports. In that case, a careful review of each food frequency questionnaire was done. Dietary data were grouped into nine food groups (cereals, fruits and vegetables, dairy, meats and eggs, legumes, fish and shellfish, high-fat foods, oils and fats, sugars and processed foods), according to dietary analysis previously reported by Bascuñán et al. [21]. Dietary data was analyzed using the software Food Processor SQL® (ESHA Research, Salem, OR, USA), to calculate the daily intake of energy and nutrients. Nutritional composition of foods was obtained using a database from the USDA National Nutrient Database for Standard Reference, which also incorporated information from locally generated nutrient composition data.

2.4. Collection and Fatty Acid Analysis from Erythrocytes and Breast Milk Samples

Blood samples were obtained at the enrollment, immediately after the delivery and at the 1st and the 6th month after lactation. The samples were immediately centrifuged to obtain the erythrocyte fraction (3000× g for 10 min at 20 °C) and then frozen at −80 °C until further analysis. Breast milk was extracted by the mothers themselves after the infant had been fed for at least 2 min and was collected in plastic vials. Breast milk samples (5 mL) were collected monthly from the 1st until the 6th month of lactation. Once collected, the samples were immediately frozen at −80 °C until further analysis. Details of the analysis of fatty acids of erythrocyte phospholipids and breast milk samples were previously described by Valenzuela et al. [15].

2.5. Statistical Analyses

Dietary data were checked by contrasting the energy/nutrient intake data composition with dietary questionnaires, identifying potential outliers. In that case, a careful review of each food frequency questionnaire was done. After a descriptive analysis, the distribution of variables was evaluated using the Shapiro–Wilk test. Results are expressed as the mean ± SD. Assessment of significant differences between mean values was performed by one-way ANOVA and with Bonferroni post-hoc test. Statistical significance was set at an alpha level of 5%. For all analyses, the statistical software used was SPSS v.24.0 (Chicago, IL, USA).

3. Results

3.1. Background and Anthropometric Characteristics of the Sample

Table 1 shows the main background characteristics of the sample (age, socio-economic status (SES), weight, BMI, nutritional status, and gestational age). 68.2% of women belonged to the SES medium. Regarding the nutritional status, 37.8% were overweight and 11.1% obese; therefore, 48.9% of women exhibited overnutrition at the study enrollment.

Table 2 shows the anthropometric characteristics of women during the pregnancy and lactation period. Significant modification was observed in the weight and BMI during the time course of the study. The weigh and BMI were higher ($p < 0.05$) than delivery compared with other times evaluated. At the beginning of the study, 4.4% were underweight. At the end of the study, 46.7% of women were overweight and 16.1% obese; therefore, 62.8% exhibited overnutrition, and no underweight was observed. The 45% of deliveries were after cesarean, condition that may modify the milk production in amount and nutritional quality (not evaluated in the present study). At 6th month of lactation, infant presented a normal increment of weight and height. An important aspect is the increase in weight of the women from the 6th month of pregnancy until the delivery (12.2 kg on average), along with the weight of infant at birth, which on average was 4.25 kg.

Table 1. Background characteristics of the women at the study enrollment.

Variable		(n = 50)
Age (Years)		29.4 ± 6.2
SES	High (%)	20.4
	Medium (%)	68.2
	Low (%)	11.4
Preconception Weight (kg)		64.9 ± 9.3
Preconception BMI (kg/m^2)		24.9 ± 3.3
Nutritional Status	Underweight (%)	4.4
	Normal Weight (%)	46.7
	Overweight (%)	37.8
	Obese (%)	11.1
Gestational Age (Weeks) *		24.2 ± 3.8

Value are shown as mean ± S.D., or as a percentage (%); SES, socioeconomic status; BMI, body mass index = kg/m^2. (*) Data taken at study enrollment.

Table 2. Anthropometric characteristics of the women during the pregnancy and lactation period.

Variable	6th Month of Pregnancy	Delivery	1th Month of Lactation	6th Month of Lactation
Weight (kg)	70.3 ± 9.0 ^{b}	82.5 ± 10.8 ^{a,c,d}	69.1 ± 9.7 ^{b}	66.2 ± 9.4 ^{b}
Height (m)	1.61 ± 0.1	1.61 ± 0.1	1.61 ± 0.1	1.61 ± 0.1
BMI (kg/m^2)	27.1 ± 3.2 ^{b}	31.9 ± 3.9 ^{a,c,d}	26.5 ± 3.5 ^{b}	25.5 ± 3.4 ^{b}
Nutritional Status				
Underweight (%)	4.4	0	0	0
Normal Weight (%)	46.7	42.2	40.8	37.2
Overweight (%)	37.8	38.3	44.4	46.7
Obese (%)	11.1	19.5	14.8	16.1
Gestational age at birth (weeks)	——	39 ± 1	——	——
Vaginal delivery (%)	——	55	——	——
Cesarean delivery (%)	——	45	——	——
Gender: male (%)	——	53	——	——
Gender: female (%)	——	47	——	——
Infant Weight (g)	——	4251 ± 489 ^{d}	4619 ± 619	7916 ± 852 ^{b}
Infant Height (cm)	——	47.9 ± 4.2 ^{d}	53.9 ± 5.8	66.9 ± 6.4 ^{b}

Values are shown as mean ± S.D., or as a percentage (%); BMI, body mass index = kg/m^2. Statistical significance ($p < 0.05$). ^{a}: Significantly different from the 6th month of pregnancy; ^{b}: significantly different at birth; ^{c}: significantly different from 1st month of lactation; and ^{d}: significantly different from the 6th month of lactation. One-way ANOVA and Bonferroni test.

3.2. *Daily Intake According to Food Groups during Pregnancy and Lactation*

Table 3 shows the dietary intake during the period studied. As expected at 6th month of lactation, a general reduction of food intake compared to the evaluation at 6th month of pregnancy was observed not produced. However, fruits and vegetables, fish and seafood, oil and fats, and sugar and processed foods consumption were reduced ($p < 0.05$) at the 1st and 6th month of lactation when compared to the 6th month of pregnancy. In addition, consumption of dairy, meat, and eggs was reduced ($p < 0.05$) at 6th month of lactation. Consumption of high-fat foods was not significantly modified during the study. A reduction ($p < 0.05$) of the ingestion of fish and seafood (39.3% at the 1st month of lactation and 54% at the 6th month of lactation) compared to the 6th month of pregnancy was observed.

Table 3. Daily intake according to the food groups consumed by the women during the pregnancy and lactation period.

	Food Groups Intake (g/Day)		
Food Groups	**6th Month of Pregnancy**	**1st Month of Lactation**	**6th Month of Lactation**
Cereals	347.0 ± 59.8	302.7 ± 40.3	299.7 ± 31.7
Fruits and Vegetables	638.9 ± 51.2 ^{b,c}	371.5 ± 54.6 ^{a}	303.6 ± 38.9 ^{a}
Dairy	461.4 ± 40.2 ^{c}	383.6 ± 38.6	332.2 ± 27.6 ^{a}
Meats and Eggs	113. 5 ± 12.5 ^{c}	112.0 ± 10.6 ^{c}	85.2 ± 8.4 ^{a,b}
Fish and Seafood	28.5 ± 6.9 ^{b,c}	17.3 ± 3.3 ^{a}	13.1 ± 2.4 ^{a}
Legumes	20.0 ± 4.4 ^{b}	10.5 ± 2.6 ^{a}	15.9 ± 4.4
High-Lipid Foods	47.1 ± 10.9	38.6 ± 9.7	37.1 ± 8.9
Oils and Fats	39.8 ± 7.3 ^{b,c}	23.5 ± 5.5 ^{a}	22.6 ± 4.4 ^{a}
Sugar and Processed Foods	537.7 ± 53.5 ^{b,c}	368.6 ± 48.6 ^{a}	390.3 ± 41.7 ^{a}

Value are shown as mean ± S.D. Statistical significance ($p < 0.05$). ^{a}: Significantly different from the 6th month of pregnancy; ^{b}: significantly different from the 1st month of lactation; and ^{c}: significantly different the 6th month of lactation. The food was organized in nine groups according to the methodology described in the text. One-way ANOVA and Bonferroni test.

3.3. *Energy, Nutrients, and Most Relevant Fatty Acid Intake during Pregnancy and Lactation*

Table 4 shows the energy, nutrients, and the most relevant fatty acids intake of the sample. At the 1st and 6th month of lactation, a significant reduction in the energy and carbohydrate intake compared to the 6th month of pregnancy was observed. No significant modification in the intake of protein, fiber, and fat was observed. Table 4 also shows the daily intake of the most relevant fatty acids during pregnancy and lactation. During the study, women had a high intake of saturated fatty acid (SFA), total *n*-6 fatty acids, LA, and AA, together with an adequate intake of total monounsaturated fatty acid (MUFA) and total polyunsaturated fatty acid (PUFA) and a low intake of total *n*-3 fatty acids ALA, EPA, and DHA. At the 1st month of lactation a significant reduction of the intake of EPA and DHA (50% and 33%, respectively) was produced, and at the 6th month this reduction was 50% for both LCPUFA, compared to the values at the 6th month of pregnancy. The rest of the most relevant fatty acids and the *n*-6/*n*-3 PUFA ratio were not significantly modified.

3.4. *Fatty Acid Composition of Erythrocyte Phospholipids*

Table 5 shows the fatty acid composition of erythrocyte phospholipids at the 6th month of pregnancy, at the delivery and at the 1st and 6th month of lactation. No significant changes were produced for SFA, MUFA, PUFA, LCPUFA, and *n*-6 LCPUFA when compared to the values for the 6th month of pregnancy and for the 6th month of lactation. However, docosapentaenoic acid (C22:5, *n*-6 DPA) was significantly increased (34.2%) and DHA and total *n*-3 LCPUFA were significantly reduced for the same period (27.6% reduction for DHA and 21.6% reduction for total *n*-3 LCPUFA, compared to the 6th month of pregnancy).

3.5. Composition of the Most Relevant Fatty Acids of Breast Milk during the First Six Months of Lactation

Data from Table 6 shows that the composition of the majority of the fatty acids from milk is maintained during the period studied, with the exception of DHA, LCPUFA, and *n*-3 LCPUFA, which were significantly reduced from the 4th month of lactation. It is interesting to mention that at the 6th month of lactation the levels of DHA, LCPUFA, and *n*-3 LCPUFA were even lower ($p < 0.05$) than the values observed at the 4th month of lactation. In addition, the DHA was reduced by 38.5% at the 4th month of lactation and by 64.1% at the 6th month of lactation, compared to the values obtained at the 1st month of lactation. The reduction of *n*-3 LCPUFA is reflected in the significant increase of the *n*-6/*n*-3 LCPUFA ratio.

4. Discussion

A woman's diet during pregnancy and lactation has a fundamental role in the adequate contribution of macro and micronutrients for her infant during the fetal life and during lactation [22,23]. The tissue levels of fatty acids in a woman during pregnancy and lactation are directly related to her diet, her reserve capacity, and her metabolic utilization of fatty acids (synthesis, oxidation, transport, etc.) [24,25]. Therefore, the diet and the metabolism of fatty acids of women during pregnancy and lactation have a relevant role in determining the levels of LCPUFA present in erythrocytes and breast milk [26,27]. The availability of LCPUFA for the infant is directly related to the transfer of these fatty acids from the mother to her offspring, first through the placenta (intra-uterine life) [28] and then through lactation [29]. Regarding AA and DHA, their availability will depend on the intake of foods that provided these fatty acids [30] and/or from the capacity of the mother to form these fatty acids from their metabolic precursors [31]. According to our results we concluded that the Chilean women evaluated have a high intake of *n*-6 PUFA, LA, and AA (Table 4), and a low intake of *n*-3 PUFA, ALA, EPA, and DHA (Table 4). In this context, is also remarkable that among LCPUFA, DHA is one the fatty acid with the most important metabolic characteristics for the physiological period studied [28,32]. The low intake of foods that are natural sources of DHA, such as fish or seafood, as was observed in our study (Table 3), added to an excessive intake of foods that are high in *n*-6 fatty acids, especially LA (e.g., consumption of soy or sunflower oil), which can produce a reduction of the capacity of the mother for transferring DHA to her offspring during pregnancy and breast feeding [13,26,27]. In our sample, DHA levels in breast milk were reduced by 38.5% at the 4th month, by 48.7% at the 5th month, and by 64.1% at the 6th month of lactation compared with the 1st month of lactation (Table 6). This situation was not produced for AA and LA in erythrocytes and breast milk because of the adequate consumption of foods considered good sources of these fatty acids (Table 3).

The reserve capacity of women for LCPUFA, particularly DHA, is sensitive to the number of pregnancies, because it is produced by a significant decrease in the tissue levels and availability of DHA after frequent pregnancies [28,30,33]. In addition, another interesting aspect to consider is the activity of the Δ-5 and Δ-6 desaturases, key enzymes for the synthesis of LCPUFA from their specific precursors [8,31]. The presence of polymorphisms in the genes encoding these enzymes may produce a lower synthesis of both *n*-6 and *n*-3 LCPUFA, but being the diet sufficient in AA, the effect of polymorphism should be more deleterious for the availability of DHA than AA [34]. Is important to emphasize that the dietary imbalance of *n*-6 to *n*-3 PUFA can lower the synthesis of *n*-3 LCPUFA, particularly DHA, because of the competition generated between the respective precursors for the active sites of desaturase enzymes [6,8,35]. An excess of *n*-6 fatty acid (such as LA) may decrease the synthesis of DHA from ALA [36]. The increment in the values for DPAn-6 (Table 5) may be a metabolic compensatory mechanism to form LCPUFA because of the reduction of the *n*-3 LCPUFA (DHA), an aspect that remains to be studied. The synthesis of LCPUFA, as well as the availability of precursors and the activity of Δ-5 and Δ-6 desaturase enzymes, is also dependent on the availability of specific nutrients, such as zinc, magnesium, calcium, vitamin B6, and vitamin C [37]. It is also interesting that while the synthesis of DHA from ALA may be sufficient for the adult human in normal physiological conditions [38], some diseases, such as non-alcoholic fatty liver, a pathology very prevalent in populations that are overweight or obese [39] (in our study, women who were overweight or obese reached 48.9% at 6th month of pregnancy), which reduces the activity of Δ-5 and Δ-6 desaturase enzymes [40], could adversely affect the synthesis of DHA, decreasing the levels of *n*-3 LCPUFA in erythrocytes and breast milk, as was observed in this work (Tables 5 and 6). Another aspect observed in this study was the increase in weight of the women from the 6th month of pregnancy until the delivery (average 12.2 kg), in addition to the high prevalence of overweight and obese women at the end of pregnancy (62.8%), along with the birth weight of children, which, on average, was 4.25 kg. In this context, previous studies suggest that Chilean women during the fertile age show a fast and growing tendency towards obesity [41], and a high prevalence of being overweight (50%) and obese (20%) is observed in pregnant Chilean women [42]. This nutritional situation has been related to (i) the increasing tendency of the Chilean newborns to have a weight at birth higher than 4.0 kg [43] and (ii) a high number of births by caesarian intervention, which are associated with overweight and obesity of pregnant women (up to 35%) [44].

In relation to the Chilean population, Bascuñán et al. [21] reported that women in the 3rd trimester of pregnancy with a low intake of DHA showed low levels of this fatty acid in erythrocyte phospholipids. In the population evaluated in this study, it was observed that DHA levels in erythrocytes were significantly decreased at the 6th month of lactation (Table 5) and the content of DHA in breast milk also decreased ($p < 0.05$), starting from the 4th month of lactation (Table 6). In this same context, Valenzuela et al. [15] reported that in Chilean pregnant women, who included in their diet chia oil ("*Salvia hispanica* L.", 60% ALA) instead of the traditionally consumed oils (soy and sunflower oil) from the 6th month of pregnancy and until the 6th month of lactation, it a significant increase of DHA levels in breast milk was produced, but only until the 3rd month of lactation, without modification of the AA levels during the 6th month of lactation. The same authors reported that AA and DHA in erythrocyte phospholipids were not modified during the dietary intervention [15], suggesting that the ingestion of oils with high content of ALA (such as chia oil) would not be entirely efficient to increase the levels of DHA in breast milk during a lactation period up to three months [15].

Concerning the actual background of *n*-3 LCPUFA, dietary strategies have been developed to improve the quality of the diet of women during pregnancy and lactation through educational programs focused on promoting consumption of foods that provide DHA (especially from marine origin) [45–47]. However, it is not easy to modify the dietary habits of women during these periods [45,47], which adds to the concern that currently exists about the contamination of foods from marine origin (heavy metals, dioxins, PGB, etc.) and the questioning in the population about "possible adverse effects" of seafood consumption [48–50]. It is remarkable that, in the present study, it was observed that women significantly decreased fish intake after the delivery (Table 3), even though they were advised by professional nutritionist that they should increase the consumption of fish and other foods from marine origin. In this regard, the decrease of DHA levels ($p < 0.05$) observed in erythrocytes and breast milk in women's sample (Tables 5 and 6) may be a concern, as it has been previously reported that higher levels of DHA in breast milk are associated with better academic performance, particularly in mathematics, in long-term studies on children [51]. Addressing this dietary and nutritional problem, various studies have used supplements containing DHA or DHA-added foods, evidencing that an increase in the intake of DHA increases the content of the fatty acid in erythrocytes and subsequently in breast milk in pregnant and lactating women [52–55]. In consistent with this same direction, the Chilean Ministry of Health has developed a food program that benefits (free of cost) all women during pregnancy and lactation, providing a dairy drink containing DHA (60 mg/200 mL of product), and recommending the intake of two daily portions (120 mg DHA/day) [56]. Although the program began in 2009, there are no current results regarding the impact of this dairy product, either on DHA levels in erythrocytes and breast milk or on scholarly performance. The results of this program are currently being assessed.

Table 4. Energy, nutrients, and most relevant fatty acid consumed by the women during the pregnancy and lactation period.

	Time of Study					
Energy/Nutrients/Fatty Acid	**6th Month of Pregnancy**	**Adequacy (%) [Φ]**	**1st Month of Lactation**	**Adequacy (%) [Φ]**	**6th Month of Lactation**	**Adequacy (%) [Φ]**
Energy (kcal)	2721.4 ± 254.5 [b,c]	126.9 ± 18.6 [b,c]	2157.6 ± 219.3 [a]	92.4 ± 8.9 [a]	2110.2 ± 231.4 [a]	96.2 ± 9.2 [a]
Protein (g)	97.1 ± 26.6	139.6 ± 35.4	86.8 ± 29.7	121.1 ± 27.5	81.4 ± 32.6	123.6 ± 27.9
Carbohydrate (g)	442.4 ± 75.8 [b,c]	121.8 ± 21.5 [b,c]	278.4 ± 61.1 [a]	83.1 ± 9.2 [a]	261.5 ± 55.9 [a]	82.1 ± 8.7 [a]
Fiber (g)	32.6 ± 12.4	116.6 ± 25.8	22.3 ± 8.1	76.8 ± 14.6	25.7 ± 11.7	79.6 ± 15.8
Fat (g)	90.9 ± 31.1	129.1 ± 23.5	82.0 ± 26.6	115.4 ± 16.8	86.9 ± 28.4	118.7 ± 19.0
SFA (g)	38.5 ± 4.8	154.5 ± 44.3	32.6 ± 3.9	135.4 ± 33.2	34.8 ± 2.8	145.1 ± 36.8
MUFA (g)	24.7 ± 3.7	102.2 ± 10.5	22.9 ± 2.9	95.8 ± 9.9	25.7 ± 2.9	101.8 ±10.1
PUFA (g)	25.6 ± 3.1	98.3 ± 9.5	24.4 ± 7.4	101.1 ± 11.4	25.3 ± 7.4	95.2 ± 10.2
n-3 fatty acid (g)	2.96 ± 0.92	59.4 ± 5.8	2.68 ± 0.5	61.9 ± 6.8	2.75 ± 0.5	47.1 ± 5.1
n-6 fatty acid (g)	22.5 ± 3.23	161.8 ± 15.4	21.4 ± 2.6	155.3 ± 18.9	22.4 ± 2.6	143.3 ± 14.4
18:2*n*-6 (LA) (g)	18.5 ± 1.27	152.2 ± 19.3	18.5 ± 2.1	168.5 ± 20.3	21.1 ± 2.2	149.1 ± 14.8
18:3*n*-3 (ALA) (g)	2.78 ± 0.90	68.7 ± 10.9	2.54 ± 0.4	71.4 ± 9.3	2.68 ± 0.6	59.4 ± 8.5
20:4*n*-6 (AA) (g)	1.57 ± 0.03	191.5 ± 23.5	1.06 ± 0.02	132.5 ± 25.4	1.12 ± 0.05	145 ± 27.5
20:5*n*-3 (EPA) (g)	0.04 ± 0.01 [b,c]	41.4 ± 8.8 [b,c]	0.02 ± 0.005 [a]	23.8 ± 5.3 [a]	0.02 ± 0.005 [a]	25.2 ± 5.0 [a]
22:6*n*-3 (DHA) (g)	0.06 ± 0.01 [b,c]	30.1 ± 3.8 [b,c]	0.04 ± 0.005 [a]	20.8 ± 2.5 [a]	0.03 ± 0.005 [a]	16.9 ± 1.8 [a]
n-6/*n*-3 PUFA ratio	7.60 ± 0.61	—	7.99 ± 0.64	—	8.15 ± 0.72	—

Values are shown as the mean ± S.D.; [Φ] adequacy: (nutrient intake/nutrient daily recommendation) × 100; for this nutrient, energy or fatty acid, the proposed recommendation is "as low possible while consuming a nutritionally adequate diet". [a]: Significantly different from the 6th month of pregnancy; [b]: significantly different from the 1st month of lactation; and [c]: significantly different from the 6th month of lactation. The food was organized in nine groups according to the methodology described in the text. One-way ANOVA and Bonferroni test. Saturated fatty acids (SFA) correspond to 6:0, 8:0, 10:0, 12:0, 14:0, 16:0, 18:0, 20:0 and 22:0, and 24:0. Monounsaturated fatty acids (MUFA) correspond to 14:1*n*-5, 16:1*n*-7, and 18:1, *n*-9. Polyunsaturated fatty acids (PUFA) correspond to 18:2*n*-6, 18:3, *n*-3, 20:4*n*-6, 20:5*n*-3, 22:5*n*-3, and 22:6*n*-3.

Table 5. Fatty acid composition in erythrocyte phospholipids of the women during the pregnancy and lactation period.

	Time of Study			
	6th Month of Pregnancy	Delivery	1st Month of Lactation	6th Month of Lactation
Fatty Acid	Fatty Acid Composition (FAME)			
C16:0	33.5 ± 3.7	32.5 ± 3.9	30.8 ± 2.9	31.4 ± 3.2
C18:0	16.2 ± 1.2	18.9 ± 1.7	17.9 ± 1.6	18.6 ± 1.7
C18:1*n*-9	11.8 ± 1.1	12.8 ± 1.6	13.5 ± 1.8	12.7 ± 1.1
C18:2*n*-6 (LA)	12.6 ± 1.0	12.8 ± 1.1	12.5 ± 1.3	12.4 ± 0.9
C18:3*n*-3 (ALA)	1.06 ± 0.1	1.09 ± 0.2	1.12 ± 0.1	1.14 ± 0.2
C20:4*n*-6 (AA)	12.9 ± 1.2	12.5 ± 1.4	12.1 ± 1.0	11.8 ± 1.3
C20:5*n*-3 (EPA)	0.98 ± 0.1	0.95 ± 0.1	1.03 ± 0.2	0.93 ± 0.2
C22:5*n*-6 (DPAn-6)	0.73 ± 0.05 [d]	0.76 ± 0.05	0.81 ± 0.1	0.98 ± 0.1 [a]
C22:5*n*-6 (DPAn-3)	0.57 ± 0.04	0.62 ± 0.05	0.67 ± 0.05	0.70 ± 0.1
C22:6*n*-3 (DHA)	4.16 ± 0.6 [d]	4.03 ± 0.4	3.96 ± 0.3	3.01 ± 0.2 [a]
SFA	52.6 ± 3.2	54.6 ± 4.3	52.8 ± 3.2	51.8 ± 3.8
MUFA	13.5 ± 1.4	15.6 ± 1.7	16.8 ± 1.9	14.6 ± 1.6
PUFA	33.9 ± 2.8	29.8 ± 2.5	30.4 ± 3.1	33.6 ± 2.9
LCPUFA	19.7 ± 1.6	19.1 ± 1.4	18.9 ± 1.2	17.6 ± 1.0
n-6 LCPUFA	13.7 ± 1.5	13.4 ± 1.2	13.1 ± 1.0	12.9 ± 1.1
n-3 LCPUFA	6.00 ± 0.6 [d]	5.70 ± 0.5	5.80 ± 0.04	4.70 ± 0.05 [a]
n-6/*n*-3 LCPUFA ratio	2.28 ± 0.05	2.35 ± 0.04	2.26 ± 0.05	2.75 ± 0.05

Data are expressed as g fatty acid per 100 g FAME and represent the mean ± SD for $n = 60$ women. Statistical significance ($p < 0.05$). [a]: Significantly different from the 6th month of pregnancy; [d]: significantly different from the 6th month of lactation. One-way ANOVA and Bonferroni test. The identification of saturated and unsaturated fatty acids and their relationships are shown in Table 4.

Table 6. Composition of most relevant fatty acid from breast milk of the women during the lactation period studied.

	Time of Study					
FA Composition	**1st Month**	**2rd Month**	**3rd Month**	**4th Month**	**5th Month**	**6th Month**
C12:0	2.75 ± 0.2	2.64 ± 0.2	2.29 ± 0.1	2.84 ± 0.2	2.55 ± 0.2	2.34 ± 0.1
C14:0	6.92 ± 0.4	6.17 ± 0.5	6.34 ± 0.4	6.19 ± 0.5	5.98 ± 0.4	5.83 ± 0.6
C16:0	25.5 ± 2.9	24.3 ± 2.5	25.1 ± 2.8	25.7 ± 3.1	24.9± 2.8	24.6 ± 2.4
C18:0	4.15 ± 0.5	4.23 ± 0.4	4.38 ± 0.6	4.56 ± 0.4	5.01± 0.5	4.09 ± 0.5
C18:1*n*-9	33.2 ± 3.9	33.1 ± 3.7	35.2 ± 4.0	37.5 ± 4.5	37.7 ± 3.5	40.7 ± 4.6
C18:2*n*-6 (LA)	18.1 ± 2.1	18.7 ± 1.9	17.2 ± 2.0	16.8 ± 1.7	17.0 ± 1.5	16.8 ± 1.3
C18:3*n*-3 (ALA)	2.12 ± 0.3	2.29 ± 0.4	1.99 ± 0.3	1.92 ± 0.4	1.85 ± 0.2	1.79 ± 0.2
C20:4*n*-6 (AA)	0.75 ± 0.1	0.79 ± 0.1	0.74 ± 0.1	0.72 ± 0.05	0.68 ± 0.1	0.70 ± 0.05
C20:5*n*-3 (EPA)	0.13 ± 0.04	0.11 ± 0.02	0.12 ± 0.03	0.09 ± 0.03	0.11 ± 0.03	0.09 ± 0.02
C22:6*n*-3 (DHA)	0.39 ± 0.04 [d,e,f]	0.37 ± 0.04 [d,e,f]	0.36 ± 0.03 [d,e,f]	0.24 ± 0.02 [a,b,c,f]	0.19 ± 0.03 [a,b,c]	0.14 ± 0.02 [a,b,c,d]
SFA	40.5 ± 4.6	39.5 ± 4.3	40.6 ± 3.9	39.5 ± 3.8	38.6 ± 4.8	36.9 ± 3.8
MUFA	36.9 ± 3.2	37.2 ± 3.8	38.9 ± 4.1	40.6 ± 4.0	40.7 ± 4.5	43.1 ± 4.8
PUFA	22.6 ± 2.7	23.3 ± 2.8	20.5 ± 2.5	19.9 ± 2.0	20.7 ± 1.8	20.0 ± 1.6
LCPUFA	1.46 ± 0.1 [d,e,f]	1.40 ± 0.1 [d,e,f]	1.36 ± 0.1 [e,f]	1.19 ± 0.1 [a,b,f]	1.08 ± 0.05 [a,b,c]	0.99 ± 0.05 [a,b,c,d]
n-6 LCPUFA	0.83 ± 0.1	0.85 ± 0.1	0.81 ± 0.1	0.78 ± 0.05	0.74 ± 0.05	0.72 ± 0.05
n-3 LCPUFA	0.63 ± 0.05 [d,e,f]	0.55 ± 0.05 [d,e,f]	0.55 ± 0.04 [d,e,f]	0.41 ± 0.03 [a,b,c,e,f]	0.34 ± 0.02 [a,b,c,d,f]	0.27 ± 0.02 [a,b,c,d,e]
n-6/*n*-3 LCPUFA ratio	1.32 ± 0.1 [b,c,d,e,f]	1.55 ± 0.1 [a,d,e,f]	1.74 ± 0.1 [a,e,f]	1.90 ± 0.2 [a,b,f]	2.18 ± 0.3 [a,b,c]	2.67 ± 0.3 [a,b,c,d]

Data are expressed as g fatty acid per 100 g FAME and represent the mean ± SD for $n = 60$ women. Statistical significance ($p < 0.05$). [a]: Significantly different from the 1st month of lactation; [b]: significantly different from the 2rd month of lactation; [c]: significantly different from the 3rd month of lactation; [d]: significantly different from the 4th month of lactation; [e]: significant difference from de 5th month of lactation; and [f]: significant difference from 6th month of lactation. One-way ANOVA and Bonferroni test. The identification of saturated and unsaturated fatty acids and their relationships are shown in Table 4.

5. Conclusions

This study shows that Chilean women during pregnancy and lactation have a low intake of foods that are natural sources of *n*-3 fatty acids (vegetable oils, fish, and seafood) and a high intake of *n*-6 fatty acid (LA and AA). This dietary situation produced a significant reduction of DHA levels in erythrocytes and breast milk. Therefore, it is necessary to promote the consumption of foods that naturally contain DHA or are fortified with *n*-3 LCPUFA. Another alternative is direct supplementation with DHA during pregnancy and lactation through products now widely available (fish oil or krill oil capsules or microcapsules).

Author Contributions: R.V., K.B., and R.C. designed the study and analyzed and interpreted the data. K.B., R.V., C.B., J.S., and C.P. performed clinical and nutritional evaluations. C.B., K.B., R.C., N.S., F.V., and M.-P.V. conducted the dietary analysis. R.V., K.B., R.C., and A.V. wrote the manuscript. All authors reviewed and approved the final version of the manuscript.

Acknowledgments: Authors are grateful to Department of Nutrition of the Faculty of Medicine of the University of Chile and the Obstetrics and Gynecology Department, Clinical Hospital of the University of Chile, for supporting this study.

References

1. Carlson, S.E.; Colombo, J. Docosahexaenoic Acid and Arachidonic Acid Nutrition in Early Development. *Adv. Pediatr.* **2016**, *63*, 453–471. [CrossRef] [PubMed]
2. Svennerholm, L.; Vanier, M.T. The distribution of lipids in the human nervous system. 3. Fatty acid composition of phosphoglycerides of human foetal and infant brain. *Brain Res.* **1973**, *50*, 341–351. [CrossRef]
3. Birch, E.E.; Hoffman, D.R.; Uauy, R.; Birch, D.G.; Prestidge, C. Visual acuity and the essentiality of docosahexaenoic acid and arachidonic acid in the diet of term infants. *Pediatr. Res.* **1998**, *44*, 201–209. [CrossRef] [PubMed]
4. Uauy, R.; Hoffman, D.R.; Peirano, P.; Birch, D.G.; Birch, E.E. Essential fatty acids in visual and brain development. *Lipids* **2001**, *36*, 885–895. [CrossRef] [PubMed]
5. González-Mañán, D.; Tapia, G.; Gormaz, J.G.; D'Espessailles, A.; Espinosa, A.; Masson, L.; Varela, P.; Valenzuela, A.; Valenzuela, R. Bioconversion of α-linolenic acid to *n*-3 LCPUFA and expression of PPAR-alpha, acyl Coenzyme A oxidase 1 and carnitine acyl transferase I are incremented after feeding rats with α-linolenic acid-rich oils. *Food Funct.* **2012**, *3*, 765–772. [CrossRef] [PubMed]
6. Nakamura, M.T.; Nara, T.Y. Structure, function, and dietary regulation of delta6, delta5, and delta9 desaturases. *Annu. Rev. Nutr.* **2004**, *24*, 345–376. [CrossRef] [PubMed]
7. Rincón-Cervera, M.A.; Valenzuela, R.; Hernandez-Rodas, M.C.; Marambio, M.; Espinosa, A.; Mayer, S.; Romero, N.; Barrera, C.; Valenzuela, A.; Videla, L.A. Supplementation with antioxidant-rich extra virgin olive oil prevents hepatic oxidative stress and reduction of desaturation capacity in mice fed a high-fat diet: Effects on fatty acid composition in liver and extrahepatic tissues. *Nutrition* **2016**, *32*, 1254–1267. [CrossRef] [PubMed]
8. Brenna, J.T.; Salem, N., Jr.; Sinclair, A.J.; Cunnane, S.C.; International Society for the Study of Fatty Acids and Lipids, ISSFAL. α-Linolenic acid supplementation and conversion to *n*-3 long-chain polyunsaturated fatty acids in humans. *Prostaglandins Leukot. Essent. Fat. Acids* **2009**, *80*, 85–91. [CrossRef] [PubMed]
9. Lauritzen, L.; Carlson, S.E. Maternal fatty acid status during pregnancy and lactation and relation to newborn and infant status. *Matern. Child Nutr.* **2011**, *7*, 41–58. [CrossRef] [PubMed]
10. Lewis, R.M.; Desoye, G. Placental Lipid and Fatty Acid Transfer in Maternal Overnutrition. *Ann. Nutr. Metab.* **2017**, *70*, 228–231. [CrossRef] [PubMed]
11. Simopoulos, A.P. An Increase in the Omega-6/Omega-3 Fatty Acid Ratio Increases the Risk for Obesity. *Nutrients* **2016**, *8*, 128. [CrossRef] [PubMed]

12. Metherel, A.H.; Lacombe, R.J.S.; Chouinard-Watkins, R.; Hopperton, K.E.; Bazinet, R.P. Complete assessment of whole-body *n*-3 and *n*-6 PUFA synthesis-secretion kinetics and DHA turnover in a rodent model. *J. Lipid Res.* **2018**, *59*, 357–367. [CrossRef] [PubMed]
13. Urwin, H.J.; Zhang, J.; Gao, Y.; Wang, C.; Li, L.; Song, P.; Man, Q.; Meng, L.; Frøyland, L.; Miles, E.A.; et al. Immune factors and fatty acid composition in human milk from river/lake, coastal and inland regions of China. *Br. J. Nutr.* **2013**, *109*, 1949–1961. [CrossRef] [PubMed]
14. Bravi, F.; Wiens, F.; Decarli, A.; Dal Pont, A.; Agostoni, C.; Ferraroni, M. Impact of maternal nutrition on breast-milk composition: A systematic review. *Am. J. Clin. Nutr.* **2016**, *104*, 646–662. [CrossRef] [PubMed]
15. Valenzuela, R.; Bascuñán, K.; Chamorro, R.; Barrera, C.; Sandoval, J.; Puigrredon, C.; Parraguez, G.; Orellana, P.; Gonzalez, V.; Valenzuela, A. Modification of Docosahexaenoic Acid Composition of Milk from Nursing Women Who Received Alpha Linolenic Acid from Chia Oil during Gestation and Nursing. *Nutrients* **2015**, *7*, 6405–6424. [CrossRef] [PubMed]
16. Atalah, E.; Castillo, C.; Castro, R.; Aldea, A. Proposalof a new standard for the nutritional assessment of pregnant women. *Rev. Med. Chile* **1997**, *125*, 1429–1436. [PubMed]
17. European Society for Opinion and Marketing Research. *The ESOMAR Standard Demographic Classification*; ESOMAR: Amsterdam, The Netherlands, 1997.
18. WHO/FAO/UNU. *Human Energy Requirements, Report of a Joint FAO/WHO/UNU Expert Consultation*; Food and Agriculture Organization: Rome, Italy, 2014.
19. Food and Nutrition Board, Institute of Medicine. *Dietary Reference Intakes: Guiding Principles for Nutrition Labeling and Fortification*; Institute of Medicine of the National Academies: Washington, DC, USA, 2001; pp. 1–224.
20. Cerda, R.; Barrera, C.; Arena, M.; Bascuñán, K.A.; Jimenez, G. *Photographic Atlas of Chilean Food and Typical Preparations. National Survey of Food Consumption*, 1st ed.; Government of Chile, Ministry of Health: Santiago, Chile, 2010.
21. Bascuñán, K.A.; Valenzuela, R.; Chamorro, R.; Valencia, A.; Barrera, C.; Puigrredon, C.; Sandoval, J.; Valenzuela, A. Polyunsaturated fatty acid composition of maternal diet and erythrocyte phospholipid status in Chilean pregnant women. *Nutrients* **2014**, *6*, 4918–4934. [CrossRef] [PubMed]
22. Kashtanova, D.A.; Popenko, A.S.; Tkacheva, O.N.; Tyakht, A.B.; Alexeev, D.G.; Boytsov, S.A. Association between the gut microbiota and diet: Fetal life, early childhood, and further life. *Nutrition* **2016**, *32*, 620–627. [CrossRef] [PubMed]
23. Innis, S.M. Metabolic programming of long-term outcomes due to fatty acid nutrition in early life. *Matern. Child Nutr.* **2011**, *2*, S112–S123. [CrossRef] [PubMed]
24. Berti, C.; Cetin, I.; Agostoni, C.; Desoye, G.; Devlieger, R.; Emmett, P.M.; Ensenauer, R.; Hauner, H.; Herrera, E.; Hoesli, I.; et al. Pregnancy and Infants' Outcome: Nutritional and Metabolic Implications. *Crit. Rev. Food Sci. Nutr.* **2016**, *56*, 82–91. [CrossRef] [PubMed]
25. Larqué, E.; Demmelmair, H.; Gil-Sánchez, A.; Prieto-Sánchez, M.T.; Blanco, J.E.; Pagán, A.; Faber, F.L.; Zamora, S.; Parrilla, J.J.; Koletzko, B. Placental transfer of fatty acids and fetal implications. *Am. J. Clin. Nutr.* **2011**, *94*, S1908–S1913. [CrossRef] [PubMed]
26. Peng, Y.; Zhou, T.; Wang, Q.; Liu, P.; Zhang, T.; Zetterström, R.; Strandvik, B. Fatty acid composition of diet, cord blood and breast milk in Chinese mothers with different dietary habits. *Prostaglandins Leukot. Essent. Fat. Acids* **2009**, *81*, 325–330. [CrossRef] [PubMed]
27. Zhang, J.; Wang, C.; Gao, Y.; Li, L.; Man, Q.; Song, P.; Meng, L.; Du, Z.Y.; Miles, E.A.; Lie, Ø.; et al. Different intakes of *n*-3 fatty acids among pregnant women in 3 regions of China with contrasting dietary patterns are reflected in maternal but not in umbilical erythrocyte phosphatidylcholine fatty acid composition. *Nutr. Res.* **2013**, *33*, 613–621. [CrossRef] [PubMed]
28. Gil-Sánchez, A.; Koletzko, B.; Larqué, E. Current understanding of placental fatty acid transport. *Curr. Opin. Clin. Nutr. Metab. Care* **2012**, *15*, 265–272. [CrossRef] [PubMed]
29. Grote, V.; Verduci, E.; Scaglioni, S.; Vecchi, F.; Contarini, G.; Giovannini, M.; Koletzko, B.; Agostoni, C.; European Childhood Obesity Project. Breast milk composition and infant nutrient intakes during the first 12 months of life. *Eur. J. Clin. Nutr.* **2016**, *70*, 250–256. [CrossRef] [PubMed]
30. Larqué, E.; Gil-Sánchez, A.; Prieto-Sánchez, M.T.; Koletzko, B. Omega 3 fatty acids, gestation and pregnancy outcomes. *Br. J. Nutr.* **2012**, *107*, S77–S84. [CrossRef] [PubMed]

31. De la Garza, A.; Montes, R.; Chisaguano, A.M.; Torres-Espínola, F.J.; Arias, M.; de Almeida, L.; Bonilla, M.; Guerendiain, M.; Castellote, A.I.; Segura, M.; et al. Association of maternal weight with FADS and ELOVL genetic variants and fatty acid levels- The PREOBE follow-up. *PLoS ONE* **2017**, *12*, e0179135. [CrossRef] [PubMed]
32. Herrera, E. Implications of dietary fatty acids during pregnancy on placental, fetal and postnatal development—A review. *Placenta* **2002**, *23*, S9–S19. [CrossRef] [PubMed]
33. Cetin, I.; Koletzko, B. Long-chain omega-3 fatty acid supply in pregnancy and lactation. *Curr. Opin. Clin. Nutr. Metab. Care* **2008**, *11*, 297–302. [CrossRef] [PubMed]
34. Glaser, C.; Lattka, E.; Rzehak, P.; Steer, C.; Koletzko, B. Genetic variation in polyunsaturated fatty acid metabolism and its potential relevance for human development and health. *Matern. Child Nutr.* **2011**, *7*, 27–40. [CrossRef] [PubMed]
35. Scholtz, S.A.; Kerling, E.H.; Shaddy, D.J.; Li, S.; Thodosoff, J.M.; Colombo, J.; Carlson, S.E. Docosahexaenoic acid (DHA) supplementation in pregnancy differentially modulates arachidonic acid and DHA status across FADS genotypes in pregnancy. *Prostaglandins Leukot. Essent. Fat. Acids* **2015**, *94*, 29–33. [CrossRef] [PubMed]
36. Lassek, W.D.; Gaulin, S.J. Linoleic and docosahexaenoic acids in human milk have opposite relationships with cognitive test performance in a sample of 28 countries. *Prostaglandins Leukot. Essent. Fat. Acids* **2014**, *91*, 195–201. [CrossRef] [PubMed]
37. Das, U.N. Essential fatty acids: Biochemistry, physiology and pathology. *Biotechnol. J.* **2006**, *1*, 420–439. [CrossRef] [PubMed]
38. Domenichiello, A.F.; Kitson, A.P.; Bazinet, R.P. Is docosahexaenoic acid synthesis from α-linolenic acid sufficient to supply the adult brain? *Prog. Lipid Res.* **2015**, *59*, 54–66. [CrossRef] [PubMed]
39. Valenzuela, R.; Videla, L.A. The importance of the long-chain polyunsaturated fatty acid *n*-6/*n*-3 ratio in development of non-alcoholic fatty liver associated with obesity. *Food Funct.* **2011**, *2*, 644–648. [CrossRef] [PubMed]
40. Araya, J.; Rodrigo, R.; Pettinelli, P.; Araya, A.V.; Poniachik, J.; Videla, L.A. Decreased liver fatty acid delta-6 and delta-5 desaturase activity in obese patients. *Obesity* **2010**, *18*, 1460–1463. [CrossRef] [PubMed]
41. Garmendia, M.L.; Alonso, F.T.; Kain, J.; Uauy, R.; Corvalan, C. Alarming weight gain in women of a post-transitional country. *Public Health Nutr.* **2014**, *17*, 667–673. [CrossRef] [PubMed]
42. Araya, B.M.; Padilla, O.; Garmendia, M.L.; Atalah, E.; Uauy, R. Prevalence of obesity among Chilean women in childbearing ages. *Rev. Med. Chile* **2014**, *142*, 1440–1448.
43. Lopez, P.O.; Bréart, G. Trends in gestational age and birth weight in Chile, 1991-2008. A descriptive epidemiological study. *BMC Pregnancy Childbirth.* **2012**, *12*, 121. [CrossRef] [PubMed]
44. Olmos, P.R.; Borzone, G.R.; Olmos, R.I.; Valencia, C.N.; Bravo, F.A.; Hodgson, M.I.; Belmar, C.G.; Poblete, J.A.; Escalona, M.O.; Gómez, B. Gestational diabetes and pre-pregnancy overweight: Possible factors involved in newborn macrosomia. *J. Obstet. Gynaecol. Res.* **2012**, *38*, 208–214. [CrossRef] [PubMed]
45. Miles, E.A.; Noakes, P.S.; Kremmyda, L.S.; Vlachava, M.; Diaper, N.D.; Rosenlund, G.; Urwin, H.; Yaqoob, P.; Rossary, A.; Farges, M.C.; et al. The Salmon in Pregnancy Study: Study design, subject characteristics, maternal fish and marine *n*-3 fatty acid intake, and marine *n*-3 fatty acid status in maternal and umbilical cord blood. *Am. J. Clin. Nutr.* **2011**, *94*, S1986–S1992. [CrossRef] [PubMed]
46. Fayet-Moore, F.; Baghurst, K.; Meyer, B.J. Four Models Including Fish, Seafood, Red Meat and Enriched Foods to Achieve Australian Dietary Recommendations for *n*-3 LCPUFA for All Life-Stages. *Nutrients* **2015**, *7*, 8602–8614. [CrossRef] [PubMed]
47. Rahmawaty, S.; Lyons-Wall, P.; Charlton, K.; Batterham, M.; Meyer, B.J. Effect of replacing bread, egg, milk, and yogurt with equivalent ω-3 enriched foods on ω-3 LCPUFA intake of Australian children. *Nutrition* **2014**, *30*, 1337–1343. [CrossRef] [PubMed]
48. Yeates, A.J.; Thurston, S.W.; Li, H.; Mulhern, M.S.; McSorley, E.M.; Watson, G.E.; Shamlaye, C.F.; Strain, J.J.; Myers, G.J.; Davidson, P.W.; et al. PUFA Status and Methylmercury Exposure Are Not Associated with Leukocyte Telomere Length in Mothers or Their Children in the Seychelles Child Development Study. *J. Nutr.* **2017**, *147*, 2018–2024. [CrossRef] [PubMed]
49. Golding, J.; Gregory, S.; Emond, A.; Iles-Caven, Y.; Hibbeln, J.; Taylor, C.M. Prenatal mercury exposure and offspring behaviour in childhood and adolescence. *Neurotoxicology* **2016**, *57*, 87–94. [CrossRef] [PubMed]
50. Gil, A.; Gil, F. Fish, a Mediterranean source of *n*-3 PUFA: Benefits do not justify limiting consumption. *Br. J. Nutr.* **2015**, *113*, S58–S67. [CrossRef] [PubMed]

51. Lassek, W.D.; Gaulin, S.J. Maternal milk DHA content predicts cognitive performance in a sample of 28 nations. *Matern. Child Nutr.* **2015**, *11*, 773–779. [CrossRef] [PubMed]
52. Smit, E.N.; Koopmann, M.; Boersma, E.R.; Muskiet, F.A. Effect of supplementation of arachidonic acid (AA) or a combination of AA plus docosahexaenoic acid on breastmilk fatty acid composition. *Prostaglandins Leukot. Essent. Fat. Acids* **2000**, *62*, 335–340. [CrossRef] [PubMed]
53. Sherry, C.L.; Oliver, J.S.; Marriage, B.J. Docosahexaenoic acid supplementation in lactating women increases breast milk and plasma docosahexaenoic acid concentrations and alters infant omega 6:3 fatty acid ratio. *Prostaglandins Leukot. Essent. Fat. Acids* **2015**, *95*, 63–69. [CrossRef] [PubMed]
54. Echeverría, F.; Valenzuela, R.; Hernandez-Rodas, M.C.; Valenzuela, A. Docosahexaenoic acid (DHA), a fundamental fatty acid for the brain: New dietary sources. *Prostaglandins Leukot. Essent. Fat. Acids* **2017**, *124*, 1–10. [CrossRef] [PubMed]
55. Atalah, S.E.; Araya, B.M.; Rosselot, P.G.; Araya, L.H.; Vera, A.G.; Andreu, R.R.; Barba, G.C.; Rodriguez, L. Consumption of a DHA-enriched milk drink by pregnant and lactating women, on the fatty acid composition of red blood cells, breast milk, and in the newborn. *Arch. Latinoam. Nutr.* **2009**, *59*, 271–277.
56. Contreras, A.; Herrera, Y.; Rodríguez, L.; Pizarro, T.; Atalah, E. Acceptability and consumption of a dairy drink with omega-3 in pregnant and lactating women of the national supplementary program. *Rev. Chil. Nutr.* **2011**, *38*, 313–320.

17

Levels of Growth Factors and IgA in the Colostrum of Women from Burundi and Italy

Daniel Munblit [1,2,3,*,†], Priya Abrol [1,†], Shreya Sheth [1], Li Yan Chow [1], Ekaterina Khaleva [3,4], Alan Asmanov [5], Silvana Lauriola [6], Ezio M. Padovani [6], Pasquale Comberiati [6], Attilio L. Boner [6], John O. Warner [1,3], Robert J. Boyle [1,3,†] and Diego G. Peroni [3,7,*,†]

1 Department of Paediatrics, Imperial College London, London W2 1NY, UK; p.abrol@doctors.org.uk (P.A.); shreyasheth@me.com (S.S.); lychow8@gmail.com (L.Y.C.); j.o.warner@imperial.ac.uk (J.O.W.); r.boyle@nhs.net (R.J.B.)
2 Faculty of Pediatrics, Sechenov University, 119991 Moscow, Russia
3 inVIVO Planetary Health, Group of the Worldwide Universities Network (WUN), 6010 Park Ave, West New York, NJ 07093, USA
4 Department of Paediatrics, Saint-Petersburg State Paediatric Medical University, 194353 Saint-Petersburg, Russia; doctor.khaleva@gmail.com
5 The Research and Clinical Institute for Pediatrics named after Academician Yuri Veltischev of the Pirogov Russian National Research Medical University, 125412 Moscow, Russia; alan-asmanov@yandex.ru
6 Department of Life and Reproduction Sciences, Section of Paediatrics, University of Verona, 37124 Verona, Italy; silvana.lauriola@ospedaleuniverona.it (S.L.); ezio.padovani@univr.it (E.M.P.); pasquale.comberiati@gmail.com (P.C.); attilio.boner@univr.it (A.L.B.)
7 Department of Clinical and Experimental Medicine, Section of Paediatrics, University of Pisa, 56126 Pisa, Italy
* Correspondence: daniel.munblit08@imperial.ac.uk (D.M.); diego.peroni@unipi.it (D.G.P.)
† These authors contributed equally to this work.

Abstract: Colostrum is produced in the first days postpartum. It is a known source of immune mediators for a newborn within the first week of life. Although it is still unclear if colostrum composition varies between populations, recent data suggest differences. Hepatocyte growth factor (HGF); transforming growth factor-β (TGF-β) 1, 2, and 3; and immunoglobulin A (IgA) are key immunological components of colostrum that stimulate neonatal gastrointestinal and immune system development. We aimed to investigate the differences in the concentration between immune markers in the colostrum of mothers living in Burundi and Italy, and to identify the factors associated with differences. In this cross-sectional birth cohort study, a total of 99 colostrum samples from Burundian ($n = 23$) and Italian ($n = 76$) women were collected at 0 to 6 days postpartum. A clinical chemistry analyser was used for IgA quantification and electro-chemiluminescence, for HGF and TGFβ1-3 assessment. A univariate analysis and multivariate linear regression model were used for statistical testing. The concentrations of TGF-β2 ($p = 0.01$) and IgA ($p < 0.01$) were significantly higher in the colostrum from the women residing in Burundi than in Italy, both in a univariate analysis and upon the adjustment for confounding factors. A similar trend is seen for HGF, reaching statistical significance upon a multivariate analysis. We found a moderate to strong positive correlation between the TGF-β isoforms and IgA concentration in both countries ($p < 0.01$), with stronger concentration in the colostrum from Burundi. The results of this study are in support of previous data, suggesting that concentration of the immune active molecules is higher in the human milk of women residing in developing countries. However, with a small sample size, caution must be applied, as the findings require further confirmation. Future work should also be focused on other factors (e.g., lipid and microbial composition), as well as the investigation into colostrum and between populations comparison, adjusting for potential confounders.

Keywords: breast milk; human milk; colostrum; IgA; HGF; TGF-β; growth factors; geographical location

1. Introduction

Human milk is a first source of nutrition for a newborn child and is globally accepted to be beneficial for the developing infant [1]. The advantages of breastfeeding include the transference of multiple immune factors, maturation of gut immunity, and anti-inflammatory effects [2]. The rising burden of non-communicable diseases increased an interest in their association with human milk (HM) cytokine composition [3,4]. It has been hypothesised that immune mediators in HM may play an important role in both the maturation of the newborn intestine and in stimulating immune system activation [5]. Previous prospective and longitudinal studies provided conflicting evidence on a breastfeeding protective effect on non-communicable [6] and communicable [7] outcomes, and have led to a suggestion that it may be due to the diversity of human milk composition between individuals [8].

Colostrum is the first human milk produced within the first days postpartum, and it allows for the transport of a high concentration of growth factors per unit volume. Hepatocyte growth factor (HGF) is secreted into human colostrum by multipotent mesenchymal stem cells [9]. HGF is expressed in BM as well as in the epithelial cells of the female reproductive tract and the gastrointestinal tract [10]. Patki et al. found greater concentrations of HGF in colostrum compared with paired umbilical cord serum samples [11]. It has been postulated that an elevated concentration of HGF in human milk is needed to maintain proliferation, angiogenesis, and intestinal tissue maturation through paracrine and endocrine signaling [9]. Additionally, HGF may regulate the proinflammatory vascular endothelial growth factor (VEGF) production from endothelial cells [12], and provide a complementary effect with VEGF on the neonatal gut [9].

Transforming growth factor-β (TGF-β) is an anti-inflammatory cytokine found in human colostrum. Throughout lactation, all three isoforms of the TGF-β superfamily (TGF-β1, TGF-β2, and TGF-β3) are produced, of which 95% is TGF-β2. The known effects of maternal TGF-β include oral and gut tolerance through the immunosuppressive action on neonatal T-lymphocytes [13,14]. Enteral exposures trigger neonatal antigen presenting cells in mucosal surfaces, to suppress inflammatory immune responses to common antigens via TGF-β2 mediated tolerance [15], which may lead to the inhibition of antigen specific T-lymphocytes' proliferation [16]. It has been shown that intact cow's milk protein (bovine alpha-S1 casein) is found in human colostrum, and a failure to tolerate this antigen could lead to a sensitisation for cow's milk protein in the infant [17]. Some authors suggest that the TGF-β presence in colostrum is of a particular importance, as it may be partially responsible for the control of inflammatory processes that could lead to atopic sensitisation [18–20].

TGF-β is also responsible for the antibodies produced by B-lymphocytes' class-switching, in particular, secretory immunoglobulin A (IgA). Japanese researchers found a correlation between the TGF-β1 concentration in human milk and IgA levels in the infant serum [21]. IgA secretion in human milk is vital to provide passive immune protection, as the newborn infant is unable to synthesise antibodies until 30 days postpartum [22]. Therefore, TGF-β mediated tolerance and IgA antibody synthesis are both key components for infant immune development.

Previous studies have highlighted the importance of maternal and environmental factors' influence on BM composition. These include both genetic and environmental factors, such as diet, psychological background, and maternal atopic status [23–26]. Very few studies have assessed the levels of immune mediators in the human milk of women from Africa and Europe; Holmlund and colleagues identified that Swedish mothers born in Mali retained higher breast milk TGF-β concentrations in comparison to women of Swedish origin [27]. The difference in association between the level of TGF-β in colostrum and ethnicity was supported further by Aihara Y. et al., explaining it by variations in the consumption of animal protein and the mode of delivery of lactating mothers in Japan and Nepal [28]. Recently, Ruiz and Espinosa-Martos et al. assessed the human milk immunological composition of women residing in different geographical locations, including Europe and Africa, showing a substantial variation within and, particularly among, human subpopulations [29].

Based on the The United Nations Children's Fund (UNICEF) reported childhood mortality rate under the age of five, in Italy, it is 4 per 1000, whereas in Burundi, the rate is 104 per 1000, with 52% of these deaths being attributable to fatal childhood infections [30,31]. We hypothesised that the levels of immune active components, which may be able to reduce neonatal infection risk, in colostrum will be higher in the colostrum of Burundi women. Evidence suggests that not only bacterial exposures, but also a large range of other maternal and environmental factors, may be attributed to changes in the growth factors and IgA concentration [32], subsequently impacting the risk of non-communicable diseases [33] or infection [34] development.

The aim of the study was to investigate the levels of all of the TGF-β isoforms (TGF-β1, 2, and 3), HGF, and IgA in the colostrum samples from Italy and Burundi, and to assess the potential factors responsible for the differences.

2. Materials and Methods

2.1. Design

This cross-sectional birth cohort study involved mother–newborn pairs recruited from postnatal wards. The inclusion criteria for the study were healthy term infants and their mothers willing to comply with the study procedures. The exclusion criteria were maternal immunosuppressive treatment during lactation, or severe illness; infants with a major birth defect, admitted to neonatal intensive care; other severe illnesses; and inability to express colostrum.

Informed consent was obtained from all of the participants who volunteered to take part, along with a colostrum sample and a questionnaire.

The investigations and sample collection were conducted following ethical approval by the ethics committees in the two countries participating in this study, the Ethical Committee of the Azienda Ospedaliera di Verona (Italy) (approval N°1288) and the Ngozi Burundi Hospital approval, which was in accordance with Italian standards.

2.2. Setting

The women were approached at postnatal wards in two very different environments, namely: in a developed country, G.B. Rossi Hospital, Verona, Italy, and in a developing country, the Hospital of Ngozi, Republic of Burundi. All of the samples were collected in the hospital by a highly skilled member of a research team. The clinical data on the participating infants and mothers were extracted from the hospital notes.

2.3. Colostrum Samples Collection

The participants were given sterile tubes to collect their own colostrum (once, in the first six days of life). Instructions were given for the collection of samples by manual expression or by collecting the drip from the contralateral breast during feeding. The colostrum samples were frozen at −20 °C in Burundi and −50 °C in Verona, within 12 h of collection, until their transfer to London. All of the samples were transported to Imperial College London, at −70 °C, where the samples were stored at −80 °C until analysis. All of the samples were analysed at Imperial College London facilities to ensure standardisation. After thawing, the samples were centrifuged at 1500× g for 15 min at 4 °C. The lipid layer was removed with a pipette tip, and the aqueous fraction was analysed for immune modulators.

2.4. Immune Mediators Measurement

We used electro-chemiluminescence to measure the immune mediators in the colostrum samples, for HGF and TGFβ1-3 (MesoScale Discovery, Rockville, MD, USA). LThe laboratory experiments were described in detail elsewhere [26]. In brief, the samples were run in duplicate, according to the manufacturer's protocol, using an 8-point standard curve. No dilution was used for the HGF, and a 1:2 dilution was used for the TGFβ assays, following pilot experiments, which showed that the TGFβ2 level in the undiluted milk samples was often greater than the upper limit of detection.

Using an Abbott Architect clinical chemistry analyser® (Abbott, Abbott Park, IL, USA.), the IgA concentration analysis was conducted as described earlier [35]. The colostrum samples were centrifuged at 3000× g for 15 min at 4 °C to remove the lipaemic interference on analysis. Then, 300 µL of the supernatant was transferred into the cuvettes using pipettes. The samples were diluted to 1:5 for the IgA quantification. The IgA analysis determined the immunoturbidity of the immune insoluble complexes formed in the presence of the reagent. The IgA analysis with the corresponding reagents was performed according to the manufacturer's protocol.

2.5. Data Analysis

Based on previously published research statistical power calculations [36], the sample size of $n = 48$ in the Italy group and $n = 22$ in Burundi group allows for 80% power at a 0.05 significance level, which would allow for detecting a 34% difference between the groups for IgA and 36% for TGF-β in the colostrum. For the purpose of this study, only those samples with all data points available were included in the statistical analysis. The differences between the concentrations of HGF; TGF-β1, 2, and 3; and IgA in the Burundian and Italian colostrum samples were calculated with GraphPad Prism, Version 6.0 (GraphPad Software, La Jolla, CA, USA), for parametric data, using an unpaired t-test, Pearson's chi-squared test, and Fisher's exact test. The Mann–Whitney U test and Kruskal–Wallis one-way analysis of variance (ANOVA) were used for the non-parametric data. The correlations between TGF-β1, 2, and 3 with IgA were determined by Spearman's rank correlation coefficient. The multivariate linear regression using a backward stepwise entry, was conducted using IBM SPSS Statistics software for Windows, Version 20 (IBM Corp, Armonk, NY, USA). The factors in the regression model included the maternal age, country of origin, animal contact, and parity. The results were considered significant when the p-values were reported at a level less than 0.05.

3. Results

3.1. Study Participants Demographics

Based on the questionnaire completed by all of the participants in the study, the demographic characteristics of the cohort have been assessed. Out of the total 117 women providing colostrum (Italy, $n = 76$; Burundi, $n = 41$), the full demographic details were available for 99 mothers only, and were included in the analysis (Italy, $n = 76$; Burundi, $n = 23$). Their demographic data is shown in Table 1. The maternal and parturition characteristics were different between the samples from Burundi and Italy. The women in Burundi were younger than the women in Italy ($p < 0.01$) and had more pregnancies ($p < 0.01$). The infants from Burundi were characterised by a lower weight and gestational age ($p < 0.01$ for both).

Table 1. Characteristics of study participants between sites of collection.

Characteristics	Burundi	Italy	p-Value
Maternal age (years), mean (SD) [1]	24.30 (5.57)	37.39 (5.38)	**<0.01**
Birth weight (grams), mean (SD) [1]	2831 (746.8)	3328 (476.9)	**<0.01**
Gestational age (weeks), mean (SD) [1]	36.48 (1.12)	39.36 (1/34)	**<0.01**
Gender (male), n (%) [2]	15/25 (60)	41/76 (54)	0.60
Mode of delivery (c-section), n (%) [3]	7/21 (33)	14/76 (18)	0.14
Parity, mean (SD) [4]	2.04 (1.15)	0.81 (0.80)	**<0.01**
Maternal smoking, n (%) [5]	2/23 (9)	3/76 (4)	0.33
Antenatal infections [6]	6/23 (26)	29/76 (38)	0.29
Regular animal contact [6]	10/23 (43)	27/76 (36)	0.49
Time of colostrum collection (hours), mean (SD) [1]	58.29 (26.4)	51.13 (32.61)	0.28

Statistical methods used: [1] Unpaired t tests. [2] Pearson chi-squared and data dichotomised into groups of female and male. [3] Pearson chi-squared test and data dichotomised into groups of vaginal delivery and caesarean section (c-section) delivery. [4] Mann–Whitney U test. [5] Fisher's exact test. [6] Pearson chi-squared test. Statistically significant results presented in bold. SD—standard deviation.

3.2. *Quantification of Factors in Colostrum Samples*

3.2.1. Univariate Analysis Results

The analysis of the TGF-β1 and TGF-β3 raw concentrations found no significant difference between the Burundian and Italian women. The HGF levels did not differ significantly, but there was a trend for higher levels in the colostrum of the Burundian women (2785 pg/mL and 697.4–10,107 vs. 1316, 785–2628, for the median and interquartile range (IQR), respectively, $p = 0.08$) (Figure 1a). The TGF-β2 concentrations in the Burundi women's colostrum were significantly higher than the colostrum samples from the Italian women (59,708 and 36,865–113,221 pg/mL vs. 33,176 and 18,046–66,520 pg/mL, for the median and interquartile range (IQR), respectively, $p = 0.01$) (Figure 1c). The principle concentration of the growth factor found in the human colostrum was dominated by TGF-β2, followed by HGF, TGF-β3, and TGF-β1, respectively.

The concentration of IgA in the colostrum from Burundian mothers was significantly higher than in the Italian colostrum samples (2.78 and 1.45–22.2 g/L vs. 1.48 and 0.89–2.67 g/L, for the median and interquartile range (IQR), respectively, $p < 0.01$) (Figure 1e).

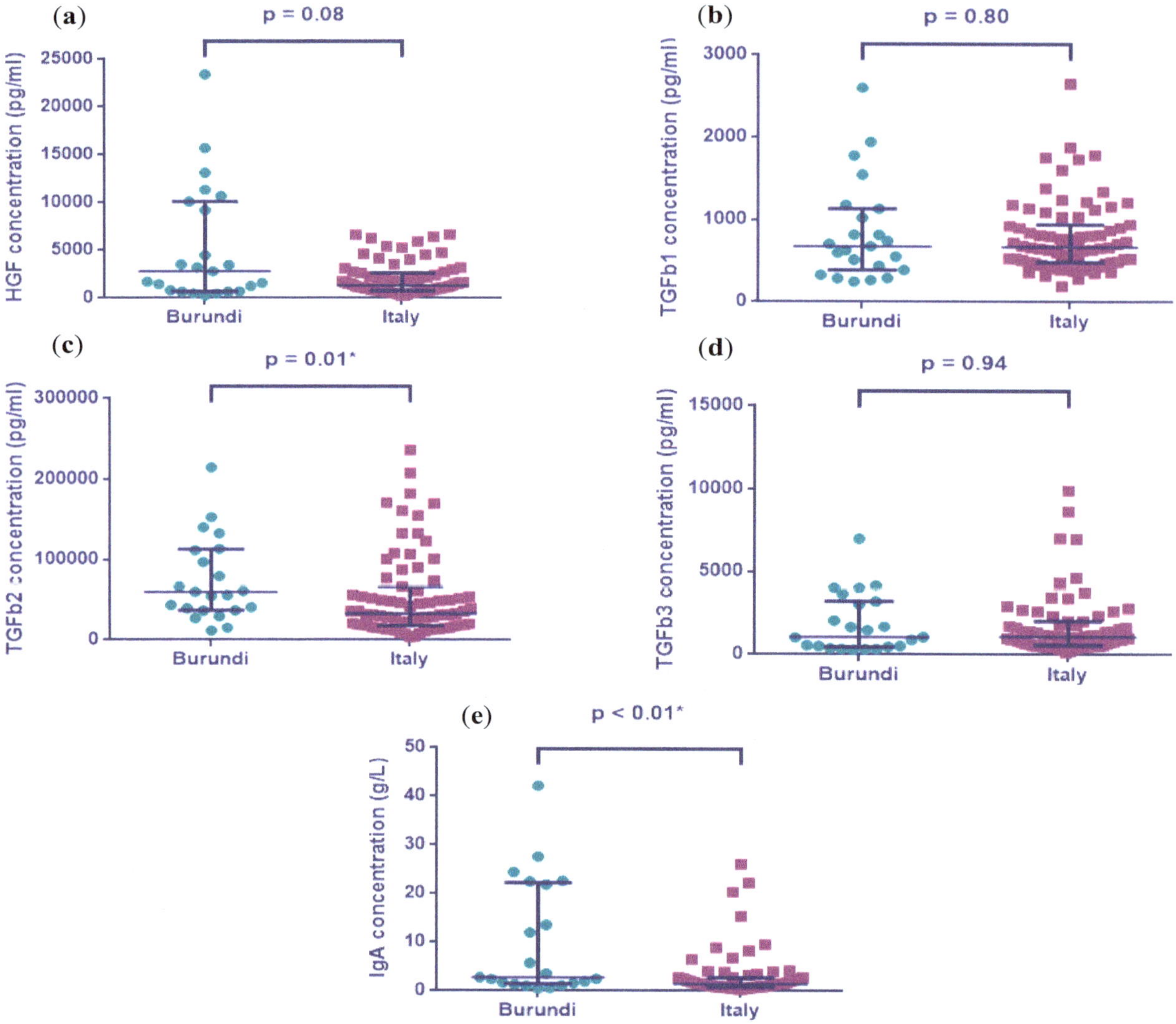

Figure 1. Comparison of growth factors: (**a**) hepatocyte growth factor (HGF), (**b**) transforming growth factor-β1 (TGF-β1), (**c**) TGF-β2, (**d**) TGF-β3, and (**e**) immunoglobulin A (IgA) raw concentrations in the colostrum samples from Burundi and Italy, using the Mann–Whitney U test. The results were considered significant when the *p*-values were reported at a level less than 0.05 *.

3.2.2. Multivariate Analysis Results

The multivariate linear regression analysis was used to adjust for the factors that may affect the immune mediator concentration in human milk. The backwards regression models calculated the most significant factors contributing to the differences in concentration, shown in Table 2. The difference in the TGF-β2 and IgA concentrations between the countries remained significant upon adjustment for potential confounders. The levels of HGF, which were at a borderline significance at the univariate analysis ($p = 0.08$), showed a significant difference upon adjustment.

Table 2. Univariate and adjusted analysis for comparison of growth factors and IgA levels in the colostrum of women from Burundi and Italy.

Immune Factor	Burundi Median (IQR)	Italy Median (IQR)	Unadjusted p-Values [1]	Adjusted Analysis [2]	
				Most Important Factor [3]	p-Value
HGF (pg/mL)	2785 (697.4–10,107)	1316 (785–2628)	0.08	Country of residence	<0.01
TGFβ1 (pg/mL)	673.1 (387.5–1133)	663 (483.1–940.4)	0.80	Parity	0.13
TGFβ2 (pg/mL)	59,708 (36,865–113,221)	33,176 (18,046–66,520)	0.01	Country of residence	0.03
TGFβ3 (pg/mL)	1056 (456.5–3212)	1066 (566.3–2038)	0.94	Parity	0.11
IgA (g/L)	2.78 (1.45–22.2)	1.48 (0.89–2.67)	<0.01	Country of residence	<0.01

[1] Statistical analysis for unadjusted comparisons between women from Italy and Burundi, using Mann–Whitney U test; [2] adjusted analysis (multivariate linear regression). Confounding factors included in the model: country of residence, parity (binary), maternal age, gestational age, and animal contact during pregnancy; [3] According to multivariate regression model; Statistically significant results (at p value < 0.05) presented in bold. interquartile range—IQR; TGF-β—transforming growth factor-β; HGF—hepatocyte growth factor; IgA—immunoglobulin A.

3.2.3. Correlation of TGF-β1, 2, and 3 with IgA Levels

To assess the correlation between the levels of TGF-β, we used Spearman's rank correlation coefficients. We found moderate positive correlations between the growth factor and IgA concentrations in the colostrum of Italian mothers ($p < 0.01$) and a moderate to strong correlation in the samples from the Burundian mothers. The growth factors correlated with IgA were apparently stronger in the colostrum samples from Burundi, as seen in Table 3.

Table 3. Correlation between levels of growth factors (TGFβ1, 2, and 3) with IgA.

Correlating Factors	Burundi (r [1])	Italy (r)
HGF/IgA	0.71 **	0.38 **
TGF-β1/IgA	0.52 *	0.28 *
TGF-β2/IgA	0.68 **	0.32 **
TGF-β3/IgA	0.72 **	0.51 **

Statistical analysis was performed using Spearman's rank correlation coefficient. [1] Spearman r values are presented; *—results are statistically significant at a level less than 0.05; **—results are statistically significant at a level less than 0.01.

4. Discussion

This study aimed to evaluate the differences in the growth factors (TGF-β isoforms and HGF) and IgA levels in the colostrum of women from two distinct cohorts, West African and a Southern European. A great variability in the microbial composition, risk of severe infections, and non-communicable disease rates is seen in these two populations. We found a few apparent differences between the sites following the unadjusted and adjusted analysis. The raw concentrations assessment identified significantly higher concentrations of TGF-β2 and IgA in the Burundian samples and a cursory trend for the HGF concentration in the colostrum samples from Burundi, which reached statistical significance upon adjustment.

Our results showed no significant difference in the TGF-β1 and 3 concentrations between the two groups of women. In contrast, a few studies previously found higher levels of TGF-β1 in the human milk of mothers from developing countries [27,37], or from those residing in a farming environment [38]. The authors suggested that maternal contact with high microbial environments was attributed to an increase of TGF-β1. As multiple factors may influence the immune marker concentration in human milk, it can be speculated that the differences between the studies are a result of ethnic and dietary differences. A major limitation of all of the abovementioned studies, as well as our own work, is a limited sample size. To fully understand the cause of the TGF-β1 variations, the assessment of the dietary and genetic profiles of mothers from different geographical locations is required.

We found higher concentrations of TGF-β2, the predominant isoform of TGF-β in human milk, and IgA in the Burundian colostrum samples. Existing differences in concentration between the sites were confirmed upon adjustment for potential confounders. This finding is in agreement with the results of the study comparing human milk samples from Estonia and Sweden, with higher secretory IgA levels found in Estonia, a country with a greater microbial burden [39]. The high bacterial and viral load in Western Africa may trigger the maternal immune responses and amplify the production of immune mediators; this induces in utero epigenetic alterations via placental Fc receptors [40]. Postnatally, the maternal immune mediators are passed to the infant through breast milk. Thus, the increased TGF-β2 and IgA concentration in the colostrum reflects their purpose, to target microbial antigens and improve mucosal barrier function [41,42]. It may be hypothesised that the elevated IgA concentrations are a potential 'compensation' for the high microbial burden in Burundi.

The surroundings in sub-Saharan Africa offer a microbial load and may possibly stimulate the elevated HGF concentration that was found in colostrum from the Burundian mothers, as a result of the immune-protective effects of HGF on the newborn mucosal barriers [11].

The gestational age of the Burundian infants was lower than their Italian peers. This could potentially result in a greater immunological need, and the mothers' milk is more likely to resemble a preterm milk composition, with higher levels of IgA and TGFβ2 [43], which could be another plausible explanation for the increased levels of these markers in the Burundian women's milk.

In Italy, a more industrialised country with fewer microbial exposures, there is decreased maternal immune stimulation and we detected lower levels of TGF-β2 and IgA in the colostrum of the Italian women. This is supported by the 'hygiene hypothesis', which associated Western lifestyles with rising non-communicable disease prevalence as a consequence of decreased microbial exposures in childhood [44]. Previously, Hawkes and colleagues established that the maternal plasma concentrations of TGF-β2 do not correlate to the levels found in paired breast milk samples [45]. It was also suggested that throughout pregnancy and lactation, the immune cells infiltrate the mammary tissue to upregulate the production of key soluble factors, including TGF-β2 [46]. These studies propose that the local mammary gland production of TGF-β2 may be responsible for the high concentrations seen in breast milk. Therefore, our results cannot unambiguously confirm that systemic immune responses due to a higher maternal microbial exposure in Burundi are a causal factor for the differences in the TGF-β2 levels between the sites. Population studies and genome wide analysis can be used to assess the relationship of host–pathogen responses in human milk components between the countries. However, our results provide additional data, improving the understanding of the selective pressures that lead to immune component variability in human milk and the factors responsible for the differences observed.

The levels of each of the TGF-β isoforms significantly correlated with the IgA concentration in the colostrum from both Burundi and Italy, with stronger correlations observed in the colostrum of the Burundi women. Correlations of immunological markers in human milk are a well-known phenomenon [47], however, it is worth noting that the strength of the correlation in different geographical locations is rarely assessed and should be considered as a potential topic of interest in the future. TGF-β is known to mediate the class-switching of antibodies and therefore regulates the production of secretory IgA [48]. Some authors have suggested that additional signaling factors are required for complete IgA differentiation and class-switching, such as interleukin (IL)-2 and IL-5 [49,50]. We are far from completely understanding the IgA production trigger, but it is necessary to consider the contributing signals for antibody class-switching. This is a possible area that may be considered for further investigation.

Understanding the immune mediator composition of human milk and its' relationships with communicable and non-communicable disease progression is an area of great interest, as it could lead to the development of various therapeutic applications. This includes manipulation with the maternal diet or the environment so as to promote 'healthier' human milk composition, as well as the fortification of formula milk for those infants unable to receive breast milk. Some animal model studies show promising outcomes [51], and there are targets for application in humans [34]. It is widely believed that airborne allergens in human milk can be used to induce TGF-β1 mediated oral tolerance [52]. This may be a possible intervention to prevent antigen-specific allergic airway diseases, but also may have applications in infectious diseases. By understanding the transfer of maternal plasma immune mediators to breast milk, there is vast potential for the development of vaccines that could immunise both mother and infant [53].

With the emergence of data showing that the differences in human milk immune composition most likely exist between the countries [26,29,38,39,54], it becomes more apparent that it should be considered as an important confounding factor in breastfeeding research. At present, most of the studies evaluating the associations between breastfeeding and health outcomes do not take differences in the breast milk composition into account, which may lead to a serious bias. This becomes particularly important when the data from the developed and developing world is compared. The diversity of the human milk composition may account for the conflicting data coming from breastfeeding studies.

More intense research of the differences between the human milk immunological composition may result in an improvement of donor human milk routine use approaches. This is particularly important for a high-income, well developed countries, when necrotizing enterocolitis (NEC) is concerned [55]. A recently published Cochrane systematic review suggests that infant formula use in preterm infants results in an almost doubled risk of NEC development, when compared with donor human milk [56]. A better understanding of human milk immune composition may help to highlight the important markers that are able to further reduce the risk of NEC development and select the most appropriate milk for the infant at risk.

Our study had several limitations; the maternal dietary patterns have not been assessed using a food frequency questionnaire and the maternal body mass index (BMI) has not been measured; we did not evaluate the maternal genotype as a potentially important determinant or modulator of human milk composition; and the small cohort size from Burundi represented another limitation within our study. Although a larger number of samples were collected from the Burundi mothers, because of missing data from the mother–newborn pairs, some data were excluded from the statistical analysis, which led to a reduced statistical power. A small sample size could potentially skew the outcomes obtained on a multivariate linear regression analysis. We sampled single colostrum specimens from each subject, which can also be considered as a limitation. The time before freezing has not been recorded, but it is extremely unlikely to have influenced the results as the samples were frozen within a few hours of collection, and it has been previously shown that the immune active molecules are very stable and do not degrade rapidly [57,58]. The difference in the initial storage conditions (−20 °C and −50 °C), for a period of less than 12 months, is also very unlikely to have had a significant effect on the immunological composition [58]. The outcomes of the statistical analysis are somewhat promising, as the univariate analysis results were subsequently confirmed when the multivariate testing was applied. Another advantage of this study is the rigorous standardisation of the sample collection and analysis, as well as the measurement of important immunological markers, using a very sensitive technique.

5. Conclusions

This cross-sectional study has found differences in the colostrum immune composition between women residing in Burundi and Italy, with higher levels and stronger correlations between the markers found in the milk of the African women. Taken together, these results suggest that differences in the environment and a higher bacterial upload in the developing countries may lead to a higher excretion of factors in to the human milk, in order to provide better protection against infections, as a compensatory mechanism. A stronger correlation between the growth factors and the IgA in colostrum of the women residing in Africa needs further investigation.

The results of this research support the idea that maternal and environmental differences between the populations may result in human milk compositional changes. However, the generalisability of these results is subject to certain limitations. For instance, a small sample size does not allow us to make definitive conclusions. What is now needed is a cross-national study involving participants from very diverse geographical locations, in order to fully determine the cause of the differences in the colostrum composition, taking into account multiple factors that may influence the outcomes.

Author Contributions: J.O.W., R.J.B., A.L.B., D.G.P., and D.M. conceived and designed the experiments; D.M., L.Y.C., P.A., and S.S. performed the experiments; S.L., P.C., and E.M.P. collected data; D.M., P.A., E.K., A.A., R.J.B., and D.G.P. wrote the paper.

Acknowledgments: We are indebted to Roberta Pigozzi for collecting the human milk samples in Verona. We are grateful to the mothers who kindly volunteered to donate their breast milk. R.J.B. is supported by the National Institute for Health Research Biomedical Research Centre (BRC). Both J.O.W. and R.J.B. have received research grant income from Danone, in relation to studies of the value of prebiotics in allergy prevention, and Airsonette, to evaluate the temperature-controlled laminar airflow for asthma. J.O.W. is on a Danone, UCB, and Airsonette scientific advisory board, and both J.O.W. and R.J.B. have given paid lectures for the companies. D.M. has received a consultancy payment from Dairy Goat Co-Operative (NZ) Ltd., and has given paid lectures for the Merck Sharp and Dohme (MSD). J.O.W. is supported by the NIHR CLAHRC for NW London and is its early years theme lead. The views expressed in this paper are those of the authors and not the NIHR or the Department of Health. The founding sponsors/pharmaceutical companies had no role in the design of the study; in the collection, analyses, or interpretation of data; in the writing of the manuscript; and in the decision to publish the results.

References

1. D'Alessandro, A.; Scaloni, A.; Zolla, L. Human milk proteins: An interactomics and updated functional overview. *J. Proteome Res.* **2010**, *9*, 3339–3373. [CrossRef] [PubMed]
2. Lawrence, R.M.; Pane, C.A. Human breast milk: Current concepts of immunology and infectious diseases. *Curr. Probl. Pediatr. Adolesc. Health Care* **2007**, *37*, 7–36. [CrossRef] [PubMed]
3. Verhasselt, V. Neonatal tolerance under breastfeeding influence. *Curr. Opin. Immunol.* **2010**, *22*, 623–630. [CrossRef] [PubMed]
4. Munblit, D.; Verhasselt, V. Allergy prevention by breastfeeding: Possible mechanisms and evidence from human cohorts. *Curr. Opin. Allergy Clin. Immunol.* **2016**, *16*, 427–433. [CrossRef] [PubMed]
5. Khodayar-Pardo, P.; Mira-Pascual, L.; Collado, M.C.; Martinez-Costa, C. Impact of lactation stage, gestational age and mode of delivery on breast milk microbiota. *J. Perinatol.* **2014**, *34*, 599–605. [CrossRef] [PubMed]
6. Lodge, C.J.; Tan, D.J.; Lau, M.X.; Dai, X.; Tham, R.; Lowe, A.J.; Bowatte, G.; Allen, K.J.; Dharmage, S.C. Breastfeeding and asthma and allergies: A systematic review and meta-analysis. *Acta Paediatr.* **2015**, *104*, 38–53. [CrossRef] [PubMed]
7. Doherty, A.M.; Lodge, C.J.; Dharmage, S.C.; Dai, X.; Bode, L.; Lowe, A.J. Human milk oligosaccharides and associations with immune-mediated disease and infection in childhood: A systematic review. *Front. Pediatr.* **2018**, *6*, 91. [CrossRef] [PubMed]
8. Munblit, D.; Peroni, D.G.; Boix-Amoros, A.; Hsu, P.S.; Land, B.V.; Gay, M.C.L.; Kolotilina, A.; Skevaki, C.; Boyle, R.J.; Collado, M.C.; et al. Human milk and allergic diseases: An unsolved puzzle. *Nutrients* **2017**, *9*, 894. [CrossRef] [PubMed]
9. Kobata, R.; Tsukahara, H.; Ohshima, Y.; Ohta, N.; Tokuriki, S.; Tamura, S.; Mayumi, M. High levels of growth factors in human breast milk. *Early Hum. Dev.* **2008**, *84*, 67–69. [CrossRef] [PubMed]
10. Galimi, F.; Brizzi, M.F.; Comoglio, P.M. The hepatocyte growth factor and its receptor. *Stem Cells* **1993**, *11*, 22–30. [CrossRef] [PubMed]
11. Patki, S.; Patki, U.; Patil, R.; Indumathi, S.; Kaingade, P.; Bulbule, A.; Nikam, A.; Pishte, A. Comparison of the levels of the growth factors in umbilical cord serum and human milk and its clinical significance. *Cytokine* **2012**, *59*, 305–308. [CrossRef] [PubMed]
12. Min, J.K.; Lee, Y.M.; Kim, J.H.; Kim, Y.M.; Kim, S.W.; Lee, S.Y.; Gho, Y.S.; Oh, G.T.; Kwon, Y.G. Hepatocyte growth factor suppresses vascular endothelial growth factor-induced expression of endothelial icam-1 and vcam-1 by inhibiting the nuclear factor-kappab pathway. *Circ. Res.* **2005**, *96*, 300–307. [CrossRef] [PubMed]
13. Cummins, A.G.; Thompson, F.M. Postnatal changes in mucosal immune response: A physiological perspective of breast feeding and weaning. *Immunol. Cell Biol.* **1997**, *75*, 419–429. [CrossRef] [PubMed]

14. Donnet-Hughes, A.; Duc, N.; Serrant, P.; Vidal, K.; Schiffrin, E.J. Bioactive molecules in milk and their role in health and disease: The role of transforming growth factor-beta. *Immunol. Cell Biol.* **2000**, *78*, 74–79. [CrossRef] [PubMed]
15. Penttila, I.A. Milk-derived transforming growth factor-beta and the infant immune response. *J. Pediatr.* **2010**, *156*, S21–S25. [CrossRef] [PubMed]
16. Tiemessen, M.M.; Kunzmann, S.; Schmidt-Weber, C.B.; Garssen, J.; Bruijnzeel-Koomen, C.A.; Knol, E.F.; van Hoffen, E. Transforming growth factor-beta inhibits human antigen-specific CD4+ T cell proliferation without modulating the cytokine response. *Int. Immunol.* **2003**, *15*, 1495–1504. [CrossRef] [PubMed]
17. Jarvinen, K.M.; Suomalainen, H. Development of cow's milk allergy in breast-fed infants. *Clin. Exp. Allergy* **2001**, *31*, 978–987. [CrossRef] [PubMed]
18. Oddy, W.H.; Rosales, F. A systematic review of the importance of milk TGF-beta on immunological outcomes in the infant and young child. *Pediatr. Allergy Immunol.* **2010**, *21*, 47–59. [CrossRef] [PubMed]
19. Morita, Y.; Campos-Alberto, E.; Yamaide, F.; Nakano, T.; Ohnisi, H.; Kawamoto, M.; Kawamoto, N.; Matsui, E.; Kondo, N.; Kohno, Y.; et al. TGF-beta concentration in breast milk is associated with the development of eczema in infants. *Front. Pediatr.* **2018**, *6*, 162. [CrossRef] [PubMed]
20. Munblit, D.; Treneva, M.; Peroni, D.G.; Colicino, S.; Chow, L.Y.; Dissanayeke, S.; Pampura, A.; Boner, A.L.; Geddes, D.T.; Boyle, R.J.; et al. Immune components in human milk are associated with early infant immunological health outcomes: A prospective three-country analysis. *Nutrients* **2017**, *9*, 532. [CrossRef] [PubMed]
21. Ogawa, J.; Sasahara, A.; Yoshida, T.; Sira, M.M.; Futatani, T.; Kanegane, H.; Miyawaki, T. Role of transforming growth factor-beta in breast milk for initiation of IgA production in newborn infants. *Early Hum. Dev.* **2004**, *77*, 67–75. [CrossRef] [PubMed]
22. Iyengar, S.R.; Walker, W.A. Immune factors in breast milk and the development of atopic disease. *J. Pediatr. Gastroenterol. Nutr.* **2012**, *55*, 641–647. [CrossRef] [PubMed]
23. Arnould, V.M.; Soyeurt, H. Genetic variability of milk fatty acids. *J. Appl. Genet.* **2009**, *50*, 29–39. [CrossRef] [PubMed]
24. Kondo, N.; Suda, Y.; Nakao, A.; Oh-Oka, K.; Suzuki, K.; Ishimaru, K.; Sato, M.; Tanaka, T.; Nagai, A.; Yamagata, Z. Maternal psychosocial factors determining the concentrations of transforming growth factor-beta in breast milk. *Pediatr. Allergy Immunol.* **2011**, *22*, 853–861. [CrossRef] [PubMed]
25. Kuitunen, M.; Kukkonen, A.K.; Savilahti, E. Impact of maternal allergy and use of probiotics during pregnancy on breast milk cytokines and food antibodies and development of allergy in children until 5 years. *Int. Arch. Allergy Immunol.* **2012**, *159*, 162–170. [CrossRef] [PubMed]
26. Munblit, D.; Treneva, M.; Peroni, D.G.; Colicino, S.; Chow, L.; Dissanayeke, S.; Abrol, P.; Sheth, S.; Pampura, A.; Boner, A.L.; et al. Colostrum and mature human milk of women from London, Moscow, and Verona: Determinants of immune composition. *Nutrients* **2016**, *8*, 695. [CrossRef] [PubMed]
27. Holmlund, U.; Amoudruz, P.; Johansson, M.A.; Haileselassie, Y.; Ongoiba, A.; Kayentao, K.; Traore, B.; Doumbo, S.; Schollin, J.; Doumbo, O.; et al. Maternal country of origin, breast milk characteristics and potential influences on immunity in offspring. *Clin. Exp. Immunol.* **2010**, *162*, 500–509. [CrossRef] [PubMed]
28. Aihara, Y.; Oh-oka, K.; Kondo, N.; Sharma, J.; Ishimaru, K.; Hara, M.; Yamagata, Z.; Nakao, A. Comparison of colostrum TGF-β2 levels between lactating women in Japan and Nepal. *Asian Pac. J. Allergy Immunol.* **2014**, *32*, 178–184. [CrossRef] [PubMed]
29. Ruiz, L.; Espinosa-Martos, I.; Garcia-Carral, C.; Manzano, S.; McGuire, M.K.; Meehan, C.L.; McGuire, M.A.; Williams, J.E.; Foster, J.; Sellen, D.W.; et al. What's normal? Immune profiling of human milk from healthy women living in different geographical and socioeconomic settings. *Front. Immunol.* **2017**, *8*, 696. [CrossRef] [PubMed]
30. UNICEF. Country Statistics-Burundi. 2013. Available online: https://www.unicef.org/infobycountry/burundi_statistics.html (accessed on 17 April 2014).
31. UNICEF. Unicef-Italy Population Statistics. 2013. Available online: https://www.unicef.org/infobycountry/italy_statistics.html (accessed on 5 April 2014).
32. Munblit, D.; Boyle, R.J.; Warner, J.O. Factors affecting breast milk composition and potential consequences for development of the allergic phenotype. *Clin. Exp. Allergy* **2015**, *45*, 583–601. [CrossRef] [PubMed]

33. Munblit, D.; Boyle, R.J. Modulating breast milk composition-the key to allergy prevention? *Int. Arch. Allergy Immunol.* **2012**, *159*, 107–108. [CrossRef] [PubMed]
34. Le Doare, K.; Bellis, K.; Faal, A.; Birt, J.; Munblit, D.; Humphries, H.; Taylor, S.; Warburton, F.; Heath, P.T.; Kampmann, B.; et al. SIgA, TGF-β1, IL-10, and TNFα in colostrum are associated with infant group B streptococcus colonization. *Front. Immunol.* **2017**, *8*, 1269. [CrossRef] [PubMed]
35. Munblit, D.; Sheth, S.; Abrol, P.; Treneva, M.; Peroni, D.G.; Chow, L.Y.; Boner, A.L.; Pampura, A.; Warner, J.O.; Boyle, R.J. Exposures influencing total IgA level in colostrum. *J. Dev. Orig. Health Dis.* **2016**, *7*, 61–67. [CrossRef] [PubMed]
36. Ismail, I.H.; Licciardi, P.V.; Oppedisano, F.; Boyle, R.J.; Tang, M.L. Relationship between breast milk scd14, TGF-beta1 and total IgA in the first month and development of eczema during infancy. *Pediatr. Allergy Immunol.* **2013**, *24*, 352–360. [CrossRef] [PubMed]
37. Amoudruz, P.; Holmlund, U.; Schollin, J.; Sverremark-Ekström, E.; Montgomery, S.M. Maternal country of birth and previous pregnancies are associated with breast milk characteristics. *Pediatr. Allergy Immunol.* **2009**, *20*, 19–29. [CrossRef] [PubMed]
38. Peroni, D.G.; Pescollderungg, L.; Piacentini, G.L.; Rigotti, E.; Maselli, M.; Watschinger, K.; Piazza, M.; Pigozzi, R.; Boner, A.L. Immune regulatory cytokines in the milk of lactating women from farming and urban environments. *Pediatr. Allergy Immunol.* **2010**, *21*, 977–982. [CrossRef] [PubMed]
39. Tomicic, S.; Johansson, G.; Voor, T.; Bjorksten, B.; Bottcher, M.F.; Jenmalm, M.C. Breast milk cytokine and iga composition differ in estonian and swedish mothers-relationship to microbial pressure and infant allergy. *Pediatr. Res.* **2010**, *68*, 330–334. [CrossRef] [PubMed]
40. Jenmalm, M.C. Childhood immune maturation and allergy development: Regulation by maternal immunity and microbial exposure. *Am. J. Reprod. Immunol.* **2011**, *66*, 75–80. [CrossRef] [PubMed]
41. Chatterton, D.E.; Nguyen, D.N.; Bering, S.B.; Sangild, P.T. Anti-inflammatory mechanisms of bioactive milk proteins in the intestine of newborns. *Int. J. Biochem. Cell Biol.* **2013**, *45*, 1730–1747. [CrossRef] [PubMed]
42. Rogier, E.W.; Frantz, A.L.; Bruno, M.E.; Wedlund, L.; Cohen, D.A.; Stromberg, A.J.; Kaetzel, C.S. Secretory antibodies in breast milk promote long-term intestinal homeostasis by regulating the gut microbiota and host gene expression. *Proc. Natl. Acad. Sci. USA* **2014**, *111*, 3074–3079. [CrossRef] [PubMed]
43. Trend, S.; Strunk, T.; Lloyd, M.L.; Kok, C.H.; Metcalfe, J.; Geddes, D.T.; Lai, C.T.; Richmond, P.; Doherty, D.A.; Simmer, K.; et al. Levels of innate immune factors in preterm and term mothers' breast milk during the 1st month postpartum. *Br. J. Nutr.* **2016**, *115*, 1178–1193. [CrossRef] [PubMed]
44. Umetsu, D.T. Early exposure to germs and the hygiene hypothesis. *Cell Res.* **2012**, *22*, 1210–1211. [CrossRef] [PubMed]
45. Hawkes, J.S.; Bryan, D.L.; Gibson, R.A. Variations in transforming growth factor beta in human milk are not related to levels in plasma. *Cytokine* **2002**, *17*, 182–186. [CrossRef] [PubMed]
46. Reed, J.R.; Schwertfeger, K.L. Immune cell location and function during post-natal mammary gland development. *J. Mammary Gland Biol. Neoplasia* **2010**, *15*, 329–339. [CrossRef] [PubMed]
47. Bottcher, M.F.; Jenmalm, M.C.; Garofalo, R.P.; Bjorksten, B. Cytokines in breast milk from allergic and nonallergic mothers. *Pediatr. Res.* **2000**, *47*, 157–162. [CrossRef] [PubMed]
48. Stavnezer, J. Regulation of antibody production and class switching by TGF-beta. *J. Immunol.* **1995**, *155*, 1647–1651. [PubMed]
49. Ehrhardt, R.O.; Strober, W.; Harriman, G.R. Effect of transforming growth factor (TGF)-beta 1 on IgA isotype expression. TGF-beta 1 induces a small increase in sIgA+ B cells regardless of the method of B cell activation. *J. Immunol.* **1992**, *148*, 3830–3836. [PubMed]
50. Sonoda, E.; Hitoshi, Y.; Yamaguchi, N.; Ishii, T.; Tominaga, A.; Araki, S.; Takatsu, K. Differential regulation of IgA production by TGF-β and IL-5: TGF-β induces surface IgA -positive cells bearing IL -5 receptor, whereas IL-5 promotes their survival and maturation into IgA-secreting cells. *Cell. Immunol.* **1992**, *140*, 158–172. [CrossRef]
51. Jain, S.K.; Baggerman, E.W.; Mohankumar, K.; Namachivayam, K.; Jagadeeswaran, R.; Reyes, V.E.; Maheshwari, A. Amniotic fluid-borne hepatocyte growth factor protects rat pups against experimental necrotizing enterocolitis. *Am. J. Physiol. Gastrointest. Liver Physiol.* **2014**, *306*, G361–G369. [CrossRef] [PubMed]

52. Verhasselt, V.; Milcent, V.; Cazareth, J.; Kanda, A.; Fleury, S.; Dombrowicz, D.; Glaichenhaus, N.; Julia, V. Breast milk-mediated transfer of an antigen induces tolerance and protection from allergic asthma. *Nat. Med.* **2008**, *14*, 170–175. [CrossRef] [PubMed]
53. Shahid, N.S.; Steinhoff, M.C.; Roy, E.; Begum, T.; Thompson, C.M.; Siber, G.R. Placental and breast transfer of antibodies after maternal immunization with polysaccharide meningococcal vaccine: A randomized, controlled evaluation. *Vaccine* **2002**, *20*, 2404–2409. [CrossRef]
54. Orivuori, L.; Loss, G.; Roduit, C.; Dalphin, J.C.; Depner, M.; Genuneit, J.; Lauener, R.; Pekkanen, J.; Pfefferle, P.; Riedler, J.; et al. Soluble immunoglobulin a in breast milk is inversely associated with atopic dermatitis at early age: The pasture cohort study. *Clin. Exp. Allergy* **2014**, *44*, 102–112. [CrossRef] [PubMed]
55. Battersby, C.; Santhalingam, T.; Costeloe, K.; Modi, N. Incidence of neonatal necrotising enterocolitis in high-income countries: A systematic review. *Arch. Dis. Child. Fetal Neonatal Ed.* **2018**, *103*, F182–F189. [PubMed]
56. Quigley, M.; Embleton, N.D.; McGuire, W. Formula versus donor breast milk for feeding preterm or low birth weight infants. *Cochrane Database Syst. Rev.* **2018**, *6*, CD002971. [CrossRef] [PubMed]
57. Lawrence, R.A. Storage of human milk and the influence of procedures on immunological components of human milk. *Acta. Paediatr. Suppl.* **1999**, *88*, 14–18. [CrossRef] [PubMed]
58. Lawrence, R.A. Milk banking: The influence of storage procedures and subsequent processing on immunologic components of human milk. *Adv. Nutr. Res.* **2001**, *10*, 389–404. [PubMed]

Permissions

All chapters in this book were first published by MDPI; hereby published with permission under the Creative Commons Attribution License or equivalent. Every chapter published in this book has been scrutinized by our experts. Their significance has been extensively debated. The topics covered herein carry significant findings which will fuel the growth of the discipline. They may even be implemented as practical applications or may be referred to as a beginning point for another development.

The contributors of this book come from diverse backgrounds, making this book a truly international effort. This book will bring forth new frontiers with its revolutionizing research information and detailed analysis of the nascent developments around the world.

We would like to thank all the contributing authors for lending their expertise to make the book truly unique. They have played a crucial role in the development of this book. Without their invaluable contributions this book wouldn't have been possible. They have made vital efforts to compile up to date information on the varied aspects of this subject to make this book a valuable addition to the collection of many professionals and students.

This book was conceptualized with the vision of imparting up-to-date information and advanced data in this field. To ensure the same, a matchless editorial board was set up. Every individual on the board went through rigorous rounds of assessment to prove their worth. After which they invested a large part of their time researching and compiling the most relevant data for our readers.

The editorial board has been involved in producing this book since its inception. They have spent rigorous hours researching and exploring the diverse topics which have resulted in the successful publishing of this book. They have passed on their knowledge of decades through this book. To expedite this challenging task, the publisher supported the team at every step. A small team of assistant editors was also appointed to further simplify the editing procedure and attain best results for the readers.

Apart from the editorial board, the designing team has also invested a significant amount of their time in understanding the subject and creating the most relevant covers. They scrutinized every image to scout for the most suitable representation of the subject and create an appropriate cover for the book.

The publishing team has been an ardent support to the editorial, designing and production team. Their endless efforts to recruit the best for this project, has resulted in the accomplishment of this book. They are a veteran in the field of academics and their pool of knowledge is as vast as their experience in printing. Their expertise and guidance has proved useful at every step. Their uncompromising quality standards have made this book an exceptional effort. Their encouragement from time to time has been an inspiration for everyone.

The publisher and the editorial board hope that this book will prove to be a valuable piece of knowledge for researchers, students, practitioners and scholars across the globe.

List of Contributors

Osita Kingsley Ezeh and Pramesh Raj Ghimire
School of Science and Health, University of Western Sydney, Locked Bag 1797, Penrith, NSW 1797, Australia

Kingsley Emwinyore Agho
School of Science and Health, University of Western Sydney, Locked Bag 1797, Penrith, NSW 1797, Australia
Translational Health Research Institute (THRI), School of Medicine, Western Sydney University, Campbell town Campus, Locked Bag 1797, Penrith, NSW 2571, Australia

Felix Akpojene Ogbo
Translational Health Research Institute (THRI), School of Medicine, Western Sydney University, Campbell town Campus, Locked Bag 1797, Penrith, NSW 2571, Australia

Garry John Stevens
Humanitarian and Development Research Initiative (HADRI), School of Social Sciences and Psychology, Western Sydney University, Locked Bag1797, Penrith, NSW 2751, Australia

Wadad Kathy Tannous
School of Business, Western Sydney University, Locked Bag 1797, Penrith, NSW 2751, Australia

Osuagwu Levi Uchechukwu
Diabetes, Obesity and Metabolism Translational Research Unit, Western Sydney University, Campbell town, NSW 2560, Australia

Carlos A. De Castro and Sagar K. Thakkar
Nestle Research Singapore Hub, Société des Produits Nestlé SA, 29 Quality Road, Singapore 618802, Singapore

Lydie Beauport, Jean-François Tolsa and Céline J. Fischer Fumeaux
Clinic of Neonatology, Department Woman Mother Child, University Hospital of Lausanne, 1011 Lausanne, Switzerland

Khalil M. Salameh
Division of Pediatrics, Al-Wakra Hospital, Hamad Medical Corporation, Doha, Qatar

Najah S. Al-Janahi
Department of Obstetrics and Gynecology, Women's Hospital, Hamad Medical Corporation, Doha, Qatar

Maria Grunewald, Christian Hellmuth, Franca F. Kirchberg, Katharina Werkstetter, Berthold Koletzko and Hans Demmelmair
Ludwig-Maximilians-Universität, Division of Metabolic and Nutritional Medicine, Dr. von Hauner Children's Hospital, University of Munich Medical Center, 80337 Munich, Germany

Maria Luisa Mearin and Sabine L. Vriezinga
Department of Paediatrics, Leiden University Medical Center, 2300 Leiden, The Netherlands

Robert K. Huston, Andi M. Markell, Elizabeth A. McCulley and Rachel L. Martin
Department of Pediatrics, Randall Children's Hospital at Legacy Emanuel, Portland, OR 97227, USA

Ilma R. Korponay-Szabo
Celiac Disease Center, Heim Pál Children's Hospital, 1089 Budapest, Hungary

Magalie Sabatier, Clara L. Garcia-Rodenas, Peter Kastenmayer, Mario Vigo, Stéphane Dubascoux, Daniel Andrey, Marine Nicolas, Janique Richoz Payot, Valentine Bordier and Michael Affolter
Nestlé Research, Société des Produits Nestlé SA, 1000 Lausanne, Switzerland

Malgorzata Witkowska-Zimny, Ewa Kamińska-El-Hassan and Edyta Wróbel
Department of Biophysics and Human Physiology, Medical University of Warsaw, Chalubinskiego 5, 02-004 Warsaw, Poland

Beatrice Letizia Crippa, Lorenzo Colombo, Daniela Morniroli, Giulia Vercesi, Lidia Zanotta, Paola Roggero, Maria Lorella Giannì and Fabio Mosca
Neonatal Intensive Care Unit, Fondazione IRCCS Cà Granda Ospedale Maggiore Policlinico, via Commenda 12, 20122 Milan, Italy
Department of Clinical Sciences and Community Health, University of Milan, Via San Barnaba 8, 20122 Milan, Italy

Veronique Demers-Mathieu and David C. Dallas
Nutrition Program, School of Biological and Population Health Sciences, College of Public Health and Human Sciences, Oregon State University, Corvallis, OR 97331, USA

Juliana C. Nunes
Laboratory of Food Science and Nutritional Biochemistry, Institute of Chemistry, Federal University of Rio de Janeiro, Rio de Janeiro 21941-909, Brazil
School of Nutrition, Federal University of the State of Rio de Janeiro, Rio de Janeiro 22290-250, Brazil

Tatiana El-Bacha
Laboratory of Food Science and Nutritional Biochemistry, Institute of Chemistry, Federal University of Rio de Janeiro, Rio de Janeiro 21941-909, Brazil
Institute of Nutrition, Federal University of Rio de Janeiro, Rio de Janeiro 21941-902, Brazil
Department of Physiology, Development and Neuroscience, University of Cambridge, Cambridge CB2 3EL, UK

Alexandre G. Torres
Laboratory of Food Science and Nutritional Biochemistry, Institute of Chemistry, Federal University of Rio de Janeiro, Rio de Janeiro 21941-909, Brazil

Alessandra Mazzocchi and Ludovica Leone
Department of Clinical Sciences and Community Health, University of Milan, 20122 Milan, Italy

Maria Lorella Giannì, Daniela Morniroli, Paola Roggero and Fabio Mosca
Department of Clinical Sciences and Community Health, University of Milan, 20122 Milan, Italy
Fondazione IRCCS Ca' Granda Ospedale Maggiore Policlinico, NICU, 20122 Milan, Italy

Carlo Agostoni
Department of Clinical Sciences and Community Health, University of Milan, 20122 Milan, Italy
Fondazione IRCCS Ca' Granda Ospedale Maggiore Policlinico, Pediatric Intermediate Care Unit, 20122 Milan, Italy

Valentina De Cosmi
Fondazione IRCCS Ca' Granda Ospedale Maggiore Policlinico, Pediatric Intermediate Care Unit, 20122 Milan, Italy

Amanda de Sousa Rebouças and Roberto Dimenstein
Department of Biochemistry, Federal University of Rio Grande do Norte, 59078-970 Natal-RN, Brazil

Ana Gabriella Costa Lemos da Silva, Amanda Freitas de Oliveira, Lorena Thalia Pereira da Silva, Vanessa de Freitas Felgueiras and Karla Danielly da Silva Ribeiro
Department of Nutrition, Federal University of Rio Grande do Norte, 59078-970 Natal-RN, Brazil

Marina Sampaio Cruz and Vivian Nogueira Silbiger
Department of Pharmacy, Federal University of Rio Grande do Norte, 59012-570 Natal-RN, Brazil

Daniela Hampel and Lindsay H. Allen
USDA/ARS Western Human Nutrition Research Center, 430 West Health Sciences Drive, Davis, CA 95616, USA
Department of Nutrition, University of California, One Shields Ave, Davis, CA 95616, USA

Setareh Shahab-Ferdows
USDA/ARS Western Human Nutrition Research Center, 430 West Health Sciences Drive, Davis, CA 95616, USA

Muttaquina Hossain, M. Munirul Islam and Tahmeed Ahmed
Nutrition and Clinical Services Division, International Centre for Diarrhoeal Disease Research, 68 Shaheed Tajuddin Ahmed Sarani, Mohakhali, Dhaka 1212, Bangladesh

Therese A. O'Sullivan
School of Medical and Health Sciences, Edith Cowan University, 270 Joondalup Drive, Joondalup, WA 6027, Australia

Aleksandra Wesolowska
Laboratory of Human Milk and Lactation Research at Regional Human Milk Bank in Holy Family Hospital, Department of Neonatology, Faculty of Health Sciences, Medical University of Warsaw, Zwirki i Wigury Str. 63A, 02-091 Warsaw, Poland

Joanna Brys
Department of Chemistry, Faculty of Food Sciences, Warsaw University of Life Sciences—SGGW, Nowoursynowska St. 166, 02-787 Warsaw, Poland

Olga Barbarska
Laboratory of Human Milk and Lactation Research at Regional Human Milk Bank in Holy Family Hospital, Department of Neonatology, Faculty of Health Sciences, Medical University of Warsaw, Zwirki i Wigury Str. 63A, 02-091 Warsaw, Poland
Department of Medical Biology, Faculty of Health Sciences, Medical University of Warsaw, 14/16 Litewska St., 00-575 Warsaw, Poland

Jiahui Yu, Tinglan Yuan, Xinghe Zhang, Qingzhe Jin, Wei Wei and Xingguo Wang
State Key Lab of Food Science and Technology, Jiangnan University, Wuxi 214122, China
International Joint Research Laboratory for Lipid Nutrition and Safety, Collaborative Innovation Center of Food Safety and Quality Control in Jiangsu Province, School of Food Science and Technology, Jiangnan University, Wuxi 214122, China

Kamila Strom and Gabriela Oledzka
Department of Medical Biology, Faculty of Health Sciences, Medical University of Warsaw, 14/16 Litewska St., 00-575 Warsaw, Poland

Jolanta Szymanska-Majchrzak
Department of Biochemistry, Second Faculty of Medicine, Medical University of Warsaw, Banacha 1b Str. 02-093 Warsaw, Poland

Katarzyna Karzel
Faculty of Psychology, Warsaw University, Stawki 5/7, 00-183 Warsaw, Poland

Emilia Pawlikowska
High Pressure Physics, Polish Academy of Science, Sokolowska 29, 01-142 Warsaw, Poland

Monika A. Zielinska and Jadwiga Hamulka
Department of Human Nutrition, Faculty of Human Nutrition and Consumer Sciences, Warsaw University of Life Sciences—SGGW, 159 Nowoursynowska St., 02-776 Warsaw, Poland

Maria Lorella Gianni, Beatrice Letizia Crippa, Daniela Morniroli, Nadia Liotto, Paola Roggero and Fabio Mosca
Fondazione IRCCS Ca' Granda Ospedale Maggiore Policlinico, NICU, via Commenda 12, 20122 Milan, Italy
Department of Clinical Sciences and Community Health, University of Milan, Via San Barnaba 8, 20122 Milan, Italy

Maria Enrica Bettinelli
Department of Clinical Sciences and Community Health, University of Milan, Via San Barnaba 8, 20122 Milan, Italy

Priscilla Manfra, Gabriele Sorrentino, Elena Bezze, Laura Plevani, Giacomo Cavallaro, Genny Raffaeli and Lorenzo Colombo
Fondazione IRCCS Ca' Granda Ospedale Maggiore Policlinico, NICU, via Commenda 12, 20122 Milan, Italy

Eduardo Villamor
Department of Pediatrics, Maastricht University Medical Center (MUMC+), School for Oncology and Developmental Biology (GROW), 6202 AZ Maastricht, The Netherlands

Agnieszka Bzikowska-Jura, Aneta Czerwonogrodzka-Senczyna and Dorota Szostak-Węgierek
Department of Clinical Dietetics, Faculty of Health Sciences, Medical University of Warsaw, E Ciolka Str. 27, 01-445 Warsaw, Poland

Céline J. Fischer Fumeaux, Lydie Beauport and Jean-François Tolsa
Clinic of Neonatology, Department Woman Mother Child, University Hospital of Lausanne, 1011 Lausanne, Switzerland

Clara L. Garcia-Rodenas
Nestlé Institute of Health Sciences, Nestlé Research, 1000 Lausanne, Switzerland

Carlos A. De Castro
Clinical Development Unit, Nestlé Research Asia, Singapore 138567, Singapore

Marie-Claude Courtet-Compondu and Michael Affolter
Nestlé Institute of Food Safety & Analytical Science, Nestlé Research, 1000 Lausanne, Switzerland

Sagar K. Thakkar
Nestlé Research Asia, Singapore 138567, Singapore

Mohèb Elwakiel
Food Quality and Design Group, Wageningen University & Research, Bornse Weilanden 9, 6708 WG Wageningen, The Netherlands
Laboratory of Food Chemistry, Wageningen University & Research, Bornse Weilanden 9,6708 WG Wageningen, The Netherlands

Sean Austin, Norbert Sprenger, Aristea Binia, Michael Affolter and Clara L. Garcia-Rodenas
Nestlé Research, Vers-Chez-Les-Blanc, 1000 Lausanne, Switzerland

Paola Agnese Mauri and Annalisa Canziani
Department of Clinical Sciences and Community Health, University of Milan, Via San Barnaba 8, 20122 Milan, Italy
Dipartimento Donna-Bambino-Neonato, Fondazione IRCCS Cà Granda Ospedale Maggiore Policlinico, via Commenda 12, 20122 Milan, Italy

Carlos A. De Castro
Nestle Research Singapore, 29 Quality Road, 618802 Singapore, Singapore

Lydie Beauport, Jean-François Tolsa and Céline J. Fischer Fumeaux
Centre Hospitalier Universitaire Vaudois, 1011 Lausanne, Switzerland

Gabriela Olędzka
Department of Medical Biology, Faculty of Health Sciences, Medical University of Warsaw, Litewska Str. 14/16, 00-575 Warsaw, Poland

Dario Consonni
Epidemiology Unit, Fondazione IRCCS Ca' Granda Ospedale Maggiore Policlinico, Via San Barnaba 8, 20122 Milan, Italy

Maria Enrica Bettinelli
Mother and Child Unit, Università degli Studi di Milano, ATS Città Metropolitana di Milano, 20122 Milan, Italy

Laura Plevani
Neonatal Intensive Care Unit, Fondazione IRCCS Cà Granda Ospedale Maggiore Policlinico, via Commenda 12, 20122 Milan, Italy

Irene Spreafico, Patrizio Sannino, Donatella Bertoli, Stefania Zorzan
Direzione Professioni Sanitarie, Fondazione IRCCS Cà Granda Ospedale Maggiore Policlinico,via Commenda 12, 20122 Milan, Italy

Daniel Munblit
Department of Paediatrics, Imperial College London, London W2 1NY, UK
Faculty of Pediatrics, Sechenov University, 119991 Moscow, Russia
in VIVO Planetary Health, Group of the Worldwide Universities Network (WUN), 6010 Park Ave, West New York, NJ 07093, USA

Priya Abrol, Shreya Sheth and Li Yan Chow
Department of Paediatrics, Imperial College London, London W2 1NY, UK

Ekaterina Khaleva
inVIVO Planetary Health, Group of the Worldwide Universities Network (WUN), 6010 Park Ave, West New York, NJ 07093, USA
Department of Paediatrics, Saint-Petersburg State Paediatric Medical University, 194353 Saint-Petersburg, Russia

John O. Warner and Robert J. Boyle
Department of Paediatrics, Imperial College London, London W2 1NY, UK
inVIVO Planetary Health, Group of the Worldwide Universities Network (WUN), 6010 Park Ave, West New York, NJ 07093, USA

Alan Asmanov
The Research and Clinical Institute for Pediatrics named after Academician Yuri Veltischev of the Pirogov Russian National Research Medical University, 125412 Moscow, Russia

Silvana Lauriola, Ezio M. Padovani, Pasquale Comberiati and Attilio L. Boner
Department of Life and Reproduction Sciences, Section of Paediatrics, University of Verona, 37124 Verona, Italy

Diego G. Peroni
in VIVO Planetary Health, Group of the Worldwide Universities Network (WUN), 6010 Park Ave, West New York, NJ 07093, USA
Department of Clinical and Experimental Medicine, Section of Paediatrics, University of Pisa, 56126 Pisa, Italy

Index

A

Aboriginal, 44, 55

Adipokines, 70-71, 73, 78, 157

Antenatal Care, 1-2, 25, 169, 181, 185

Antibiotic Use, 27, 116

B

Bioactive Factors, 39, 119, 133-134, 156

Birth Cohort, 23, 54, 67, 69, 168, 225, 227

Body Composition, 70-72, 75, 77-79, 117, 157-158

Breastfeeding, 1-5, 8-9, 12-18, 22, 26, 38, 42-45, 47-49, 51-59, 65 68, 70, 72, 77-79, 81-82, 84, 93-101, 103-104, 118-119, 137-150, 156-158, 160-170, 173-174, 177-178, 181-186, 197, 226, 233-234

Breastfeeding Cessation, 42, 48-49, 137-139, 141-144, 146-147, 161, 186

Breastfeeding Difficulties, 22, 166

Breastfeeding Discontinuation, 55, 160, 166

Breastfeeding Frequency, 65, 158

Breastfeeding Issues, 160, 166

Breastfeeding Mothers, 100, 138, 147-148, 184

Breastfeeding Support, 43, 51, 147, 160, 166, 168

C

Caesarean Section, 7, 11, 13, 16, 46, 48, 50, 84, 102-103, 112-113, 115, 117-118, 176, 180, 229

Choline, 61-62, 64-65, 68, 106, 116

Chromatography, 29, 68, 122, 125, 211

Colostrum, 27, 40, 66, 69, 121, 149, 188, 195, 197-199, 206-207, 225-230, 232-236

Confidence Intervals, 4, 9, 45, 142-143, 162, 172-173

Cortisol, 83, 153, 159

Culturally And Linguistically Diverse, 42-43, 47, 54, 186

D

Daily Intake, 72, 213, 215

Dietary Intake, 23, 59, 65, 133-134, 156, 211-213, 215

Donor Milk, 71, 123, 126, 133-136, 201, 207

E

Early Breastfeeding Cessation, 137-138, 142-144, 147, 161

Epithelial Cells, 82, 95, 116, 187, 226

Exclusive Breastfeeding, 15-16, 42-43, 48-49, 54-56, 66, 81, 97-98, 104, 137-140, 142-148, 162-165, 167-170, 173-174, 177-178, 184-186, 197

Extrahepatic Tissues, 221

F

Fatigue, 166

Fatty Acids, 59, 66, 103, 106, 109, 111, 116, 118, 122, 124-127, 129-132, 134-136, 211-213, 215-216, 218-223, 235

Fortification, 26, 36, 100, 189, 201, 222, 232

G

Galactagogues, 81-86, 91, 93-98

Gestation, 35, 86-87, 91, 94, 97, 101, 167, 222

Gestational Age, 2, 19-20, 26, 28, 30, 35, 40, 70, 90, 96, 118, 138, 153, 161, 166, 187, 189, 191-194, 196-201, 210, 212-214, 223, 228-229, 232, 234

Ghrelin, 70-73, 76-77, 79-80, 157

Glycerophosphocholine, 62, 64

Growth Trajectory, 70, 136

H

Health Care Professionals, 161-162, 166

Hemorrhage, 2

Homeostasis, 68, 77, 197, 236

Hormonal Function, 77

Hormones, 68, 70-72, 75-80, 82-83, 150, 158

Human Milk, 26-29, 36-41, 43, 54, 58-59, 61, 63-69, 78-80, 82, 95, 97, 99-100, 102-103, 109, 112-124, 126-127, 130-136, 149, 156-158, 187-201, 203, 205-206, 209-210, 222-223, 225-226, 230, 232-237

Human Milk Oligosaccharides, 26, 38-41, 59, 116, 120-121, 234

Hypothalamus, 77, 83

I

Immune Development, 66, 226

Immunoglobulins, 59, 187-188, 197-198, 200, 209

Infancy, 14, 59, 68, 78, 80, 82, 103, 118, 187, 197, 236

Infant Growth, 43, 59, 65-66, 70-73, 78-80, 116, 118, 149, 153, 158

Infant Mortality, 1, 12, 170

Infant Outcomes, 58, 150, 156

Infectious Diseases, 1-2, 43, 187, 197, 233-234

Influenza Vaccine, 203, 208

Initiation Of Breastfeeding, 1, 4-5, 8-9, 13-16, 184, 186

L

Lactating Women, 17-18, 21-22, 25, 69, 73, 88, 184, 217, 224, 235-236

Lactation, 17-18, 22-26, 28-30, 33-41, 59, 65-66, 68, 70, 72, 77-79, 81-86, 88, 90-101, 103, 116-120, 122-123, 134, 136, 149-150, 156-159, 161-167, 187, 197-198, 200, 203, 210-221, 223, 226-227, 232, 234

Lactose, 27, 40-41, 58-59, 61-62, 64-68, 95, 105, 107, 116, 120, 151
Leptin, 70-73, 75-77, 79-80, 153, 156-157
Lipidome, 122, 124-125, 133, 136
Lipoproteins, 105-106, 109, 116

M

Macronutrient, 69-70, 95, 103, 149, 153, 156, 158
Magnesium, 216
Mammary Gland, 65, 68, 78-79, 83, 94, 101, 116-117, 121, 157, 198, 208, 232, 236
Mature Milk, 27, 40, 104, 149, 156, 195
Milk Metabolome, 41, 58-59, 66-68, 102, 112, 115, 118-120
Monoacylglycerols, 129, 132
Monounsaturated Fatty Acid, 127, 215

N

Negative Breastfeeding Experience, 166
Nutrition For Infants, 26
Nutritional Needs, 26
Nutritional Status, 18, 22, 24, 213-214

O

Oxidation, 124, 127, 131-133, 135, 216

P

Passive Immunization, 200, 208
Plasma, 17-21, 24-25, 65, 68, 73, 80, 89, 92, 106-107, 111, 114, 120, 136, 156-157, 188, 224, 232-233, 236
Polyunsaturated Fatty Acids, 103, 116, 122, 127, 131-132, 134, 211, 218, 221
Pooled Human Milk, 29, 37, 135, 195
Post-delivery, 48, 75
Postmenstrual Ages, 38
Postnatal Period., 42, 44-45, 51, 73, 77
Postpartum Age, 26, 30, 33, 36, 38
Predominant Breastfeeding, 162-163
Pregnancy, 1-2, 12, 14-25, 44-45, 48, 51, 55-56, 68, 81-82, 84, 94, 98, 101, 118, 136, 148, 158, 167, 184-185, 198, 203, 207-209, 211-212, 214-219, 221-223, 232, 235
Prematurity, 2, 53, 82, 133, 165, 187-188, 198, 200, 210
Preterm Infants, 16, 26-30, 32-33, 36, 38-40, 55, 82, 84-85, 91-92, 94-100, 123, 133, 135-136, 160-161, 165-168, 186-189, 191-198, 200-202, 204-207, 209-210, 233
Preterm Milks, 37
Protease Inhibitors, 198
Proteases, 191, 194-195, 198

R

Respiratory Infection, 15, 22, 157
Retinol, 54

S

Sampling Point, 37
Secretor, 26-27, 40, 118
Selenium, 25
Serum Leptin, 77, 80
Sialic Acids, 35, 41
Sialyltransferase, 35, 37

V

Vaginal Delivery, 12, 14, 103, 112-113, 115, 177, 214, 229

W

Water-based Drinks, 162

www.ingramcontent.com/pod-product-compliance
Lightning Source LLC
LaVergne TN
LVHW080954210926
848485LV00004B/833